E. Raz (Ed.)

Immunostimulatory DNA Sequences

Springer-Verlag Berlin Heidelberg GmbH

E. Raz (Ed.)

Immunostimulatory DNA Sequences

With 22 Figures and 16 Tables

Springer

Eyal Raz, MD

University of California, San Diego
Dept. of Medicine-0663
9500 Gliman Drive
La Jolla, CA 92093
USA
e-mail: eraz@ucsd.edu

ISBN 978-3-642-63212-9

Cip-Data applied for
Die Deutsche Bibliothek -CIP-Einheitsaufnahme

ISBN 978-3-642-63212-9 ISBN 978-3-642-56866-4 (eBook)
DOI 10.1007/978-3-642-56866-4

Originally published by Springer-Verlag Berlin Heidelberg New York in 2001
Softcover reprint of the hardcover 1st edition 2001

Production: PRO EDIT GmbH, 69126 Heidelberg, Germany
Cover Design: design & production, 69126 Heidelberg, Germany
Printed on acid-free paper SPIN: 10773980 27/3130So - 5 4 3 2 1 0

Preface

To Ofra, Hillel,
Miriam and Ariel

The immunological properties of bacterial DNA represent an emerging field in biology, which attract the interest and attention of scientists and physicans in academic institutes, hospitals as well as in the biotech-based industry.

Bacterial DNA is enriched in immunostimulatory sequences (ISS) which contain an unmethylated CpG dinucleotide core in a particular base context (CpG motifs). Their immunostimulatory properties are attributed, in part, to their ability to activate innate immunity in a fashion described with other microbial by-products such as LPS or dsRNA. ISS, usually used in a form of a single stranded oligonucleotide (ODN), stimulate the production of type-1 cytokines such as IL-12 and IFNs from dendritic cells, macrophages and NK cells. Furthermore, ISS enhance the expression of various co-stimulatory ligands such as B7, CD40, ICAM-1 on antigen presenting cells. This consorted set of activities contributes to the reported systemic Th1 and CTL induction as well as to the mucosal adjuvant effects of ISS.

Methylation at the C-5 position of the cytosine of the CpG basepair (^{methyl}CpG) in the ISS abolishes its immunostimulatory activity. This phenomenon is particularly interesting as vertebrate genomic DNA contains highly methylated cytosines in the CpG basepairs (90%) while bacteria usually do not methylate the cytosines of the CpG basepair in their genome to any large degree (only 15%). These differences between bacterial and mammalian DNA led to the hypothesis that the mammalian innate immune system has evolved to respond to this structural pattern (i.e., CpG motif) by a unique and yet unknown pattern-recognition- receptor. Thus, it is speculated that the putative ISS-ODN receptor would detect the DNA of invading microbial pathogens, elicit the *immunological danger/alarm signal* and initiate protective immunity in the mammalian host

The signaling pathways that mediate the immunostimulatory properties of ISS-ODN have also been investigated. It has been reported that bacterial DNA and ISS-ODNs do not induce tyrosine phosphorylation or increased inositol triphosphate or calcium ion levels. In contrast, the NF-kB , p38 and JNK pathways have been shown to be activated. However, the molecular link that leads to ISS-ODN-induced signaling remains to be elucidated.

The potential applications of ISS are mainly related, but not limited, to the field of vaccination. The ISS, as an adjuvant, have to date been used with a variety of clinical relevant antigens, by different immunization schemes. These include: ISS antigen co-delivery, ISS delivery prior to antigen administration (pre-priming), delivery of ISS-ODN conjugated to the antigen of interest and in the case of gene vaccination by co-delivery or by sub-cloning ISS to the immunization vector. ISS-based clinical trials are in-progress and will provide useful information whether the data generated in animal models can be translated to humans.

Finally, this volume is a product of a collaborative effort and attempts to provide a wide and up-to-date coverage of topics on the biology and on the applications of immunostimulatory DNA. I wish to thank all the authors for their contributions, Jane Uhle for her superb secretarial help and the editors for their support and determination in getting this book to press in a relative short time.

La Jolla, California, May 2000 EYAL RAZ

Contents

Introduction to immunostimulatory DNA sequences

John Van Uden, Eyal Raz

126C Stein Clinical Research Building, MC 0663, UCSD, Department of Medicine,
9500 Gilman Dr., La Jolla, USA

Defining immunostimulatory DNA sequences

Complete Freund's adjuvant (CFA) consisting of mycobacterial extract in oil immersion was initially characterized 60 years ago [7] as an immune adjuvant. Although it contains many immunologically active substances, it has recently been shown that much of the immunostimulatory ability of CFA is attributable to the bacterial DNA fraction (discussed by S. Yamamoto et al. in this volume). Tokunaga and coworkers discovered that DNA purified from *Bacillus Calmette-Guerin* (BCG) induced an innate antitumor activity that appeared to be mediated through its ability to activate NK cells and induce production of interferons (IFNs) α/β/γ [26]. A variety of synthetic 45-mer oligodeoxynucleotides (ODNs) corresponding to various coding regions of three BCG proteins were synthesized. The ODNs that induced IFN secretion and augmented NK cell activity included CpG dinucleotides within a palindromic hexamer (also known as CpG motifs), e.g., 5'-GACGTC-3', 5'-AGCGCT-3' and 5'-AACGTT-3' [27]. Furthermore, only bacterial and not vertebrate DNA produced the NK-immunostimulatory effect. This initial observation demonstrated for the first time that DNA carries information about its originating organism in addition to its genetic blueprints (discussed by D. Pisetsky in this volume). A consensus motif of rrCGyy (where r = purine and y = pyrimidine) has been proposed [12]; however, this CpG motif is only a loose rule: there are sequences that are stimulatory that do not follow the motif and sequences that would be included within the consensus that are not stimulatory. Recent work proposes that the optimal human immunostimulatory sequences are 5'-rTCGyy-3' or a shortened version, 5'-TCG-3'(discussed by H. Liang et al.in this volume). However, we have found that the sequence 5'-AACGTTCG-3' has pronounced stimulatory ability in both mouse and human systems. Some DNA sequences without CpG have stimulatory ability, which is why we prefer the functionally defined name immunostimulatory DNA sequence (ISS) to the structurally defined name CpG motif. Table 1 gives an annotated list of the sequences that have been demonstrated to have potent immunostimulatory activity to date.

Correspondence to: J. Van Uden

Table 1. Potent immunostimulatory DNA sequences

Sequence	Notes	References
Stimulatory activity shown reproducibly by several groups		
AACGTT	One of the first sequences discovered; we and others use this sequence frequently;stimulates human cells	[1, 10, 13, 19, 27, 28]
AACGTTCG	More active than AACGTT in our hands; this is the sequence we use most often	[18, 19]
AGCGCT	One of the first sequences discovered	[12, 13, 19, 27]
GACGTC	One of the first sequences discovered; active as a 6-mer ODN; stimulates human cells	[19, 21, 27, 28]
GACGTT	Active as a 6-mer ODN; stimulates human cells; modified flanking sequences can give good response with low TNF-α; this sequence has been used in many studies	[5, 15, 16, 21]
Limited reports of stimulatory activity		
AACGAT	Moderate B cell activation	[12]
AACGCT		[10, 12]
ACGCGT	Active as a 6-mer ODN	[21]
AGCGTT		[32]
ATCGAT	Active as a 6-mer ODN	[13, 21]
CACGTG	Active as a 6-mer ODN	[1, 21]
CACGTT		[30]
CTCGAC		[12]
CTCGCA	From acute retrovirus genome	[14]
CTCGTA	From acute retrovirus genome	[14]
GACGAT		[30]
GACGCT		[30]
GACGTA		[30]
GACGTG		[30]
GGCGTT		[30]
GTCGAC	Active as a 6-mer ODN	[21]
GTCGAT		[1, 31]
GTCGCT	Stimulates human cells	[15, 31, 32]
GTCGTC	Stimulates human cells	[15]
GTCGTT	Stimulates human cells	[1, 9, 32]
TACGTA	Active as a 6-mer ODN	[21]
TACGTT		[30]

Table 1. Continued

Sequence	Notes	References
TCGCGA	Active as a 6-mer ODN	[13, 21]
TGACGTT	Version of GACGTT that is claimed to be optimal mouse B cell stimulatory sequence	[32]
Conflicting reports of stimulatory ability		
CGCGCG	Has been shown to be stimulatory [13], has been shown to be inhibitory [11]	[11, 13]
GACGGT	Demonstrated activity[1, 32], demonstrated lack of activity [30]	[1, 30, 32]
GCGCGC	Has been shown to be stimulatory [13], has been shown to be inhibitory [11]	[11, 13]
GGCGCC	Report likely activity [24], but not as 6-mer ODNs [21]	[21, 24]
GGCGGT	Demonstrated moderate activity [32], demonstrated lack of activity [30]	[30, 32]
GTCGGT	Demonstrated low stimulatory ability [1], demonstrated high stimulatory ability [12, 32]	[1, 12, 32]
TGCGCA	Report likely activity [24], but not as 6-mer ODNs[21]	[21, 24]

Central core sequences of ODNs shown to be immunostimulatory are given; however, except where noted that the 6-mer ODN is stimulatory, the actual ODN used was longer than this core sequence. Indirect evidence suggests that these core sequences constitute the fundamental stimulatory units (see text for details). Note that most of these studies used different assays for immune stimulation under different treatment conditions; the most common assays include induction of proliferation (B cells), cytokines (APCs and NK cells), or cytolytic activity (mostly NK cells, some macrophages) upon incubation of murine splenocytes with short (12–30-mer) ps-modified ODNs. The work to define the exact motifs required for immune stimulation is still in progress; this table is not meant to be a final and authoritative listing, only as a guide to what has been shown to date. This table is reproduced in a modified form from [25] with permission from the publisher.

DNA methylation is an important epigenetic mechanism. It has been widely shown that methylation within promoters and enhancers shuts down transcriptional activity, and is used in long-term gene regulation, X-chromosome inactivation, and suppression of invading and endogenous viruses and transposons [2, 4]. One theory holds that methylation is responsible for the drastic reduction in frequency of CpG in the vertebrate genome. ^{me}CpG is a hotspot for mutation to TpG during replication, and organisms with low CpG tend to have more TpG and its complement CpA than expected. It has been shown that ISS lose their stimulatory effects upon methylation at the 5' position of the cytosine at the CpG core [12]. This is particularly interesting because vertebrates methylate about 70% of their CpG DNA (which is already reduced about fivefold in frequency) [3]. Not all CpGs are ISS, and we have found that the frequencies of active ISS are even further reduced in mammalian genomes and are altered in pathogen genomes (Van Uden and Raz, manuscript in preparation) beyond dinucleotide CpG frequencies.

While ISS are generally considered by researchers in this field to be modular 6-mer units, it has been difficult to determine the minimum stimulatory motif length. One study showed that a minimum length of 18 bases was required, but that a length of 22 bases gave greater activity [29]. Another study demonstrated good activity with a 15-mer ODN [1]. Still another study used cationic lipid transfection to show a stimulatory effect with 6-mer ODNs [21]. Phosphorothioate (ps) ODNs are nuclease resistant, and therefore are as much as 200-fold more potent than natural po-ODNs, while apparently maintaining the original sequence specificity and spectrum of stimulation. Phosphorothioate-based ISS-ODNs were shown to have activity when as short as 8 bases [12]. It is possible that the minimum active motif is around 6 bases, but that exonucleases within target cells destroy short ODNs before they can mediate their activities.

Activation of innate and cell-mediated immunity by ISS

The innate immune response to an invading pathogen involves the effective and rapid recognition of highly conserved and repeated foreign structures such as polysaccharides, lectins, lipids, LPS or double-stranded (ds) RNA. The presence of ISS in microbial genomes appears to impart a signature that the immune system can recognize, as it does for dsRNA. ISS is then apparently perceived as a marker for dangerous intracellular invasion, and this may help us to understand why ISS is such a potent activator of type 1 cytokine release (IFNs and IL-12) and induction of cell-mediated immunity (CMI).

NK cell activation

Activation of NK tumoricidal activity was the first effect of ISS that was described (discussed by S. Yamamoto et al. in this volume), and it has subsequently been shown that ISS-activated NK cells represent over 90% of the early IFN-γ-producing cells [6]. Purified NK cells are not directly activated by ISS; the IL-12, TNF-α, and IFN-α/β produced by monocytes/macrophages or other antigen-presenting cells (APCs) are required [1].

Macrophage and dendritic cell activation

ISS directly activate macrophages and macrophage-like cell lines but indirect activation via IFN-γ (released by NK cells) appears to account for the majority of quantitative activation of macrophages in mixed cell cultures and in vivo systems [27]. ISS-activated macrophages become cytotoxic and produce the type 1 cytokines IL-12, IL-18, and IFN-α/β as well as TNF-α. More recently it has been appreciated that the antigen-processing and -presentation apparatus of macrophages is also augmented upon ISS stimulation. Bone marrow-derived macrophages treated with ISS up-regulate their expression of class I MHC, CD40, B7, ICAM-1, and CD16/32 (IgG receptor for bound antigen internalization and antibody-dependent cellular cytotoxicity), and consequently function more effectively as APCs [17].

Dendritic cells are similarly activated by ISS (discussed by J. Vogel et al. in this volume). They produce IL-12, IL-6 and TNF-α in response to ISS, and they increase their MHC class II and B7–2 levels [8, 22]. ISS-treated dendritic cells also function better as APCs in allogeneic mixed lymphocyte reactions and with superantigen stimulation [22], and may be particularly important in ISS-stimulated responses in vivo due to the proposed role of dendritic cells in the priming of immune responses. Thus, the two most important classes of professional APCs are potently stimulated by ISS.

B cell activation

Although B cells are a major component of adaptive immunity, they are also directly stimulated by ISS in an antigen-independent fashion (discussed by H. Liang et al.). ISS have a profound B cell mitogenic effect and induce polyclonal IgM antibodies independent of T cell help or antigen exposure [12]. Furthermore, ISS rescue B cells from surface IgM cross-linking-induced apoptosis and activate B cells to produce IL-6 and IL-12 [10, 30] (discussed by A. Krieg et al. in this volume). B cell proliferation is independent of IL-6 production (as determined with blocking antibodies and with knockout mice), but neutralization of IL-6 reduces IgM production by 90% in pure B cell cultures stimulated by ISS, suggesting autocrine stimulation [10]. The surface molecule expression profile of B cells is also drastically altered by ISS activation. MHC class I, MHC class II, B7-1, B7-2, CD40, CD16/32, ICAM-1, IFN-γR, and IL-2R are up-regulated in vivo or in vitro, while CD23 (the low-affinity IgE receptor) is down-regulated [17].

Induction of CMI

Unlike B cells, T cells are not directly activated by ISS, although their indirect activation (discussed by S. Sun et al. in this volume) is crucial to development of the Th1-dominated response to ISS in vivo. Plasmid DNA vaccine administration or antigen/ISS coinjection induces type 1 cytokines (IFNs, IL-12 and IL-18) and the up-regulation of a distinct profile of cell surface molecules on APCs that are likely to mediate the potent generation of Th1-biased responses and CTL activity [5, 18, 19]. Furthermore, the administration of ISS up to 2 weeks prior to antigen administration (pre-priming) generates a Th1 response to subsequently injected antigens more potently than with ISS/antigen co-vaccination (discussed by H. Kobayashi et al.). Another promising way to induce CMI is to chemically conjugate the antigen to the ISS-ODN. Thus, ISS co-delivered with or conjugated to an antigen generates an immune response similar to that induced by genetic vaccination (Raz, submitted). Indeed, the Th1 and CTL responses observed in gene-vaccinated animals are at least

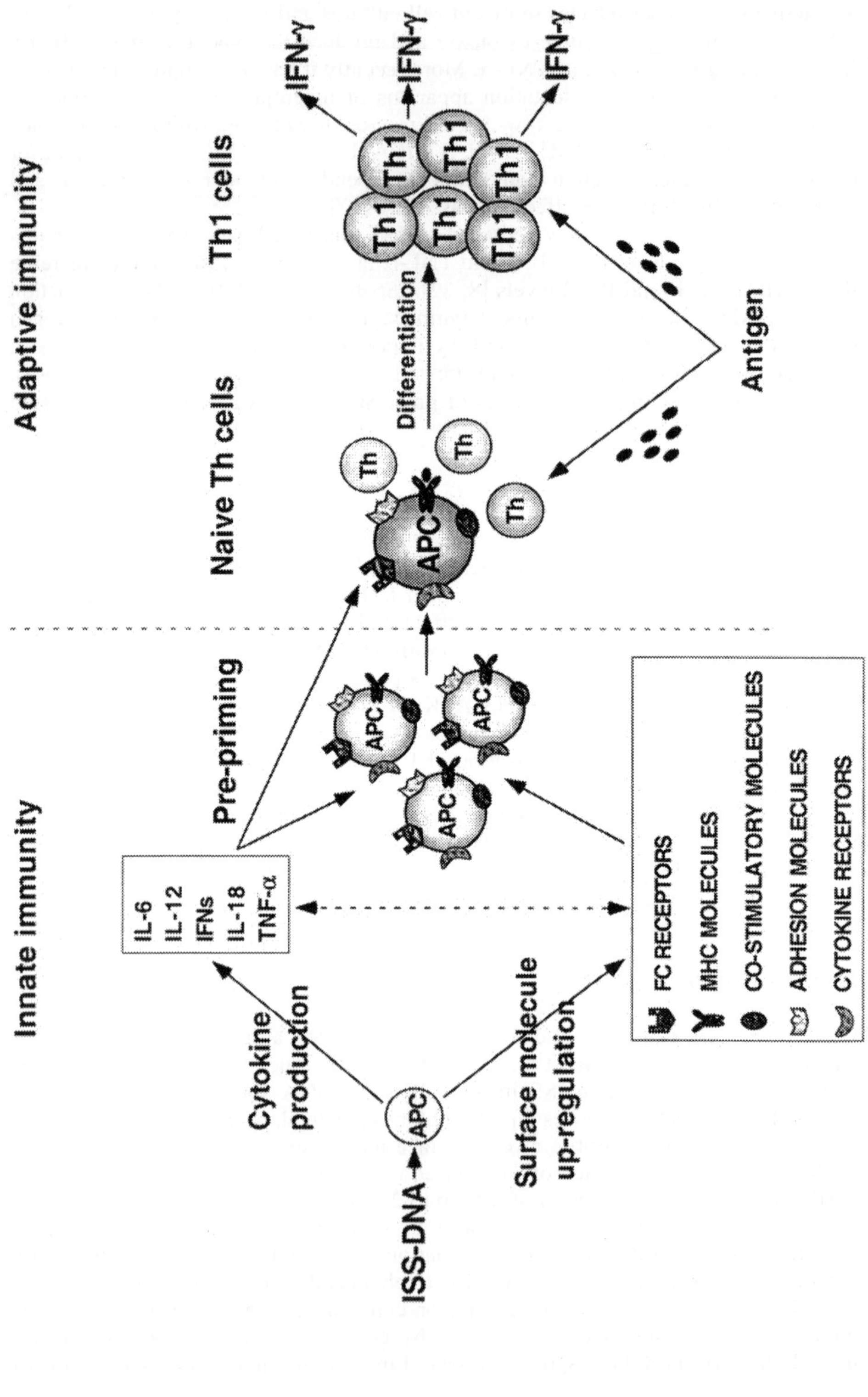
Innate immunity
Adaptive immunity
ISS-DNA
APC
Cytokine production
Surface molecule up-regulation
IL-6
IL-12
IFNs
IL-18
TNF-α
Pre-priming
APC
Naive Th cells
Th
Differentiation
Th1 cells
Th1
IFN-γ
Antigen
FC RECEPTORS
MHC MOLECULES
CO-STIMULATORY MOLECULES
ADHESION MOLECULES
CYTOKINE RECEPTORS

largely due to the presence of ISS in the backbone of most plasmids, which are bacterially derived (discussed by M. McCluskie et al.). The basic mechanisms driving ISS-induced Th1 responses are depicted in Fig. 1.

Based on its ability to secrete type 1 cytokines and to promote Th1 differentiation, ISS has been used to modulate allergic reactions in a variety of animal models. Indeed, it inhibits IgE responses, while reducing airway hyper-reactivity and eosinophilic lung inflammation in a mouse model of asthma (discussed by D. Broide et al.). Furthermore, ISS administration inhibits the induction of the immediate and late phases of the allergic reaction in a murine model of allergic conjunctivitis (M. Magone et al., in press, European Journal of Immunology). Thus, ISS exerts powerful immunomodulatory properties, which may even be able to regulate established allergic responses.

Future directions

The molecular pathways and mechanisms of ISS activation are areas of active investigation (discussed by A. Krieg). NF-κB has been shown to be activated, and is apparently necessary for ISS stimulation. The mitogen-activated protein kinase (MAPK) and stress kinase pathways are also activated by ISS. Specifically, c-Jun NH2-terminal kinase (JNK), JNK kinase 1 (JNKK1), p38, activating transcription factor-2, c-Jun, MAPK-activated protein kinase-2, and activator protein-1 have been implicated in ISS signaling. The p38 pathway appears to be crucial, as its blockade results in a lack of downstream signaling component activation as well as inhibition of cytokine production. In contrast, several other pathways have been shown to not be involved, including tyrosine phosphorylation, inositol triphosphate (IP_3) generation, calcium ion flux, protein kinase C activation, protein kinase A activation, and nitric oxide production.

Perhaps the most important undiscovered piece of the ISS signaling puzzle is identification of the mechanism directly responsible for sensing ISS in or on responsive cells. It seems likely that there is one or more sequence-specific DNA binding protein(s) that function(s) as the ISS receptor. There is some evidence that ISS need to be internalized for activity. Whether the Toll family of receptors, which have been recently shown to mediate activation of other branches of innate immunity, is involved is yet to be explored.

There is a broad spectrum of potential clinical applications where the ability of ISS to induce the innate anti-pathogen response, CTL, Th1, and mucosal immunity (discussed by A. Horner et al.), while suppressing Th2 responses could be useful. These include the design of infectious disease-targeting vaccines or chemotherapeutic protocols, cancer-targeting vaccines (discussed by G. Weiner) or chemotherapeu-

◀ **Fig. 1.** Innate and adaptive immunity interactions mediated by ISS. This simplified schematic shows the main events involved when ISS-DNA induces the immune response to generate a Th1 response to an antigen. Note that the direct effects of ISS are apparently limited to stimulation of professional APCs (e.g., dendritic cells and macrophages) and B cells (not shown) in an antigen-independent fashion (innate immunity). Although not shown, NK cells are stimulated by APC-generated cytokines and are important for the early production of IFN-γ. The production of cytokines, induction of cell surface molecules involved in cognate interactions, and stimulation of antigen processing and presentation drive the pre-priming effects of ISS (discussed by H. Kobayashi et al.) and the characteristic Th1 development in the antigen-specific arm (adaptive immunity) (*ISS* immunostimulatory DNA sequences, *APC* antigen-presenting cell)

tic protocols, and immunomodulatory protocols for allergic diseases. A recent study demonstrated activation of human fibroblasts by ISS [23], opening up the possibility for applications outside of the currently appreciated arena of immunomodulation.

The potential side effects of ISS have to be considered and there is always the possibility of unwanted effects due to the powerful immune stimulation ISS delivers (discussed by D. Klinman et al.). Indeed, it has been shown that mice given ISS followed by sublethal doses of LPS die of shock at an increased frequency (discussed by H. Wagner et al.). Some autoimmune diseases are Th1 in nature, and the danger exists of precipitating disease in genetically or environmentally predisposed individuals. In the mouse model experimental allergic encephalomyelitis (EAE), ISS-stimulated, antigen-specific T cells could transfer disease to recipient mice, raising the possibility of activation of quiescent autoreactive T cell clones in vivo [20]. The generation of anti-DNA antibodies is also a matter of concern (discussed by D. Pisetsky et al.). Normal healthy mice make anti-DNA antibodies and even develop low levels of proliferative glomerulonephritis and proteinuria when immunized with modified bacteria DNA. However, there still are no examples of ISS directly causing any type of autoimmune disease in animal models.

Finally, most of the work on ISS has been in mice, but it is clear that human cells also respond. It may be important to optimize ISS for potency and consistency in humans as it is already clear that the best sequences in mice are not necessarily the best in people. ISS hold great promise for influencing the immune response and we anticipate that the high efficacy and low toxicity observed in animal models will translate into success in a variety of human clinical applications.

References

1. Ballas ZK, Rasmussen WL, Krieg AM (1996) Induction of NK activity in murine and human cells by CpG motifs in oligodeoxynucleotides and bacterial DNA. J Immunol 157:1840
2. Bestor TH (1998) The host defence function of genomic methylation patterns. Novartis Found Symp 214:187; discussion 195
3. Bird AP (1980) DNA methylation and the frequency of CpG in animal DNA. Nucleic Acids Res 8:1499
4. Bird AP (1993) Functions for DNA methylation in vertebrates. Cold Spring Harb Symp Quant Biol 58:281
5. Chu RS, Targoni OS, Krieg AM, Lehmann PV, Harding CV (1997) CpG oligodeoxynucleotides act as adjuvants that switch on T helper 1 (Th1) immunity. J Exp Med 186:1623
6. Cowdery JS, Chace JH, Yi AK, Krieg AM (1996) Bacterial DNA induces NK cells to produce IFN-gamma in vivo and increases the toxicity of lipopolysaccharides. J Immunol 156:4570
7. Freund J, Casals J, Hosmer EP (1937) Sensitization and antibody formation after injection of tubercule bacilli and paraffin oil. Proc Soc Exp Biol Med 37:509
8. Häcker H, Mischak H, Miethke T, Liptay S, Schmid R, Sparwasser T, Heeg K, Lipford GB, Wagner H (1998) CpG-DNA-specific activation of antigen-presenting cells requires stress kinase activity and is preceded by non-specific endocytosis and endosomal maturation. EMBO Journal 17:6230
9. Hartmann G, Weiner GJ, Krieg AM (1999) CpG DNA: a potent signal for growth, activation, and maturation of human dendritic cells. Proc Natl Acad Sci, USA 96:9305
10. Klinman DM, Yi AK, Beaucage SL, Conover J, Krieg AM (1996) CpG motifs present in bacteria DNA rapidly induce lymphocytes to secrete interleukin 6, interleukin 12, and interferon gamma. Proc Natl Acad Sci USA 93:2879
11. Krieg AM, Wu T, Weeratna R, Efler SM, Love-Homan L, Yang L, Yi AK, Short D, Davis HL (1998) Sequence motifs in adenoviral DNA block immune activation by stimulatory CpG motifs. Proc Natl Acad Sci USA 95:12631
12. Krieg AM, Yi AK, Matson S, Waldschmidt TJ, Bishop GA, Teasdale R, Koretzky GA, Klinman DM (1995) CpG motifs in bacterial DNA trigger direct B-cell activation. Nature 374:546

13. Kuramoto E, Yano O, Kimura Y, Baba M, Makino T, Yamamoto S, Yamamoto T, Kataoka T, Tokunaga T (1992) Oligonucleotide sequences required for natural killer cell activation. Jpn J Cancer Res 83:1128
14. Lapatschek MS, Gilbert RL, Wagner H, Miethke T (1998) Activation of macrophages and B lymphocytes by an oligodeoxynucleotide derived from an acutely pathogenic simian immunodeficiency virus. Antisense Nucleic Acid Drug Dev 8:357
15. Liang H, Nishioka Y, Reich CF, Pisetsky DS, Lipsky PE (1996) Activation of human B cells by phosphorothioate oligodeoxynucleotides. J Clin Invest 98:1119
16. Lipford GB, Sparwasser T, Bauer M, Zimmermann S, Koch ES, Heeg K, Wagner H (1997) Immunostimulatory DNA: sequence-dependent production of potentially harmful or useful cytokines. Eur J Immunol 27: 3420
17. Martin-Orozco E, Kobayashi H, Van Uden J, Nguyen M-D, Kornbluth RS, Raz E (1999) Enhancement of antigen-presenting cell surface molecules involved in cognate interactions by immunostimulatory DNA sequences. Int Immunol 11:1111
18. Roman M, Martin-Orozco E, Goodman JS, Nguyen MD, Sato Y, Ronaghy A, Kornbluth RS, Richman DD, Carson DA, Raz E (1997) Immunostimulatory DNA sequences function as T helper-1-promoting adjuvants. Nat Med 3:849
19. Sato Y, Roman M, Tighe H, Lee D, Corr M, Nguyen MD, Silverman GJ, Lotz M, Carson DA, Raz E (1996) Immunostimulatory DNA sequences necessary for effective intradermal gene immunization. Science 273:352
20. Segal BM, Klinman DM, Shevach EM (1997) Microbial products induce autoimmune disease by an IL-12-dependent pathway. J Immunol 158:5087
21. Sonehara K, Saito H, Kuramoto E, Yamamoto S, Yamamoto T, Tokunaga T (1996) Hexamer palindromic oligonucleotides with 5'-CG-3' motif(s) induce production of interferon. J Interferon Cytokine Res 16:799
22. Sparwasser T, Koch ES, Vabulas RM, Heeg K, Lipford GB, Ellwart JW, Wagner H (1998) Bacterial DNA and immunostimulatory CpG oligonucleotides trigger maturation and activation of murine dendritic cells. Eur J Immunol 28:2045
23. Takeshita A, Imai K, Hanazawa S (1999) CpG motifs in Porphyromonas gingivalis DNA stimulate interleukin-6 expression in human gingival fibroblasts. Infect Immun 67:4340
24. Tokunaga T, Yano O, Kuramoto E, Kimura Y, Yamamoto T, Kataoka T, Yamamoto S (1992) Synthetic oligonucleotides with particular base sequences from the cDNA encoding proteins of *Mycobacterium bovis* BCG induce interferons and activate natural killer cells. Microbiol Immunol 36:55
25. Van Uden J, Raz E (1999) Immunostimulatory DNA and applications to allergic disease. J Allergy Clin Immunol 104:902
26. Yamamoto S, Kuramoto E, Shimada S, Tokunaga T (1988) In vitro augmentation of natural killer cell activity and production of interferon-alpha/beta and -gamma with deoxyribonucleic acid fraction from *Mycobacterium bovis* BCG. Jpn J Cancer Res 79:866
27. Yamamoto S, Yamamoto T, Kataoka T, Kuramoto E, Yano O, Tokunaga T (1992) Unique palindromic sequences in synthetic oligonucleotides are required to induce IFN and augment IFN-mediated natural killer activity. J Immunol 148:4072
28. Yamamoto T, Yamamoto S, Kataoka T, Komuro K, Kohase M, Tokunaga T (1994) Synthetic oligonucleotides with certain palindromes stimulate interferon production of human peripheral blood lymphocytes in vitro. Jpn J Cancer Res 85:775
29. Yamamoto T, Yamamoto S, Kataoka T, Tokunaga T (1994) Ability of oligonucleotides with certain palindromes to induce interferon production and augment natural killer cell activity is associated with their base length. Antisense Res Dev 4:119
30. Yi AK, Chang M, Peckham DW, Krieg AM, Ashman RF (1998) CpG oligodeoxyribonucleotides rescue mature spleen B cells from spontaneous apoptosis and promote cell cycle entry. J Immunol 160:5898
31. Yi AK, Hornbeck P, Lafrenz DE, Krieg AM (1996) CpG DNA rescue of murine B lymphoma cells from anti-IgM-induced growth arrest and programmed cell death is associated with increased expression of c-myc and bcl-xL. J Immunol 157:4918
32. Yi AK, Klinman DM, Martin TL, Matson S, Krieg AM (1996) Rapid immune activation by CpG motifs in bacterial DNA. Systemic induction of IL-6 transcription through an antioxidant-sensitive pathway. J Immunol 157:5394

The discovery of immunostimulatory DNA sequence

Saburo Yamamoto[1], Toshiko Yamamoto[1], Tohru Tokunaga[2]

[1] Department of Bacterial and Blood Products, National Institute of Infectious Diseases, 4-7-1 Gakuen, Musashimurayama, Tokyo 208-0011, Japan
[2] Fukuoka Jo-Gakuin University, Fukuoka, Japan

Antitumor activity of a fraction extracted from BCG

Since the 1960s, *Mycobacterium bovis* BCG has been investigated widely within the scope of cancer immunotherapy of experimental animals and humans [10, 19, 20]. Efforts have also been made to isolate the bacterial component possessing antitumor activity from BCG. While trying to obtain water-soluble components of BCG, we found that BCG cytoplasm precipitated by streptomycin sulfate contained substances strongly active against Line-10 hepatoma of Strain-2 guinea pigs [17, 21]. The streptomycin sulfate precipitate of BCG was a complex of various components, protein, nucleic acid, lipid and sugar. Repeated injections of this fraction into guinea pigs caused severe anaphylactic shock. In one approach, we tried to extract fractions of streptomycin sulfate precipitate with hot water and found that the heat extract contained substances that strongly inhibited tumor growth. This fraction was further purified with multi-step procedures, and a final fraction designated MY-1 was obtained. The chemical composition of MY-1 and the other fractions obtained in the process of isolating MY-1, as well as that of an RNase digest of MY-1 and a DNase digest of MY-1 was examined. MY-1 was composed of 98% nucleic acid (70% DNA, 28.0% RNA) and only 1.3% protein. The sugar content of MY-1 was 0.2% when measured by gas-liquid chromatography. The RNase digest of MY-1 contained mostly DNA (97.0%), and the DNase digest of MY-1 was composed of RNA (98.5%). MY-1 did not contain any unusual amino acids. The diaminopimeric acid content was less than 0.01% and no hexosamines were detected. Of the neutral sugars, only glucose was detected at 0.20%. These results suggested that contamination of MY-1 with cell wall components or polysaccharides was negligible. The base composition of the RNase digest of MY-1 and of the DNA extracted and purified from BCG by the method of Marmur were examined. The GC contents were 69.8% and 71.5%, respectively, and their base compositions were similar. The DNA contained in MY-1 was single stranded as judged by the results of an ultracentrifuge analysis, chromatography on a hydroxy apatite column, and measurement of temperature absorbance. When guinea pigs were given subcutaneous injections of 2 mg MY-1 three times a week for

Correspondence to: S. Yamamoto

2 weeks and then challenged with a single intraveneous injection of 5 mg MY-1 2 weeks later, they did not show anaphylactic shock, suggesting that the MY-1 contained a negligible amount of anaphylactic substances. MY-1 showed stronger antitumor activity than the streptomycin sulfate precipitate. Although a typical delayed-type inflammatory reaction was observed at the site of BCG injection, no macroscopic inflammatory change was observed at the injection sites of MY-1. The DNA contained in MY-1 was essential for the activity because the RNase-digested fraction of MY-1 showed higher antitumor activity than MY-1, while the DNase-digested MY-1 containing mostly RNA had reduced activity. MY-1 showed strong antitumor activity when injected intralesionally, and an antitumor effect against many kinds of mouse tumors and guinea pig tumor when administered intralesionally. Many reports exist on mycobacterial components possessing antitumor activity [1–3, 6, 12, 13, 24, 28]. However, MY-1 is unique because its component is mostly nucleic acid and its activity is ascribed to DNA. No direct cytotoxicity of MY-1 was observed in three different kinds of experiments. The in vitro growth and viability of cells of 11 cultured cell lines were not influenced by incubation of 1,000 μg MY-1/ml, judged by a trypan blue dye exclusion test and by the uptake of tritiated thymidine, uridine, or glucosamine by the cells. In addition, tumor cells preincubated with MY-1 grew progressively in vivo as did control tumor cells treated in the same way without MY-1. These results suggested that antitumor activity of MY-1 is due to a host-mediated mechanism.

Oligonucleotide sequences contained in MY-1

A gel filtration column chromatography indicated that MY-1 contained molecules with a broad range of molecular size; the elution peak corresponded to 45 bases. To determine whether the immunostimulatory activity of MY-1 was dependent on base sequence, 13 different 45-mer single-stranded oligodeoxynucleotides (ODNs) were synthesized [23]. Sequences were selected from the known cDNA encoding 64-kDa protein (antigen-A), MPB-70 protein or alpha-antigen. To evaluate the immunostimulatory activity of each ODN, the ability of the ODN to augment NK cell activity of normal mouse spleen cells was assayed. Of the 13 ODNs, 6 (BCG-A3, BCG-A4, BCG-A6, BCG-A7, BCG-M3 and BCG-alpha-1) showed strong activity, while the others did not (Table 1). Two ODNs, BCG-A4 and BCG-A2 were selected as representative of active and inactive ODN, respectively. The cytotoxicity of the spleen cells was elevated remarkably by BCG-A4 in a dose-dependent manner, while the cells incubated with BCG-A2 showed no significant change in activity at any concentration. To determine the minimal sequence required for NK cell activation by BCG-A4, seven types of ODN (30 bases or 15 bases) were synthesized from different parts of BCG-A4 (Table 2). Of each of these ODN 100 μg was incubated with mouse spleen cells, and the NK cell activity was assayed. The supernatants of the cultures were examined for IFN activity. BCG-A4a, a 30-mer ODN corresponding to the sequence beginning at the 5′ terminus of BCG-A4, activated NK cells and induced IFN as efficiently as BCG-A4. The activity of BCG-A4b, a 30-mer fragment of the 3′ terminus of BCG-A4, was much less than that of BCG-A4a. All of the 15-mer fragments showed almost no activity. Mixing the three kinds of 15-mer nucleotides, BCG-A4c, BCG-A4d and BCG-A4e, did not reconstitute the NK activity. These results suggest that BCG-A4a contained an active sequence, and that a molecular size

Table 1. Augmentation of NK activity by the oligonucleotides

Name	Base sequence (5′–3′)	NK activity (%)
BCG-A1	AACGAGGGGC ATGACCCGGT GCGGGGCTTC TTGCACTCGG CATAG	6.5
BCG-A2	AAAAGAAGTG GGGTGCCCCC ACGATCACCA ACGATGGTGT GTCCA	5.5
BCG-A3	TCCATCGCCA AGGAGATCGA GCTGGAGGAT CCGTACGAGA AGATC	33.4
BCG-A4	ACCGATGACG TCGCCGGTG CGGCACCACG ACGGCCACCG TGCTG	42.1
BCG-A5	TATGCGGTTC GACAAGGGCT ACATCTCGGG GTACTTCGTG ACCGA	10.4
BCG-A6	ACGAGACCAC CATCGTCGAG GGCGCCGGTG ACACCGACGC CATCG	30.4
BCG-A7	GCCGAGAAGG TGCGCAACCT GCCGGCTGGC CACGGACTGA ACGCT	32.4
BCG-A8	ACCGAGAACA GCCACGCAGT CGTGTAGGCA ACCTTTGGCC GCTGT	11.6
BCG-M1	GGCGATCTGG TGGGCCCGGG CTGCGCGGAA TACGCGGCAG CCAAT	6.1
BCG-M2	TCGGTGCAGG GAATGTCGCA GGACCCGGTC GCGGTGGCGG CCTCG	9.5
BCG-M3	ACGCCGACGT CGTCTGTGGT GGGGTGTCTA CCGCCAACGC GACGG	26.9
BCG-alpha 1	CGACTACAAC GGCTGGGATA TCAACACCCC GGCGTTCGAG TGGTA	65.6
BCG-alpha 2	GACCCGGCAT GGGAGCGCAA CGACCCTACG CAGCAGATCC CCAAG	10.5

Table 2. Augmentation of NK activity and induction of interferon by the 30-mer and 15-mer oligonucleotide fragments of BCG-A4 (*ND* not detectable)

Name	Base sequence (5′–3′)	NK activity (%)	IFN (IU)
BCG-A4	ACCGAT*GACG TC*GCCGGTGA CGGCACCACG ACGGCCACCG TGCTG	41.6	256
BCG-A4a	ACCGAT*GACG TC*GCCGGTGA CGGCACCACG	42.0	256
BCG-A4b	GGTGA CGGCACCACG ACGGC CACCGTGCTG	17.0	16
BCG-A4c	ACCGAT*GACG TC*GCC	22.4	<8
BCG-A4d	GGTGA CGGCACCACG	14.6	<8
BCG-A4e	ACGGCCACCG TGCTG	18.8	<8
BCG-A4f	*TGACG TC*GCCGGTGA	16.7	ND
BCG-A4g	TCGCCGGTGA CGGCA	19.6	ND

of nearly 30-mer bases is required for ODN to augment the NK cell activity. IFN-inducing activity was paralleled with these results, suggesting that some stereochemical structures constructed by particular sequences are required for expressing the immunostimulatory activity. Five kinds of 30-mer ODN were selected from the cDNA encoding BCG or human proteins [25]. The ability of these ODNs to augment NK cell varied. Three ODN with a 5′-GACGTC-3′ palindrome strongly stimulated the NK activity, whereas two ODN with no palindrome did not. Further, four kinds of 30-mer ODN with a palindrome other than 5′-GACGTC-3′ were also chosen from the cDNA encoding another human protein. None of the ODN with either 5′-TGTACA-3′, 5′-AATATT-3′, 5′-TGATCA-3′, or 5′-GCGCGC-3′ exhibited the potency to augment NK cell activity. Next, the 5′-GACGTC-3′ sequence was introduced into different sites of an ODN, BCG-M2a, which was an inactive ODN with no palindrome. In contrast to the parental ODN, the analogue of BCG-M2a, with the 5′-GACGTC-3′ sequence, strongly stimulated the NK cell activity. ODN having palindromic sequences of either 5′-GACGTC-3′, 5′-AGCGCT-3′ or 5′-AACGTT-3′ were active, while ODN with 5′-ACCGGT-3′ were inactive. The importance of the integrity of palindromic sequence was tested by exchanging two neighboring mononucleotides within or outside the palindromic sequence. BCG-A4a-M1, in which G and T were exchanged within the palindrome (5′-GACGTC-3′) of BCG-A4a, had much reduced activity as compared to the unmodified BCG-A4a, whereas BCG-A4a-M2, in which G and A were exchanged out side the palindrome, retained the activity. Similarly, the exchange of G and T within the palindrome of active ODN, BCG-M3a and BCG-M4a, formed inactive ODNs, BCG-M3a-M1 and BCG-M4a-M1, respectively. The NK cell activity of mouse spleen cells was assayed after the incubation with BCG-M2a-AAC for 20 h in the presence of 500 neutralization U/ml of either anti-IFN-α/β antibody, anti-IFN-β antibody, or anti-IFN-γ antibody. Presence of anti-IFN-α/β antibody, but not of anti IFN-β antibody or anti-IFN-γ antibody, inhibited the augmentation of NK cell activity by BCG-M2a-AAC. On the other hand, production of macrophage-activating factor (MAF) from the spleen cells stimulated with BCG-M2a-AAC was abolished with anti-IFN-γ antibody, but not with anti-IFN-α/β antibody or anti-IFN-β antibody.

The palindromic sequence (5′-GACGTC-3′) of BCG-A4a, an active ODN, the sequence of which is 5′-accgatGACGTCgccggtgacggcaccacg-3′, was replaced with each of the 63 theoretically possible 6-mer palindromic sequences. The resulting BCG-A4a analogues were tested for their ability to enhance NK cell activity. More than 100% relative activity was observed in the 8 ODNs with one of the following palindromic sequences: AACGTT, AGCGCT, ATCGAT, CGATCG, CGTACG, CGCGCG, GCGCGC and TCGCGA. All the potent palindromes included one or more 5′-CG-3′ motif(s). In contrast, palindromes composed entirely of adenine (A) and thymine (T) and those with a sequence of either Pu (purine)-Pu-Pu-Py (pyrimidine)-Py-Py or Py-Py-Py-Pu-Pu-Pu were generally unfavorable for activity. To examine the role of the extra-palindromic sequence, the NK-augmenting activity was compared among four types of 30-mer homo-oligomers with one of the potent palindromic sequences, AACGTT, CGATCG or ATCGAT, at the center position. No activity was found in the homo-oligomers without a palindrome. Oligo-guanylate (oligo-G) showed the highest activity irrespective of the palindromic sequence included, but oligo-adenylate gave only marginal activity. This was also true of the homo-oligomers including the GACGTC palindrome. In contrast, no activity was found in the 30-mer oligo-G containing an ACCGGT palindrome. These results indicate the independent and cooperative effects of the palindromic sequence and the extra-palindromic sequence on the activity of ODNs. Next, the effect of palindrome size on the activity was investigated. The CGATCG palindrome in the ODNs with having extra-palindromic oligo-G sequences was expanded or truncated. Among these ODNs, one containing the 10-mer palindrome GACGATCGTC showed the highest activity, and those with a palindrome smaller than CGATCG had no activity. Essentially the same results were obtained with the AACGTT palindrome. Finally, the effects of the number and the location of the palindrome sequences on the activity were investigated. Among the ODNs containing a different number of AACGTT palindromes and extra-palindromic oligo-G sequences, an ODN with one palindrome showed the highest activity. The ODNs with an AACGTT palindrome at the 5′ or the 3′ end showed slightly stronger activity than ODNs with it in the center, although the activity was influenced more drastically by the number of palindromes than by the location.

The relationship between the sequence and the activity of the palindrome is not clear at present. The stacking stability between guanine and cytosine is higher than that between adenine and thymine. Stacking between pyrimidines is less stable than that between purines or that between purine and pyrimidine. Thus, the stable helical structure formed by the palindromes including the 5′-CG-3′ but without Py-Py-Py sequence may be favorable for the activity. However, this does not quite explain the inactivity of some of the ODNs with a palindromic sequence including the 5′-CG-3′. Studies are necessary on the target molecule(s) of the palindromic sequences.

These results suggest distinct and cooperative roles of the palindromic and the extra-palindromic sequences in the mechanism of NK cell activation by ODNs. The reduced activity of the ODNs with shorter oligo-G sequence supports this assumption. Since the mixture of a palindrome-including fragment of BCG-A4a and another fragment without it had a reduced activity as compared to BCG-A4a, the palindromic and the extra-palindromic sequence should be present in the same molecule to act cooperatively. It is unlikely that the cooperativity between the palindromic and the extra-palindromic sequences is due to some secondary structure(s), such as bulges or hairpin-loops possibly formed in these sequences, for the following reasons. First, the thermostability of secondary structures was not correlated with the activity of ODNs as judged by temperature gradient gel electrophoresis. Second, there was no correlation between the activity and the preferred secondary structure of the ODN as predicted by thermodynamic calculation. Third, the activity of the single-stranded BCG-A4a was comparable to that of the double-stranded counterpart, although the latter is less likely to form secondary structure than the former.

Immunostimulatory activity of the DNA prepared from various sources

We found that DNA-rich fractions from various species of bacteria exhibited an immunostimulatory activity similar to MY-1, but DNA extracted from calf thymus and salmon testis did not [26]. At first we thought the different procedures employed for DNA extraction and purification might have resulted in DNA possessing different activity, and we prepared DNA fractions from six species of bacterium, *Streptomyces aureofaciens*, *Mycobacterium bovis* BCG, *Pseudomonas putida*, *Escherichia coli*, *Bacillus subtilis* and *Staphylococcus aureus,* and those from two species of animals, calf thymus and salmon testis, by exactly the same procedures as used in the preparation of MY-1, and examined their immunostimulatory activity. The DNA fraction from all of the bacteria yielded remarkable elevation of NK activity of the spleen cell, and induced generation of both MAF and IFN by the spleen cells in a concentration-dependent manner. However, the DNA fractions from calf thymus and salmon testis did not lead to any stimulation at any of the concentrations used.

In addition to these DNA fractions from the 8 different sources, all prepared by the same method as used for MY-1, 23 other DNA samples were extracted and purified by the Marmur's method. The concentrations of the samples were adjusted for their DNA content, and their abilities to augment NK activity and to induce IFN production in mouse spleen cells were examined. Each of the DNA samples from *Mycrococcus lysodeikticus*, *Mycobacterium bovis* BCG, *E. coli*, and *Mycoplasma pneumoniae* strongly augmented NK activity and induced IFN. The biological activities of the DNA samples from *Clostridium perfringens* were relatively low, but were statistically significant. The DNA sample from phaiX 174 phage showed strong activity, and that from adenovirus exhibited less but significant activity. From the DNA samples from 4 invertebrate species, the sample from silkworm showed strong activity, and those from sea urchin, lobster and mussel showed less but significant activities. In contrast, all DNA samples from 10 different vertebrate species (including 5 mammals) and from 2 plant species exhibited no activity.

To explain such a difference in immunostimulatory activity among DNA from different sources, we set up the following six hypotheses: (1) the bacterial DNA fraction might be contaminated with biologically active substance(s) like LPS; (2) the molecular size of DNA contained in the DNA fractions might be different between bacteria and vertebrates, resulting in the different activities; (3) the DNA from vertebrates might be more sensitive than bacterial DNA to DNase prepared from vertebrate animals, so that the bacterial DNA would persist longer in the cultures of mouse spleen cells; (4) the (G+C) content might influence the activities; (5) the majority of CpG motifs are known to be methylated in vertebrates, but not in bacteria, and the presence of methyl cytosine might obstruct the activity of CpG motifs; and/or (6) the frequency of particular base sequence essential for biological activity of the DNA might be different. We examined all of these six possibilities. The respective results were as follows:

1.) The activity of the bacterial DNA fractions was not influenced by the presence of polymixin B, an inhibitor of LPS, and was observed even in the spleen cells from LPS-insensitive C3H/HeJ mice, indicating that the activity could not be attributable to possible LPS contamination.
2.) The profiles of agarose gel electrophoresis were essentially the same in all of the DNA fractions from eight different sources.
3.) UV absorbance at 260 nm of MY-1 and the DNA from calf thymus decreased to the same proportion by DNase treatment, suggesting that the third possibility may not be the case.
4.) The (G+C) content of the bacterial DNA used varied from more than 70% to less than 30%, all of which were active, and those of calf and salmon DNA were 50.2% and 40.2%, respectively. No correlation between (G+C) content and immunostimulatory activity of DNA was found.
5.) We previously reported that a synthetic single-stranded poly(dG,dC) is immunostimulatory in vitro [22]. We synthesized poly(dG,dC), in which all of the cytosines were substituted with methyl cytosines. Poly(dG,methyl-dC) augmented NK activity and induced IFN as effectively as the unsubstituted poly (dG,dC). Furthermore, we tested a 30-mer nucleotide with a 5′-AACGTT-3′ sequence, and its analogue in which C was replaced with methyl cytosine; both ODNs induced IFN equally effectively. These results led us to mis-judge and neglect the fifth hypothesis. In 1994 we found that certain hexamer ODNs alone could induce IFN when they were encapsulated in liposome [27]. Using this liposome system, we discovered that methylation of the cytosine of AACGTT resulted in a significant decrease of its activity [18]. We also found that the incubation of *E. coli* DNA with CpG methylase reduced the IFN-inducing activity after an incubation period. Therefore, we think now that hypothesis (5) must be one of the reasons for the difference in activity between the DNA of vertebrates and non-vertebrates.
6.) We surveyed the incidence frequency of the nine potent palindromic sequences in some of the cDNA sequences in the GenBank DNA database. We chose one or more sequences at will from the cDNA of 17 species. The summed incidences of the potent palindromic sequences in all of the cDNA sequences from vertebrates and plants were less than 1.0 in 1,000 base pairs, while those from most of the

bacteria, viruses, and silkworm were greater than 1.0. There were some exceptions; the incidence, for instance, in the cDNA sequences from *Mycoplasma pneumoniae* and *Clostridium perfringens* was very low (0.4–0.2) but their activity was high. These discrepancies may be due to our limited analysis of only the tiny parts of the huge genomic DNA. The incidence of particular 8-, 10- or 12-mer palindromic sequences, which show stronger immunostimulatory activity than a particular 6-mer [18], was not taken into account either. Bird described that CpG in bulk vertebrate DNA occurs at about one-fifth of the expected frequency [4]. We think that the different frequency of potent sequences in DNA between vertebrate and invertebrate DNA must be another reason for the difference in activities.

Antitumor activity of immunostimulatory ODNs

The antitumor activity of each ODN was also examined [7]. A cell suspension of IMC tumor cells was mixed with each test sample containing 100 μg of the ODN, and the mixtures were intradermally inoculated into CDF1 mice. As a control, saline alone was used. At 35 days after the inoculation, all mice were killed and the tumors were resected and weighed. When tumor cells were mixed with BCG-A4 ODN, the tumor growth was markedly suppressed, but BCG-A2 ODN did not significantly affect the tumor growth. Next, the effects of repeated injections of the ODNs into established tumors were also examined. IMC tumor cells (5×10^5) were inoculated intradermally into CDF1 mice. The ODN test samples (100 μg each) dissolved in 0.1 ml saline were injected into the tumor lesion twice a week from the 5th day of the tumor inoculation. At 35 days after the tumor inoculation, all the mice were killed and the tumors were resected and weighed. Of the 11 ODNs tested, 6 (BCG-A3, BCG-A4, BCG-A6, BCG-A7, BCG-M3 and BCG-alpha1) inhibited tumor growth significantly, while the others did not. The antitumor activity of the active ODNs correlated well with the NK-augmenting activity and IFN-inducing activity. It is noteworthy that the inactive ODNs, BCG-A1, BCG-A2, BCG-A5 and BCG-A8, do not contain a hexameric palindrome, while the active ODNs do possess such a sequence, i.e., GACGTC, GGCGCC or TGCGCA. The exception is that an inactive ODN, BCG-M1, contains an overlapping palindrome sequence (GGGCCCGGG). To test in vivo effect of the bacterial DNA fraction, mice bearing intradermal IMC tumors were treated with intralesional injections of the DNA fraction. In the group given phosphate-buffered saline alone, tumors grew progressively; on the 35th day, the mean tumor weight was 3.82±1.55 g. In the groups given DNA fraction from either of the bacteria species, tumor growth was significantly inhibited. For instance, the mean tumor weight in the mice given the DNA fraction from *Streptomyces aureofaciens* was 0.39±0.45 g and the growth inhibition was 90%. Seven mice were cured out of 8 in this group. The DNA fractions from all of the other bacteria were also effective and showed more than 85% tumor growth inhibition. On the other hand, little effect was observed in the DNA fractions from vertebrate cells. The DNA fraction from salmon testis showed moderate tumor growth inhibition, but no mouse was cured. Although data are not shown here, the bacterial DNA fraction digested with DNase completely lost antitumor activity; digestion with RNase had no influence.

Conclusions

The concept of immunostimulatory DNA sequence was born in a long series of studies on BCG-mediated tumor resistance. DNA purified from BCG inhibited the growth of various animal tumors, augmented cell activity and induced IFN from mouse spleen cells. Further, we found two remarkable facts (1) DNA from bacteria, but not animals and plants, showed the above-mentioned immunogical activity, and (2) the activity was completely dependent on particular base sequences having CpG motifs. Research interests of immunostimulatory DNA sequences were galvanized in 1995 by the report of Krieg showing murine B cell activation with bacterial DNA containing CpG motifs [9]. Within a short period of time, a huge number of papers have been published in this field, and the study has expanded rapidly and widely. Now, it includes a number of research fields, for example, host-defense mechanisms against infection, allergy, autoimmune diseases, cytokine networks, plasmid vaccination, and therapeutic application of certain diseases [5, 8, 11, 15, 16, 29]. The response of higher animals against immunostimulatory DNA must be the most primitive but important mechanism for self-nonself discrimination against foreign DNA.

References

1. Adam A, Ciobaru R, Pett J-F, Lederer E (1972) Isolation and properties of a macromolecular, water-soluble, immunoadjuvant fraction from the cell wall of *Mycobacterium smegmatis*. Proc Natl Acad Sci USA 69:851
2. Azuma I, Ribi EE, Meyer TJ, Zbar B (1974) Biological active components from mycobacterial cell walls. I. Isolation and composition of cell wall skeleton and component P3. J Natl Cancer Inst 52:95
3. Baldwin RW, Hopper DG, Pimm MV (1976) Bacillus Calmette-Guerin contact immunotherapy of local and metastatic deposits of rat tumors. Ann NY Acad Sci 277:124
4. Bird AP (1986) CpG-rich islands and the function of DNA methylation. Nature 321:209
5. Goodman JS, Van Uden JH, Kobayashi H, Broide D, Raz E (1998) DNA immunotherapeutics: new potential treatment modalities for allergic disease. Int Arch Allergy Immunology 116:177
6. Hiu IJ (1972) Water-soluble and lipid free fraction from BCG with adjuvant and antitumor activity. Nature 238:241
7. Kataoka T, Yamamoto S, Yamamoto T, Kuramoto E, Kimura Y, Yano O, Tokunaga T (1992) Antitumor activity of synthetic oligonucleotides with sequences from cDNA encoding proteins of *Mycobacterium bovis* BCG. Jpn J Cancer Res 83:244
8. Krieg AM, Love-Homan L, Yi A-K, Harty J T (1998) CpG DNA induces sustained IL-12 expression in vivo and resistance to *Listeria monocytogenes* challenge. J Immunol 161:2428
9. Krieg AM, Yi A-K, Matson S, Waldschmidt TJ, Bishop GA, Teasdale R, Koretzky GA, Klinman DM (1995) CpG motifs in bacterial DNA trigger direct B cell activation. Nature 374:546
10. Lamoureux G, Turcotte R, Portelance V (eds) (1976) BCG in cancer immunotherapy. Grune, New York
11. Lowrie DB, Tascon RE, Bonato VLD, Lima VMF, Faccioli LH, Stavropoulos E, Colston MJ, Hewinson RG, Moelling K, Silva CL (1999) Therapy of tuberculosis in mice by DNA vaccination. Nature 400:269
12. Millman I, Maguire HC, Pass N, Youmans AS, Youmans GP (1976) Mycobacterial RNA: a comparison with intact mycobacteria for suppression of murine tumor growth. J Exp Med 7:249
13. Millman I, Scott AW, Halbherr T, Youmans AS (1976) Mycobacterial cell wall fractions for regression of murine tumor growth. Infect Immun 14:929
14. Morton DL, Eilber FR, Holmes EC (1974) BCG immunotherapy of malignant melanoma: summary of a seven-year experience. Ann Surg 180: 635
15. Pisetsky DS (1996) Immune activation by bacterial DNA: a new genetic code. Immunity 5:303
16. Sato Y, Roman M, Tighe H, Lee D, Corr M, Nguyen M-D, Silverman GJ, Lotz M, Carson DA, Raz E (1996) Immunostimulatory DNA sequences necessary for effective intradermal gene immunization. Science 273:352

17. Shimada S, Yano O, Inoue H, Kuramoto E, Fukuda T, Yamamoto H, Kataoka T, Tokunaga T (1985) Antitumor activity of the DNA fraction from *Mycobacterium bovis* BCG. II. Effects on various syngeneic mouse tumors. J Natl Cancer Inst 74:681
18. Sonehara K, Saito H, Kuramoto E, Yamamoto S, Yamamoto T, Tokunaga T (1996) Hexamer palindromic oligonucleotides with 5'-CG-3' motif(s) induce production of interferon. J Interferon Cytokine Res 16:799
19. Southam CM, Friedman H (eds) (1976) International conference on immunotherapy of cancer. Ann NY Acad Sci 277:60, 94
20. Terry WD, Yamamura Y (eds) (1979) Immunobiology and immunotherapy of cancer; developments in immunology, vol 6. Elsevier/North-Holland, New York
21. Tokunaga T, Yamamoto H, Shimada S, Abe H, Fukuda T, Fujisawa Y, Furutani Y, Yano O, Kataoka T, Sudo T, Makiguchi N, Sugamura T (1984) Antitumor activity of deoxyribonucleic acid fraction from *Mycobacterium bovis* BCG. I. Isolation, physico-chemical characterization and antitumor activity. J Natl Cancer Inst 72:955
22 Tokunaga T, Yamamoto S, Namba K (1988) A synthetic single-stranded DNA, poly(dG,dC), induces interferon-alpha/beta and -gamma, augments natural killer activity, and suppresses tumor growth. Jpn J Cancer Res 79:682
23. Tokunaga T, Yano O, Kuramoto E, Kimura Y, Yamamoto T, Kataoka T, Yamamoto S (1992) Synthetic oligonucleotides with particular base sequences from the cCNA encoding proteins of *Mycobacterium bovis* BCG induce interferons and activate natural killer cells. Microbiol Immunol 36:55
24. Weiss DW, Bonhag RS, Parks JA (1964) Studies on the heterologous immunogenicity of a methanol-insoluble fraction of attenuated tubercle bacilli (BCG). J Exp Med 119:53
25. Yamamoto S, Yamamoto T, Kataoka T, Kuramoto E, Yano O, Tokunaga T, (1992) Unique palindromic sequences in synthetic oligonucleotides are required to induce IFN and augment IFN-mediated natural killer activity. J Immunol 148:4072
26. Yamamoto S, Yamamoto T, Shimada S, Kuramoto E, Yano O, Kataoka T, Tokunaga T (1992) DNA from bacteria, but not from vertebrates, induces interferons, activates natural killer cells and inhibits tumor growth. Microbiol Immunol 36:983
27. Yamamoto T, Yamamoto S, Kataoka T, Tokunaga T (1994) Lipofection of synthetic oligodeoxyribonucleotides having a palindromic sequence of AACGTT to murine splenocytes enhances interferon production and natural killer activity. Microbiol Immunol 38:831
28. Zbar B, Ribi E, Kelly M, Granger D, Evans C, Rapp HJ (1976) Immunologic approaches to the treatment of human cancer based on a guinea pig model. Cancer Immunol Immunother 1:127
29. Zimmermann S, Egeter O, Hausmann S, Lipford, GB, Rocken M, Wagner H, Heeg K (1998) CpG oligodeoxynucleotides trigger protective and curative Th1 response in lethal murine leishmaniasis. J Immunol 160:3627

Mechanisms of immune stimulation by bacterial DNA

David S. Pisetsky

Division of Rheumatology, Allergy and Clinical Immunology,
Durham VA Medical Center and Duke University Medical Center, Box 151G, Room E-1008,
508 Fulton Street, Durham, NC 27705, USA

Introduction

DNA is a complex macromolecule whose immunological properties result from sequence microheterogeneity. Although mammalian DNA is immunologically inert, DNA from bacterial sources displays powerful immunostimulatory activities that rival those of endotoxin in their range and potency. These activities result from short sequence motifs, termed CpG motifs or immunostimulatory sequences (ISSs), that occur much more commonly in bacterial than mammalian DNA. Since these sequences can activate the innate immune system, bacterial DNA may serve as a "danger signal" to stimulate host defense during infection [25].

The activities of bacterial DNA have attracted great interest among immunologists because of their implications for host defense as well as the burgeoning use of DNA to prevent and treat disease. DNA forms the basis of a variety of novel therapeutic approaches, including antisense therapy, DNA vaccination, DNA adjuvants as well as tumor immunotherapy. Some of these approaches are already in clinical trial, with the development of DNA vaccines and DNA adjuvants likely to accelerate in the coming years.

Despite the rapid introduction of DNA into the clinical arena, the mode of action of immunostimulatory DNA is still not well understood. Many questions remain about the structure-function relationship of ISSs, the mechanisms of cell uptake and signaling mechanisms operative in different cell types. Furthermore, although human use of immunostimulatory DNA is clearly in the offing, much of the basic biology of this system has involved animal models. Whether conclusions drawn from animal studies will apply to man will require much further investigation.

To provide a perspective on the role of DNA in host defense and immunotherapy, this chapter will review information on the mechanisms of cell activation by immunostimulatory DNA, focusing on three main issues: (1) cellular targets of immunostimulatory DNA; (2) structure-function relationships of immunostimulatory DNA; and (3) signal transduction mechanisms. As this account will indicate, immune properties of DNA result from short sequence motifs that can directly or indirectly trigger B cells, T cells, NK cells, macrophages and dendritic cells. The consequence of these activities is the stimulation of host defense mechanisms important in the eradication of infection and possibly malignancy.

Cellular targets of immunostimulatory DNA

The original observations establishing the immunostimulatory properties of bacterial DNA came from experiments to define the anti-tumor activity of an extract of *Mycobacterium bovis* BCG. This extract, called MY-1, could promote the in vivo rejection of transplantable tumors in mice. As shown by biochemical fractionation, this extract was predominantly DNA. Furthermore, digestion of the extract by DNase could eliminate activity, suggesting that mycobacterial DNA itself could cause tumor rejection. Since the extract did not directly affect tumor cell growth, an action on the immune system provided the most likely explanation for the observed effects in vivo [27, 28, 35].

Subsequent studies demonstrated that the MY-1 extract augmented NK cell activity, although this activation was secondary to cytokine production by an adherent cell population. As shown by assays of cytokines as well as the effects of anti-cytokine antibodies, IFN-α/β was a major factor leading to NK cell activation. Since the induction of IFN-α/β and NK cell activity was a property of DNA from bacterial, but not mammalian sources, these seminal experiments clearly showed that bacterial DNA can exert immunostimulatory properties that do not simply reflect its polyanionic nature [42].

To delineate the structural basis of immunostimulatory DNA, the in vitro activity of sequences from cloned mycobacterial DNA was tested. These studies demonstrated that stimulation of NK cell activity results from a variety of sequence motifs that in general center on a CpG motif and have features of a palindrome. Importantly, these motifs are active in the form of short oligonucleotides (30 bases or less) and in vitro can mimic the effects of intact bacterial DNA in terms of stimulation of IFN production as well as NK cell activation [18, 36].

As shown in in vitro experiments using murine cell preparations, the activity of bacterial DNA extends to B cells. Thus, DNA from a variety of bacterial DNA species can induce in vitro mitogenesis and polyclonal B cell activation. This activity is sensitive to DNase but resistant to polymixin B. Furthermore, the mitogenic activity is T cell independent since elimination of T cells by anti-T cell reagents is without effect. Since cells from endotoxin-resistant C3H/HeJ mice show similar responses as those of other strains, these findings suggest that bacterial DNA can directly activate B cells by a pathway distinct from that of LPS [21].

Subsequent studies on B cell mitogenesis explored the sequence requirements for B cell activation using synthetic oligonucleotides as in vitro stimulants. By searches for common features of active compounds, Krieg and colleagues demonstrated that a 6-base motif centered on a CpG dinucleotide is immunostimulatory and can elicit both polyclonal B cell activation and antibody production. This sequence has the general structure of two 5' purines, an unmethylated CpG dinucleotide, and two 3' pyrimidines (Pu-Pu-CpG-Pyr-Pyr) and closely resembles the sequence responsible for IFN induction [16, 22].

The active sequence, defined either as a palindrome or CpG motif, provides an explanation for how bacterial DNA can be recognized as foreign and stimulate immunity. Thus, bacterial DNA and mammalian DNA differ markedly in their content of CpG motifs. At least two reasons account for the differences in the content of CpG motifs in eukaryotic and prokaryotic DNA. In mammalian DNA, cytosine and guanosine occur in tandem much less commonly than predicted by the base composition of DNA. This phenomenon is known as CpG suppression. Furthermore, in mammalian DNA, cytosine is commonly methylated in this position [10]. The result of these two features leads to a major quantitative difference in the presence of immunostimulatory sequences in eukaryotic and prokaryotic DNA.

While the basis of CpG suppression is not known, cytosine methylation has been considered an important regulatory element in determining the transcriptional activity of genes during differentiated cells function. The delineation of immune potential of CpG DNA, however, has suggested that CpG suppression and cytosine methylation may have evolved in concert as an immunological recognition system to allow bacterial DNA to signal the presence of infection [6]. This function of this alternative genetic code is speculative at present, but this line of thought has given impetus to elucidate mechanisms of immune activation by DNA.

Although the exact sequences of ISSs remain a matter of inquiry (see below), these findings have nevertheless suggested that short, synthetic oligonucleotides (oligos) can be used to elucidate immune activation by bacterial DNA. These synthetic compounds facilitate analysis of structure-function relationships and eliminate potentially confounding factors from contamination by material such as endotoxin. In the use of synthetic oligos, both phosphodiester (Po) and phosphorothioate (Ps) compounds have been used. Phosphorothioate compounds are DNA derivatives in which one of the non-bridging oxygens in the phosphodiester backbone is replaced by a sulfur atom [31]. These compounds are resistant to nuclease and may have a greater potency both in vitro and in vivo than phosphodiesters.

Analysis of immune activation by DNA has variously used natural DNA, Po oligos and Ps oliogs. Although these DNA sources may not be identical in either mode of action or structure-function relationships, they exhibit sufficient similarity to allow results obtained with these different stimulants to be interpreted together. A subsequent section will consider differences among these compounds. For convenience, these DNA molecules will be called CpG DNA.

Cellular effects of CpG DNA

CpG DNA exerts direct or indirect effects on all major cellular elements of the immune system, leading to enhanced activity of B, T and NK cells as well as macrophages and dendritic cells as described below.

Macrophages

Similar to endotoxin, CpG DNA powerfully activates macrophages and induces cytokines whose downstream actions influence other cellular responses. The cytokines stimulated by CpG DNA include IFN-α/β, IL-1β, IL-6, TNF-α and IL-12. In addition to the production of cytokines, macrophages stimulated by CpG show enhanced expression of inducible nitric oxide synthase (iNOS) as measured by both mRNA as well as protein production. In the induction of iNOS by CpG DNA, IFN-γ may be required at least in certain cell lines used as models for this response [8, 30, 33].

Although stimulation of macrophages by CpG DNA and endotoxin leads to a similar array of inflammatory mediators, these responses are distinct. Evidence for this conclusion comes from the ability of endotoxin-resistant C3H/HeJ mice to respond to DNA. Furthermore, among macrophage cell lines, responses to CpG DNA and endotoxin are not invariably linked. The differences in activation by CpG DNA and endotoxin are also apparent in the pattern of IL-12 p40 transcription [5].

B cells

CpG DNA is mitogenic for murine B cells and can induce polyclonal immunoglobulin production. These responses are independent of T cells as shown by the responses of T-depleted cultures and B cell lines. Immunoglobulin production by B cells may result from the effects of IL-6 which is also induced by CpG DNA. This cytokine may function in an autocrine fashion since anti-IL-6 can eliminate production of Ig, although this treatment does not affect proliferation [16, 21, 44].

The effects of CpG extend to the process of apoptosis. In the WEHI-231 B cell line, CpG oligos protect against apoptosis resulting from stimulation by anti-IgM. In primary B cells, CpG DNA can protect CD40 ligand-stimulated B cells from Fas mediated cytotoxicity induced by either cytotoxic T cells or anti-Fas antibodies. This protection may result from down-regulation of Fas as demonstrated by FACS measurement of cell surface Fas expression. Although CpG DNA up-regulates IL-6, the anti-apoptotic effects are independent of this cytokine since neither IL-6 nor supernatants of CpG DNA-stimulated cells reproduce the effects of the DNA [37, 45].

NK cells

Since purified NK cells do not respond directly to CpG DNA, induction of cytotoxicity and IFN-γ production by these cells appears to be the consequence of downstream effects of cytokines induced by this stimulant. Among these cytokines, IFN-α/β, IL-12, TNF-α, all inducible by CpG DNA, can activate NK cells to cytotoxicity and IFN-γ production. Similar to findings with other cell types, CpG DNA may interact with other stimulants (e.g., cytokines) to promote cellular responses. Thus, NK cells in the presence of IL-12 may have an augmented response to CpG DNA [1, 4, 40].

T cells

T cells alone do not appear to respond directly to CpG DNA, although their activity can be influenced by cytokines produced by other cell types (e.g., macrophages) activated by CpG DNA. In addition, CpG DNA may co-stimulate T cells that have been activated through their T cell receptor. In in vitro systems in which antigen-presenting cells (APCs) are eliminated, CpG DNA can induce IL-2 production, IL-2 receptor expression and proliferation of purified T cells stimulated by anti-CD3. This stimulation occurs in both CD4 and CD8 cells and can be inhibited by cyclosporine A. Since T cells from CD28 knockout mice show proliferation by CpG DNA and anti-CD3, CpG may be able to substitute for CD28 co-stimulation [2].

Dendritic cells

Like macrophages, dendritic cells appear to respond directly to CpG DNA. As shown using dendritic cells derived from bone marrow cultures, CpG DNA can stimulate both immature and mature populations as determined by flow cytometry. For both populations, CpG DNA can induce up-regulation of MHC class II, CD40, and CD86 cell surface molecules, although expression of CD80 is not affected. Furthermore, CpG DNA can stimulate both mature and immature populations to produce IL-12, IL-6 and TNF-α. As a consequence of these effects, dendritic cells activated by CpG DNA demonstrate enhanced APC function in mixed lymphocytes reactions as well as induction of T cell responses by staphylococcal enterotoxin B [29].

Together, these observations indicate that CpG DNA can promote immune responses of the Th1 kind through direct effects on APCs and B cells as well as indirect effects on other cytokines, most notably IFN-γ. Since these effects are central to the use of CpG DNA either alone or as part of a DNA vaccine, elucidating these mechanisms has become a major investigative priority. Two important questions must be addressed to refine the use of CpG DNA: (1) What are the structures of DNA key to immunomodulation? and (2) What are the intracellular mechanisms for immune activation? The subsequent sections will review these topics.

Structure-function relationships of immunostimulatory DNA

The sequences of ISSs have been investigated intensively since defining their structure-function relationship is an important prelude to characterizing any receptors or binding molecules that interact with CpG and lead to activation. In this endeavor, synthetic oligonucleotides have become a mainstay. At this point, hundreds if not thousands of different oligos have been tested in vitro or in vivo. While this mass of information should provide clarity on this issue, important questions remain concerning the structure of motifs conferring activity.

At least two groups have extensively investigated structure-function relationships of CpG DNA. Tokunaga, Yamamoto and colleagues originally tested oligonucleotides bearing sequences from mycobacterial genes and determined common features associated with activity. These investigators then systematically varied these sequences in the form of 30-mer oligonucleotides in which flanking sequences were held invariant. Using NK cell activity as an assay, palindromic sequences showed the greatest potency in vitro. In general, these sequences had the Pur-Pur-CpG-Pyr-Pyr structure, although there were exceptions to this rule. Thus, the sequences CGATCG and ATCGAT both showed activity [12, 18, 41].

In contrast to this approach, Krieg and colleagues derived rules for activity by inspection of a large panel of oligonucleotides tested for activity primarily using B cell proliferation assays [16]. On the basis of these data, these investigators identified the Pur-Pur-CpG-Pyr-Pyr motif as the most critical for activity. While this motif accommodates many palindromes, a palindromic sequence was not found to be essential for activity. In studies by both groups, methylation of the cytosine residue was associated with loss of activity. Furthermore, at least some sequences identified on the basis of murine studies were also active in humans, using cytokine production and NK cell activation as readouts. Human B cells, however, do not seem to respond to either bacterial DNA or Po oligos [19].

Since compounds designed on the basis of either motif produce useful immunostimulants, the difference in interpretation of this issue relates to understanding mechanisms of stimulation. The studies by Tokunaga, Yamamoto and colleagues suggest that a higher order base-paired structure may be the stimulatory moiety. In contrast, the studies of Krieg and colleagues point to a linear sequence that may or may not have the capacity for base pairing.

Several aspects of this controversy bear comment. First, the focus on the 6-base motif minimizes the contribution of the flanking regions. These flanking regions may affect the conformation of the 6-base motif or exert other effects on the motif's activity. Comparing oligos that differ in length as well as flanking sequence may, therefore, lead to confusion about the intrinsic activity of the 6-base motif. Furthermore, while it is generally assumed that the structure-function relationships for stimulation of B cells are the same as for macrophages, this point has not been rigorously evaluated. Indeed, there is evidence that certain sequences can stimulate IL-12 but not TNF-α [20]. Some of the differences in structure-function relationships of compounds may, therefore, relate to the cell system used for assay.

Another issue in evaluating the structure of ISSs concerns the use of Ps oligos as test compounds. These compounds, which have the substitution of a sulfur for one of the non-bridging oxygens in the DNA backbone, differ from Po compounds in properties such as nuclease resistance, melting temperature, protein binding and cellular uptake. Available data suggests that rules for activity of Po and Ps oligos differ, since some Ps and Po oligos of the same sequence vary in their capacity to stimulate cells. Furthermore, even a limited stretch of Ps sequence in a Po oligos may alter the activity of an ISS and in some instances inhibit responses [1, 9].

In view of structural and pharmacological differences of Po and Ps compounds, any assessment of structure-function relationship must consider the impact of backbone chemistry. B cells responses provide a telling example of this point. Thus, in mouse, stimulation of murine B cells by Ps oligos is not directly related to the content of CpG motifs and can occur in their absence [3, 23]. This finding suggests primacy of the backbone in certain systems. Similarly, in humans, Ps compounds are mitogenic for highly purified B cells, whereas Po compounds are inactive; optimal activity also does not require a CpG motif for these cells [19].

Adding to the complexity of this system, recent data indicate the existence of DNA sequences that can neutralize or inhibit the immunostimulatory activity of CpG motifs. These sequences were discovered in studies on the immune activity of adenoviral DNA, which showed that, while type 12 adenoviral DNA is active, type 2 and type 5 DNA fails to stimulate responses of human peripheral blood. Since type 2 and type 5 DNA both contain CpG dinucleotides, their lack of activity suggested the presence of other DNA sequences that could neutralize or block stimulation. The ability of the non-stimulatory adenoviral DNA to block the response to *Escherichia coli* DNA supported that possibility. As shown by sequence comparisons of adenoviral DNA and as well as the effect of synthetic oligos, neutralizing sequences may result from direct repeats of CpG dinucleotides as well as CpG motifs preceded by a C or followed by a G [15]. While suggesting a strategy for viruses to subvert host defense, these motifs are also relevant in the design of DNA vectors for vaccination or gene therapy.

These considerations suggest that immune stimulation by DNA is the summation of stimulatory and inhibitory activities that is not solely related to the presence of CpG motifs. For example, unmethylated mammalian DNA fails to stimulate cells despite its content of CpG motifs, possibly because neutralizing or inhibitory sequences prevent activity [32]. Similarly, among bacterial DNA, potency of immune stimulation varies markedly depending on species, with some DNA having only limited ability to induce mitogenesis or cytokine production despite the presence of CpG

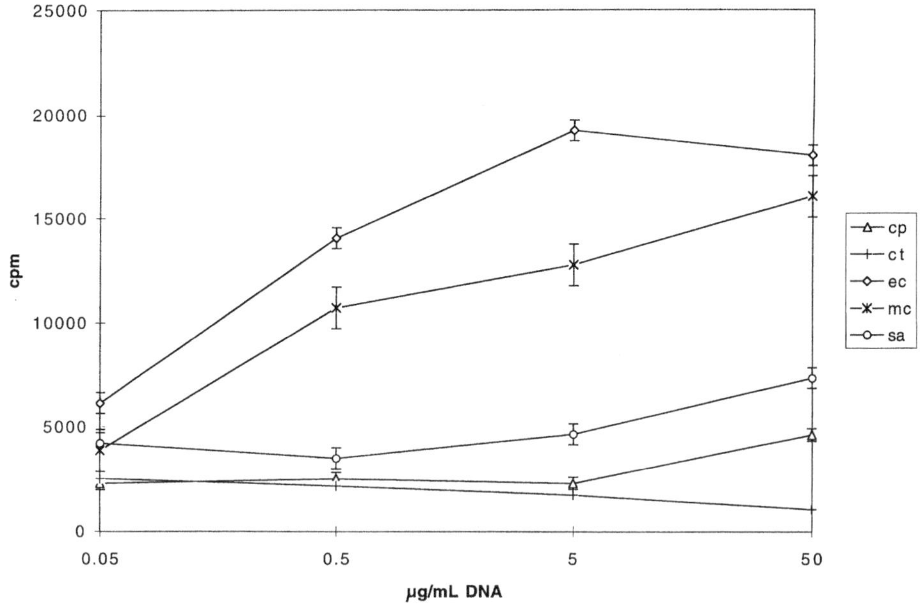

Fig. 1. Stimulation of in vitro proliferation by bacterial DNA. In vitro mitogenic activity of bacterial DNA was assessed by proliferation assays of murine spleen cells. DNA tested included *Clostridium perfringens* (*CP*), calf thymus (*CT*), *E. coli* (*EC*), *Micrococcus lysodeikticus* (*MC*) and *Staphylococcus aureus* (*SA*). Reproduced with permission from [24]

motifs [24]. Figure 1 illustrates this point. Until structure-function relationships of immunostimulatory DNA are better defined, these observations suggest caution in equating CpG content with stimulation and assuming that bacterial DNA are uniform in activating potential.

Influence of base sequence on cell binding and DNA uptake

Several lines of evidence suggest that immune activation by CpG DNA requires DNA internalization. This evidence includes the following observations; (1) DNA attached to beads fails to stimulate cells; (2) agents such as lipofectin that can promote cellular uptake of DNA augment immunostimulation; (3) cell binding of CpG and non-CpG DNA is the same; and (4) the ability of CpG DNA to stimulate different immune cell populations may be related to extent of cell binding and of endocytosis [14, 43]. Thus, resting T cells, which are unresponsive to oligos unless they receive another activating signal, are nonendocytic and show lower cell surface binding of oligos than B cells.

While the uptake and trafficking of DNA are not well understood, receptor-mediated endocytosis appears to be the predominant mechanism by which DNA enters cells. In general, this process has been considered to be sequence nonspecific and, therefore, not a factor influencing immune activation by DNA. Studies on both synthetic and natural DNA indicate, however, that certain DNA sequences can promote uptake of DNA and can significantly influence the activity of CpG DNA.

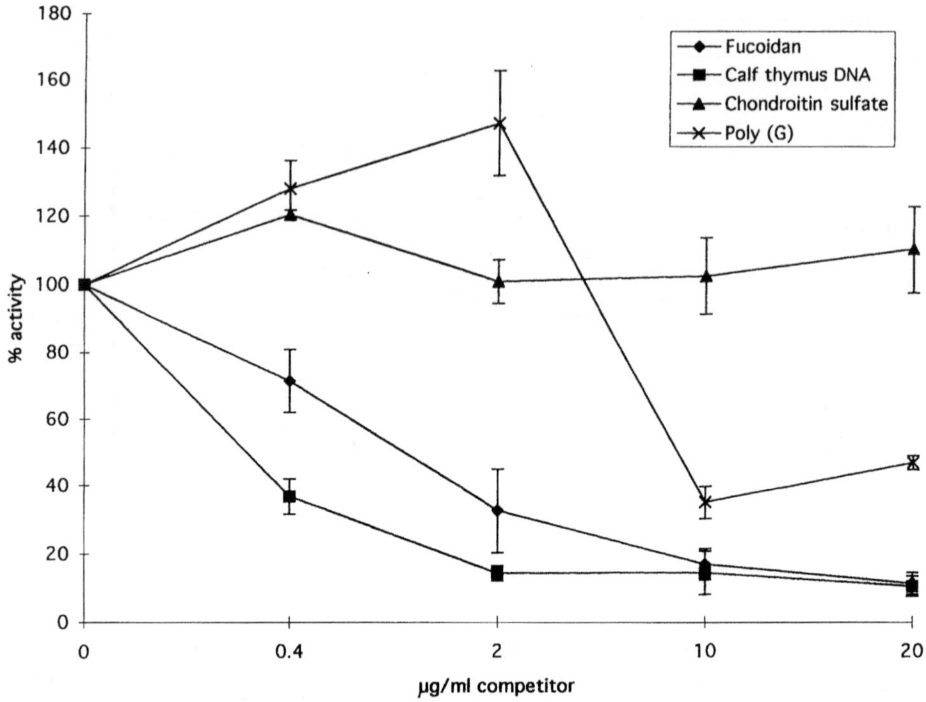

Fig. 2. Effects of MSR ligands on in vitro IL-12 responses induced by plasmid DNA. The effects of MSR ligands on IL-12 production were assessed in cultures of murine spleen cells stimulated with pCMV-β plasmid. Results are reported in terms of % activity of uninhibited cultures. Reproduced with permission from [39]

Furthermore, certain cell surface receptors may have enhanced binding to DNA on the basis of sequence, pointing to another factor determining the structure-function relationship to CpG DNA.

The clearest evidence for the impact of sequence on binding comes from observations on the effects of flanking bases on the activity of the palindromic sequence AACGTT embedded in 30-mer oligos in which the flanks consisted of single bases. In oligos of this structure, dG flanks led to the highest activity when assessed using NK cell activation as a measure. Other flanks (e.g., dT) caused appreciable activity, although dA flanks were inactive. Since extended runs of each base were inactive, these findings suggest that flanks can modify the activity of a CpG motif without themselves displaying causing immunostimulation [13].

While a variety of mechanisms could account for the ability of dG runs to enhance immunostimulation by a CpG motif, enhanced cell binding and uptake appears most likely. Extended runs of dG, by virtue of their ability to base pair with each other, can form four strand arrays called G-quartets or quadruplex DNA. In these arrays, strands can align in either the parallel or anti-parallel orientation. Such a structure may exist at telomeres where the concentration of dG runs is high [38].

Enhanced binding of dG runs to cells may relate to binding to both surface receptors as well as the phospholipid bilayer. Among macrophage cell surface molecules, the type A macrophage scavenger receptor (MSR) displays a broad pattern of polyan-

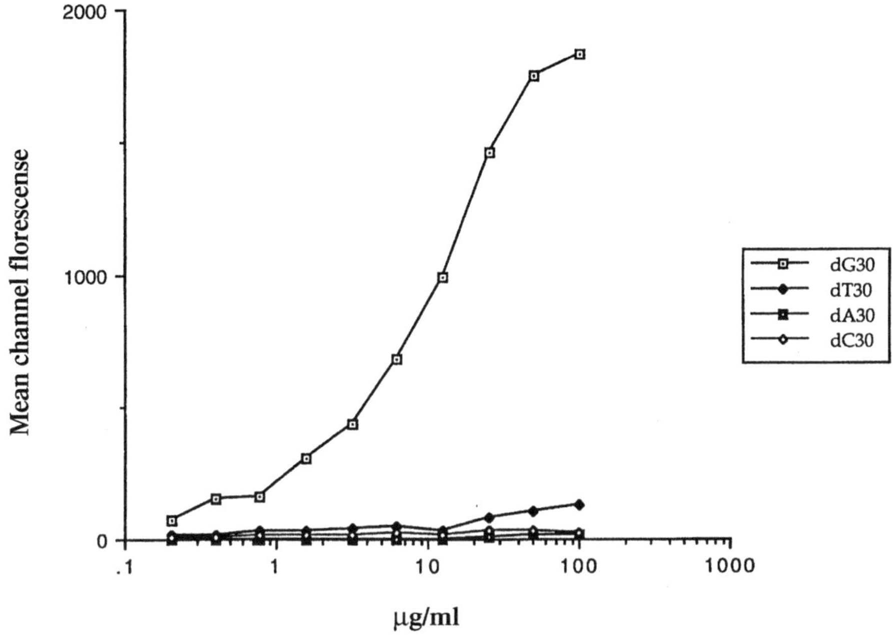

Fig. 3. Flow cytometry analysis of oligonucleotide binding to murine spleen cells. The binding of fluoresceinated single-base 30-mer oligonucleotides to murine spleen cells was assessed. Results are reported in terms of mean channel fluorescence. Reproduced with permission from [26]

ion binding and has specificity for oxidized low-density lipoprotein (LDL), acetylated LDL, dextran sulfate, fucoidan, LPS and poly I and poly G. This receptor may serve as a pattern recognition molecule and take up either foreign or damaged self proteins for elimination. Although LPS binds the MSR, it does not cause cell activation suggesting the role of the MSR as a clearance rather than triggering molecule [17].

In in vitro culture, the MSR appears to play a role in the response to CpG DNA. Thus, short oligos with dG residues show enhanced binding to macrophages and can cause activation by a mechanism that is blocked by other MSR ligands. Furthermore, although the MSR has strong preference for dG runs, it can also bind natural DNA [34, 39]. Thus, similar to effects of oligos, MSR ligands can block the response of macrophages to bacterial as well as plasmid DNA (Fig. 2). At present, it appears that the role of the MSR is to promote uptake of DNA into cells rather than signal activation since MSR ligands other than CpG DNA did not cause cytokine production.

The effects of dG residues also extends to B cells, although these cells lack the type A MSR. In contrast to results with macrophages, dG oligonucleotides, even in the absence of CpG motifs, can cause B cell proliferation and antibody production under conditions in which other single-base oligos are inactive [22]. Furthermore, among 30-base compounds with CpG motifs, dG flanks cause the highest level of cell activation. The extent of activity is correlated with cell surface binding. As shown by flow cytometry (Fig. 3), dG oligos (with or without a CpG motif) show the highest level of binding [26].

Studies with synthetic phosphorothioates indicate that dG oligos have greater interaction with phospholipid micelles than other single-base oligos. This finding suggests that increased cell binding of dG runs could reflect either binding to receptors or the lipid bilayer [11]. While indicating clearly that base composition can influence the magnitude of cell binding of DNA, these findings also demonstrate differences in the activation requirements for macrophages and B cells and the ability of non-CpG sequences to trigger activation in at least certain cell types.

Signal transduction pathways

As this account indicates, DNA signals a cell in a sequence-(or structure-) specific manner following internalization. This internalization involves maturation of an endosomal compartment, since inhibitors of endosomal acidification such as chloroquine and related compounds can block the ability of CpG DNA to induce secretion of IL-6 or prevent apoptosis induced by anti-IgM. Furthermore, while activation of IL-6 does not involve protein kinase C, protein kinase A or nitric oxide, it is associated with the generation of reactive oxygen species (ROS). The generation of ROS, which can also be blocked by chloroquine, appears to be an important step in transcriptional activation since antioxidants such as PDTC are also inhibitory [46, 49].

As shown in cell lines as well as bone marrow macrophages, CpG DNA can increase NK-κB binding activity as shown by EMSA as well as the transcriptional activity of luciferase reporter genes under the control of the HIV-1 LTR. Similarly, in J774 cells, CpG DNA can induce NF-κB as well as prevent the degradation of IκBα and IκBβ. The importance of NF-κB in activation is further demonstrated by the effects of various inhibitors of steps in NF-κB activation. PDTC, an inhibitor of IκB phosphorylation;TPCK, a protease inhibitor of IκB degradation; and gliotoxin, an inhibitor of IκB degradation can all block the induction of cytokines such as IL-6. Since anti-oxidants block the activation of NF-κB induced by CpG DNA, these findings suggest that ROS generation precedes NF-κB activation and is required for its expression [30, 46, 47, 49]. The mechanisms for ROS generation cannot be delineated from these experiments.

While NF-κB activation could explain some of the observed activation by CpG DNA, other pathways appear to be critically involved in this process. In murine macrophages and dendritic cells, CpG DNA can induce the phosphorylation of Jun N-terminal kinase (JNK) kinase 1 and subsequent activation of stress kinases JNK 1/2 and p38. Furthermore, as shown using reporter gene constructs, the activation of stress kinases is associated with an increase in AP-1 transcription activity and the phosphorylation of c-Jun. Since inhibitors of p38 kinase activity can inhibit the expression of TNF-α and IL-12, this pathway must also contribute to transcriptional activity by CpG ODN. As in the case of NK-κB, the stimulation of stress kinases is dependent on the endosomal maturation and can be inhibited by chloroquine and bafilomycin [7, 48].

While NF-κB and stress kinase pathways account for transcriptional activation by CpG motifs, they do not yet explain the sequence specificity of triggering. The activity of DNA of only certain structures (sequence or palindrome) has suggested the existence of a binding protein(s) that could serve as proximal element in signal transduction, coupling internalization of DNA with activation of NF-κB or stress kinases. With identification of such binding and coupling molecules, the activation pathways will greatly clarify and allow the development of more potent activators or inhibitors of this system.

Conclusion

Bacterial DNA promotes powerful immune system activation because of its content of characteristic sequence motifs. These sequences induce cellular changes that promote inflammation and the generation of Th1 responses. This activation involves internalization of DNA as well as the activation of NF-κB and stress kinases. Future studies will identify DNA-binding molecules that are key to these activation events and may serve as targets for novel immunomodulatory agents.

References

1. Ballas ZK, Rasmussen WL, Krieg AM (1996) Induction of NK activity in murine and human cells by CpG motifs in oligodeoxynucleotides and bacterial DNA. J Immunol 157:1840
2. Bendigs S, Salzer U, Lipford GB, Wagner H, Heeg K (1999) CpG-oligodeoxynucleotides co-stimulate primary T cells in the absence of antigen-presenting cells. Eur J Immunol 29:1209
3. Branda RF, Moore AL, Lafayette AR, Mathews L, Hong R, Zon G, Brown T, McCormack JJ (1996) Amplification of antibody production by phosphorothioate oligodeoxynucleotides. J Lab Clin Med 128:329
4. Chace JH, Hooker NA, Mildenstein KL, Krieg AM, Cowdery JS (1997) Bacterial DNA-induced NK cell IFN-γ production is dependent on macrophage secretion of IL-12. Clin Immunol Immunopathol 84:185
5. Cowdery JS, Boerth NJ, Norian LA, Myung PS, Koretzky GA (1999) Differential regulation of the IL-12 p40 promoter and of p40 secretion by CpG DNA and lipopolysaccharide. J Immunol 162:6770
6. Doerfler W (1991) Patterns of DNA methylation – evolutionary vestiges of foreign DNA inactivation as a host defense mechanism. A proposal. Biol Chem Hoppe-Seyler 372:557
7. Hacker H, Mischak H, Miethke T, Liptay S, Schmid R, Sparwasser T, Heeg K, Lipford GB, Wagner H (1998) CpG-DNA-specific activation of antigen-presenting cells requires stress kinase activity and is preceded by non-specific endocytosis and endosomal maturation. EMBO J 17:6230
8. Halpern MD, Kurlander RJ, Pisetsky DS (1996) Bacterial DNA induces murine interferon-γ production by stimulation of interleukin-12 and tumor necrosis factor-α. Cell Immunol 167:72
9. Halpern MD, Pisetsky DS (1995) In vitro inhibition of murine IFNγ production by phosphorothioate deoxyguanosine oligomers. Immunopharmacology 29:47
10. Hergersberg M (1991) Biological aspects of cytosine methylation in eukaryotic cells. Experientia 47:1171
11. Hughes JA, Avrutskaya AV, Juliano RL (1994) Influence of base composition on membrane binding and cellular uptake of 10-mer phosphorothioate oligonucleotides in Chinese hamster ovary (CH^RC5) cells. Antisense Res Dev 4:211
12. Kataoka T, Yamamoto S, Yamamoto T, Kuramoto E, Kimura Y, Yano O, Tokunaga T (1992) Antitumor activity of synthetic oligonucleotides with sequences from cDNA encoding proteins of *Mycobacterium bovis* BCG. Jpn J Cancer Res 83:244
13. Kimura Y, Sonehara K, Kuramoto E, Makino T, Yamamoto S, Yamamoto T, Kataoka T, Tokunaga T (1994) Binding of oligoguanylate to scavenger receptors is required for oligonucleotides to augment NK cell activity and induce IFN. J Biochem 116:991
14. Krieg AM, Gmelig-Meyling F, Gourley MF, Kisch WJ, Chrisey LA, Steinberg AD (1991) Uptake of oligodeoxyribonucleotides by lymphoid cells is heterogeneous and inducible. Antisense Res Dev 1:161
15. Krieg AM, Wu T, Weeratna R, Efler SM, Love-Homan L, Yang L, Yi A-K, Short D, Davis HL (1998) Sequence motifs in adenoviral DNA block immune activation by stimulatory CpG motifs. Proc Natl Acad Sci USA 95:12631
16. Krieg AM, Yi A-K, Matson S, Waldschmidt TJ, Bishop GA, Teasdale R, Koretzky GA, Klinman DM (1995) CpG motifs in bacterial DNA trigger direct B-cell activation. Nature 374:546
17. Krieger M (1997) The other side of scavenger receptors: pattern recognition for host defense. Curr Opin Lipidol 8:275
18. Kuramoto E, Yano O, Kimura Y, Baba M, Makino T, Yamamoto S, Yamamoto T, Kataoka T, Tokunaga T (1992) Oligonucleotide sequences required for natural killer cell activation. Jpn J Cancer Res 83:1128

19. Liang H, Nishioka Y, Reich CF, Pisetsky DS, Lipsky PE (1996) Activation of human B cells by phosphorothioate oligodeoxynucleotides. J Clin Invest 98:1119
20. Lipford GB, Sparwasser T, Bauer M, Zimmermann S, Koch E-S, Heeg K, Wagner H (1997) Immunostimulatory DNA: sequence-dependent production of potentially harmful or useful cytokines. Eur J Immunol 27:3420
21. Messina JP, Gilkeson GS, Pisetsky DS (1991) Stimulation of in vitro murine lymphocyte proliferation by bacterial DNA. J Immunol 147:1759
22. Messina JP, Gilkeson GS, Pisetsky DS (1993) The influence of DNA structure on the in vitro stimulation of murine lymphocytes by natural and synthetic polynucleotide antigens. Cell Immunol 147:148
23. Monteith DK, Henry SP, Howard RB, Flournoy S, Levin AA, Bennett CF, Crooke ST (1997) Immune stimulation – a class effect of phosphorothioate oligodeoxynucleotides in rodents. Anticancer Drug Des 12:421
24. Neujahr DC, Reich CF, Pisetsky DS (1999) Immunostimulatory properties of genomic DNA from different bacterial species. Immunobiology 200:106
25. Pisetsky DS (1996) Immune activation by bacterial DNA: a new genetic code. Immunity 5:303
26. Pisetsky DS, Reich CF III (1998) The influence of base sequence on the immunological properties of defined oligonucleotides. Immunopharmacology 40:199
27. Shimada S, Yano O, Inoue H, Kuramoto E, Fukuda T, Yamamoto H, Kataoka T, Tokunaga T (1985) Antitumor activity of the DNA fraction from *Mycobacterium bovis* BCG. II. Effects on various syngeneic mouse tumors. J Natl Cancer Inst 74:681
28. Shimada S, Yano O, Tokunaga T (1986) In vivo augmentation of natural killer cell activity with a deoxyribonucleic acid fraction of BCG. Jpn J Cancer Res 77:808
29. Sparwasser T, Koch E-S, Vabulas RM, Heeg K, Lipford GB, Ellwart JW, Wagner H (1998) Bacterial DNA and immunostimulatory CpG oligonucleotides trigger maturation and activation of murine dendritic cells. Eur J Immunol 28:2045
30. Stacey KJ, Sweet MJ, Hume DA (1996) Macrophages ingest and are activated by bacterial DNA. J Immunol 157:2116
31. Stein CA, Cheng Y-C (1993) Antisense oligonucleotides as therapeutic agents – is the bullet really magical? Science 261:1004
32. Sun S, Beard C, Jaenisch R, Jones P, Sprent J (1997) Mitogenicity of DNA from different organisms for murine B cells. J Immunol 159:3119
33. Sweet MJ, Stacey KJ, Kakuda DK, Markovich D, Hume DA (1998) IFN-γ primes macrophage responses to bacterial DNA. J Interferon Cytokine Res 18:263
34. Takagi T, Hashiguchi M, Mahato RI, Tokuda H, Takakura Y, Hashida M (1998) Involvement of specific mechanism in plasmid DNA uptake by mouse peritoneal macrophages. Biochem Biophys Res Commun 245:729
35. Tokunaga T, Yamamoto H, Shimada S, Abe H, Fukuda T, Fujisawa Y, Furutani Y, Yano O, Kataoka T, Sudo T, Makiguchi N, Suganuma T (1984) Antitumor activity of deoxyribonucleic acid fraction from *Mycobacterium bovis* BCG. I. Isolation, physicochemical characterization, and antitumor activity. J Natl Cancer Inst 72:955
36. Tokunaga T, Yano O, Kuramoto E, Kimura Y, Yamamoto T, Kataoka T, Yamamoto S (1992) Synthetic oligonucleotides with particular base sequences from the cDNA encoding proteins of *Mycobacterium bovis* BCG induce interferons and activate natural killer cells. Microbiol Immunol 36:55
37. Wang Z, Karras JG, Colarusso TP, Foote LC, Rothstein TL (1997) Unmethylated CpG motifs protect murine B lymphocytes against fas-mediated apoptosis. Cell Immunol 180:162
38. Williamson JR (1994) G-quartet structures in telomeric DNA. Annu Rev Biophys Biomol Struct 23:703
39. Wloch MK, Pasquini S, Ertl HCJ, Pisetsky DS (1998) The influence of DNA sequence on the immunostimulatory properties of plasmid DNA vectors. Hum Gen Ther 9:1439
40. Yamamoto S, Kuramoto E, Shimada S, Tokunaga T (1988) In vitro augmentation of natural killer cell activity and production of interferon-α/β and -γ with deoxyribonucleic acid fraction from *Mycobacterium bovis* BCG. Jpn J Cancer Res 79:866
41. Yamamoto S, Yamamoto T, Kataoka T, Kuramoto E, Yano O, Tokunaga T (1992) Unique palindromic sequences in synthetic oligonucleotides are required to induce IFN and augment IFN-mediated natural killer activity. J Immunol 148:4072
42. Yamamoto S, Yamamoto T, Shimada S, Kuramoto E, Yano O, Kataoka T, Tokunaga T (1992) DNA from bacteria, but not from vertebrates, induces interferons, activates natural killer cells and inhibits tumor growth. Microbiol Immunol 36:983

43. Yamamoto T, Yamamoto S, Kataoka T, Tokunaga T (1994) Lipofection of synthetic oligodeoxyribonucleotide having a palindromic sequence of AACGTT to murine splenocytes enhances interferon production and natural killer activity. Microbiol Immunol 38:831
44. Yi A-K, Chace JH, Cowdery JS, Krieg AM (1996) IFN-γ promotes IL-6 and IgM secretion in response to CpG motifs in bacterial DNA and oligodeoxynucleotides. J Immunol 156:558
45. Yi A-K, Hornbeck P, Lafrenz DE, Krieg AM (1996) CpG DNA rescue of murine B lymphoma cells from anti-IgM induced growth arrest and programmed cell death is associated with increased expression of *c-myc* and $bcl\text{-}x_l$. J Immunol 157:4918
46. Yi A-K, Klinman DM, Martin TL, Matson S, Krieg AM (1996) Rapid immune activation by CpG motifs in bacterial DNA. Systemic induction of IL-6 transcription through an antioxidant-sensitive pathway. J Immunol 157:5394
47. Yi A-K, Krieg AM (1998) CpG DNA rescue from anti-IgM-induced WEHI-231 B lymphoma apoptosis via modulation of IκBα and IκBβ sustained activation of nuclear factor-κB/c-Rel. J Immunol 160:1240
48. Yi A-K, Krieg AM (1998) Cutting edge: rapid induction of mitogen-activated protein kinases by immune stimulatory CpG DNA. J Immunol 161:4493
49. Yi A-K, Tuetken R, Redford T, Waldschmidt M, Kirsch J, Krieg AM (1998) CpG motifs in bacterial DNA activate leukocytes through the pH-dependent generation of reactive oxygen species. J Immunol 160:4755

Activation of NK cell (human and mouse) by immunostimulatory DNA sequence

Saburo Yamamoto[1], Toshiko Yamamoto[1], Sumiko Iho[2], Tohru Tokunaga[3]

[1] Department of Bacterial and Blood Products, National Institute of Infectious Diseases, 4-7-1 Gakuen, Musashimurayama, Tokyo 208-0011, Japan
[2] Department of Immunology and Medical Zoology, Faculty of Medicine, Fukui Medical University, Fukui, Japan
[3] Fukuoka Jo-gakuin University, Fukuoka, Japan

In vivo augmentation of mouse NK cell activity with BCG-DNA

A purified nucleic acid fraction extracted from *Mycobacterium bovis* BCG and designated MY-1, which was composed of 70.0% DNA and 28.0% RNA, 1.3% protein, 0.27% hexose and 0.1% lipid with no detectable amounts of cell wall components possesses strong antitumor activity against various syngeneic mouse and guinea pig tumors. This fraction showed no direct cytotoxicity in vitro against these tumors. MY-1 after digestion with RNase contained 97.0% single-stranded DNA with a guanine-cytosine content of 69.8%, and showed stronger antitumor activity than undigested MY-1, while MY-1 digested with DNase contained 97.0% RNA, and had reduced activity [15, 19]. Peritoneal cells from BALB/c mice injected intraperitoneally with MY-1 (100 μg) 3 h, 1 day, 2 days, 4 days or 7 days before, were tested for cytotoxic activity. An intraperitoneal injection of MY-1 1 day earlier rendered mouse peritoneal cells strongly cytotoxic to YAC-1 cells in vitro, but those obtained 3 h and 4 days after MY-1 showed only weak cytotoxicity. Those obtained 2 days after MY-1 injection induced moderate cytotoxicity. The effector cells were non-adherent to plastic dishes. No cytotoxicity of the adherent cell fraction was observed. Nonadherent cells activated by MY-1 were not cytotoxic against P815 cells even in a 16-h ^{51}Cr release assay. The activity was destroyed by treatment with anti-asialo-GM1 antiserum plus complement or carrageenan in vitro, but not with carbonyl-iron or anti-Thy 1.2 antiserum, suggesting that the cells are NK cel. In vivo augmentation of NK activity was dependent on MY-1 dose, and reached a peak 1 day after MY-1 injection. Since NK activity in lipopolysaccharide (LPS)-nonresponder mice could be augmented by MY-1, the possibility that LPS contaminated the MY-1 augmented-NK cell activity was excluded. MY-1 digested preliminarily with DNase lost its NK-inducing activity suggesting that the DNA entity of MY-1 was essential for the activity. When mice were pretreated with anti-asialo-GM1 or carrageenan, MY-1 could not render the peritoneal cells cytotoxic. Antitumor activity of MY-1 was also abolished if the animals were pretreated with asialo GM1 antiserum or carrageenan suggesting that the activity can be ascribed mainly to activated NK cells [16].

S. Yamamoto

In vitro augmentation of mouse NK cell activity

MY-1 also augmented NK cell activity of mouse spleen cells in vitro, and produced factors which showed antiviral activity and rendered normal macrophages cytotoxic towards tumor cells. Spleen cells from normal BALB/c mouse were incubated for 20 h with various concentrations of MY-1, and the NK activity of the cells and the IFN and macrophage-activating factor (MAF) activities of the culture supernatants were measured. All of the NK, IFN and MAF activities were elevated remarkably after the incubation with MY-1 in a dose-dependent manner. The activities reached the highest level after 6 h of incubation. A significant elevation of NK activity was seen after 1 h, while neither IFN nor MAF activity was observed within 3 h. RNase-digested MY-1 induced cellular responses similar to those of MY-1, but no activity was seen in the DNase-digested MY-1, indicating that the DNA in MY-1 was essential for the responses. The MAF function was destroyed by treatment with a small amount of anti-γ antiserum or under acidic condition (pH 2), but not by treatment with anti-IFN-α/β, while the antiviral activity in the culture supernatants was almost completely destroyed by treatment with anti-IFN-alpha/beta antiserum. It appears that DNA from BCG stimulated mouse spleen cells in vitro, resulting in augmentation of NK activity and production of IFN-α/β and IFN-γ [21].

In vitro augmentation of NK activity of peripheral blood cells from cancer patients by BCG-DNA

There are several lines of evidence showing that NK cells play important roles in the elimination of tumor cells from the blood. The NK activity, however, of peripheral blood cells or tumor-associated lymphocytes of patients with malignant diseases has been reported to be depressed, especially in those with widely disseminated tumors. It is known that the NK activity is augmented by biological-response modifiers such as muramyl dipeptide, staphylococcal protein A, BCG, and *Brucella abortus*. To determine whether the NK activity of human peripheral blood lymphocytes (PBL) can be augmented in vitro by MY-1, NK activity of PBL from healthy donors, patients with gastric cancer, patients with colon cancer and patients with uterine cancer were studied. Lymphocyte-rich fractions from healthy donors and cancer patients were obtained by the Conray-Ficoll gradient centrifugation method. The lymphocyte suspensions were adjusted to a concentration of 2×10^6 cells/ml and incubated in the presence or absence of MY-1 at various concentrations for 20 h. Nonadherent cells were harvested and 3-h ^{51}Cr-release assay was performed. MY-1 (100 μg/ml) was not cytotoxic to either the lymphocytes or K562 cells when measured by the trypan blue dye exclusion test. The NK activity of PBL from healthy donors was augmented by addition of 10 or 100 μg/ml of undigested MY-1, and was further augmented when MY-1 digested with RNase (1 μg/ml, 10 μg/ml or 100 μg/ml) was used. On the other hand, MY-1 digested with DNase was not effective in augmenting the NK activity of PBL. The effect on the NK activity of PBL from the cancer patients was also examined. Specific ^{51}Cr release in PBL from the patients with gastric, colon, or uterine cancer was 32.7±24.4%, 20.7±11.1%, and 12.6±8.4%, respectively. The NK activity of PBL from the patients with gastric cancer was augmented by addition of MY-1 (1 or 10 μg/ml) in PBL in a dose-dependent manner. The NK activity of PBL from the patients with uterine cancer was also augmented by addition of 10 μg/ml but not by 1 μg/ml MY-1. Although the degree of augmentation varied depending upon the source of PBL, the NK activity in vitro was augmented in the PBL of all of the patients examined on addition of MY-1, irrespective of the stage of cancer in the patient [11].

In situ infiltration of NK-like cells induced by intradermal injection of BCG-DNA

MY-1 possesses strong antitumor activity against various experimental tumors. The antitumor activity of MY-1 depends on the particular DNA component. Since MY-1 has no cytotoxic effect on cultured tumor cell lines in vitro, the host's immune system is intimately involved in the antitumor mechanism(s) of MY-1. One of the possible explanations for the findings is that MY-1 exhibits its antitumor effects by activating the local immune system surrounding the tumor. To elucidate the response of the local immune system to MY-1, we analyzed mouse skin previously injected intradermally with MY-1 by histological methods, and found that many mononuclear cells and some histiocytes had conspicuously infiltrated the injection site after 1–3 days. The cell infiltration was more evident in the subcutaneous tissue than in the epidermis and corium. Immunohistochemical staining revealed that the majority of the mononuclear cells induced by the injection of MY-1 were positive for asialo-GM1. In contrast, asialo-GM1-positive cells were rare in normal skin except for some dendritic cells in the epidermis. The asialo-GM1-positive cells appeared as early as 6 h after injection, were the most abundant after 1–2 days, but disappeared within a week, when the skin almost completely returned to the normal state. PBS alone occasionally induced limited infiltration, but the magnitude was invariably smaller than that induced by MY-1. MY-1 caused significant cell infiltration at a dose of as low as 1 μg. Nonimmune rabbit IgG in place of anti-asialo GM1 IgG produced no immunoreactivity. To define more precisely the phenotypes of asialo-GM1-positive cells, simultaneous staining for asialo-GM1 and other markers was carried out. All of the asialo-GM1-positive cells were also positive for Ly-5. Some of the asialo-GM1-positive cells were also positive for Thy-1.2, but others were not. Mac-1 antigen was weakly present or absent. None of the asialo-GM1-positive cells were positive for Lyt, Lyt-2, L3T4, μ chain, Ia or Fc receptor II [9].

Particular base sequences in BCG-DNA are required for NK activation

The DNA molecules comprising MY-1 showed a wide range of molecular size from 10 to 350 bases, with the peak position estimated to be 45 bases. The analyses were performed on five different lots of MY-1, and the results gave essentially the same elution profile. We synthesized 13 kinds of 45-mer single-stranded ODN each having a sequence randomly chosen from cDNA sequence encoding BCG proteins such as antigen-A, MPB-70 or alpha-antigen. Ability of these ODNs to augment NK cell activity of normal mouse spleen cells was assayed. Interestingly only 6 of the 13 ODNs showed strong activity, while the others did not. IFN-inducing activity paralleled the NK activity, suggesting that particular sequences are required for expression of biological activity. We could not find any relationship between their biological activities and the features in sequences, such as guanine-cytosine ratio or purine-pyrimidine ratio. However, we noticed that all of the active ODNs contained one or more palindrome sequence(s), while the inactive ODNs did not, with some exception. We focused on one particular ODN with 45-mer, BCG-A4, to clarify the sequence responsible for the activity. The ability of two fragments of BCG-A4 spanning 30 bases to augment NK activity was examined, one was active (BCG-A4a), but the other was inactive (BCG-A4b). Since BCG-A4a has a palindrome sequence (GACGTC), while BCG-A4b does not, the possible importance of the palindromic sequence was again suggested for the active ODNs [20].

A variety of 30-mer single-stranded ODNs were synthesized, and their NK-stimulatory activity was examined. First, we found the activity of ODNs with a GACGTC palindromic sequence was stronger than that of ODNs without GACGTC, which suggested the necessity of this palindromic sequence for activity. Second, when the GACGTC palindrome was introduced into the sequence of inactive ODNs, the modified ODNs acquired the NK-stimulatory activity, irrespective of the position in the sequence at which the palindrome was introduced. ODNs with a palindromic sequence of GACGTC, AGCGCT or AACGTT were active, whereas those with ACCGGT were inactive. When a portion of the sequence of the inactive ODN was substituted with a GACGTC, AGCGCT or AACGTT palindromic sequence, but not with ACCGGT, the ODN acquired biological activity. A similar ability of these palindromes to confer NK-stimulatory activity on ODNs was also observed in completely distinct sequences. Finally, ODNs lost their activity after nucleotide exchange within, but not outside the active palindromic sequence [22].

Based on the previous finding that 30-mer single-stranded ODNs with particular 6-mer palindromic sequences could induce IFN-α and IFN-γ, and enhance NK activity, a study was carried out to clarify the entire relationship between the activity and the sequence of 30-mer ODNs. The results indicated that the activity depended critically on the presence of particular palindromic sequences including the 5′-CG-3′ motif(s). The size and number of palindromes as well as the extra-palindromic sequences also influenced activity. All the active ODNs included a palindromic sequence, such as GACGTC, AGCGCT and AACGTT, whereas the inactive ones did not. When a portion of an inactive ODN was substituted with a palindromic sequence from an active ODN, the ODN acquired ability to enhance NK activity. In contrast, a sequence substitution with an ACCGGT palindrome did not give rise to activity. Furthermore, the active ODNs lost activity after an exchange or a deletion of bases within, but not outside, the 6-mer palindromic sequence. Taken together, these findings indicate that some, but not all, of the 6-mer palindromic sequences are essential for the activity of ODNs. Extra-palindromic sequences also appear to be necessary, because trimming an active 45-mer ODN molecule to 15-mer, while keeping the palindromic sequence intact, resulted in decreased activity. The palindromic sequence (5′-GACGTC-3′) of the active ODN BCG-A4a, the sequence of which is 5′-accgatGACGTCfccggtgacggcaccacg-3′, was replaced with each of the 63 theoretically possible 6-mer palindromic sequences. More than 100% relative activity was observed in the eight ODNs with one of the following palindromic sequences: AACGTT, AGCGTC, ATCGAT, CGATCG, CGTACG, CGCGCG, GCGCGC and TCGCGA. All the potent palindromes included one or more 5′-CG-3′ motif(s). In contrast, palindromes composed entirely of adenosine (A) and thymine (T) and those with a sequence of either Pu-Pu-Pu-Py-Py-Py or Py-Py-Py-Pu-Pu-Pu(Pu, purine; py, pyrimidine) were generally unfavorable for activity [10].

Antitumor activity of ODNs correlates with NK-augmenting activity

Thirteen kinds of 45-mer or 30-mer ODNs with sequences randomly selected from the cDNA encoding three kinds of proteins of BCG were tested for their antitumor activity in a murine tumor system. Of the 13 single-stranded ODNs which contained one or more hexameric palindromic sequences, 6 showed strong antitumor activity while the others without palindromic structure did not. Repeated intralesional injection of 100 μg of the 6 ODNs caused regression of the established tumor but the others were ineffective. When tumor cells were mixed with 100 μg of an effective ODN and injected into mice, tumor growth was markedly suppressed. These results suggested that the palindromic structure is essential for antitumor activity of the ODNs. To evaluate the antitumor activity of each ODN, 0.05 ml of a cell suspension containing 5×10^5 IMC tumor cells was mixed with 0.05 ml of test sample containing 100 μg ODN, and inoculated intradermally into CDF1 mice. At 35 days after the inoculation, all mice were killed and the tumors were resected and weighed. When IMC tumor cells were premixed with BCG-A4 or BCG-A4a ODN, including GACGTC palindromic sequence, the tumor growth was markedly suppressed, while the other ODN without the palindrome did not significantly affect the tumor growth. The effect of repeated injections of the ODNs into IMC tumors was also examined. IMC tumor cells were inoculated intradermally into CDF1 mice. One hundred μg of each ODN in 0.1 ml saline were injected into the tumor lesion twice a week from the 5th day after tumor inoculation. At 35 days after the tumor inoculation, all mice were killed and the tumors were resected and weighed. Of the 11 ODNs tested, 6 inhibited the tumor growth significantly, while the others did not. Thus, the antitumor activity of the ODNs correlated well with the NK-augmenting activity. Furthermore, these activities also correlated with the IFN-inducing activity [5].

Binding of oligoguanylate to scavenger receptors

The possible target molecules of the ODNs were investigated. Oligo-B, a 30-mer single-stranded ODN with an oligo-G sequence next to the active palindromic sequence (AACGTT), had more activity than the ODN with oligo-A, oligo-C or oligo-T sequence. The activity of oligo-B was inhibited by a guanine homo-oligomer (G30), a dextran sulfate and polyvinyl sulfate. Oligo-B bound to plastic-adherent mouse splenocytes, and this binding was inhibited by G30, dextran sulfate or polyvinyl sulfate. Oligo-B inhibited acetyl-low-density hypoprotein binding to the scavenger receptor on mouse splenocytes. These findings suggest that the binding of an extra-palindromic sequence to the scavenger receptor is required for the immunostimulatory activity of oligo-B [6]. The intracellular mechanism of immunostimulation by ODNs is still unclear. We have shown that the scavenger receptors of mouse macrophages may be the binding site on the cell surface in the particular case of G-homo-oligomers with an AACGTT sequence. In addition, we observed that bone marrow cells from a scavenger receptor knockout mouse could also be stimulated with the active ODN. On the other hand, it has been reported that Mac-1 protein is an ODN-binding protein on polymorphnuclear cells, although requirement on the base sequence of ODN is unclear [2].

Ability of ODNs with palindromes to augment NK activity is associated with base length

To clarify the required minimal size of the ODNs, ten kinds of 12- to 30-mer nucleotides were examined. To prepare the various-length ODNs possessing the AACGTT palindromic sequence, the extra-palindromic sequence of a potent ODN, AAC-30, was trimmed stepwise. Trimming two nucleotides from the 3′ end of the AAC-30 ODN resulted in AAC-28. By repeating this procedure, AAC-26, AAC-24, AAC-22, AAC-20, AAC-18, AAC-16, AAC-14 and AAC-12 were selected. In these cases, only the extra-palindromic sequences were trimmed and the 6-mer palindrome of AACGTT was maintained. The activity of these ODNs in augmenting NK activity was examined by co-culture of mouse spleen cells with each of these ODNs. The immunostimulatory activity of the ODNs with 18 or more bases was proportional to the base length, with a maximum at 22–30 bases. On the other hand, ODNs with 16 or fewer bases were not active even if they possessed certain palindromic sequences. These results indicate that for ODNs with certain palindromes to have immunostimulatory activity they require at least 18 bases [25].

Lipofection of an ODN with a palindromic sequence to murine splenocytes enhances NK activity

A synthetic 22-mer ODN with an AACGTT palindrome, AAC-22, induced IFN production and augmented the NK activity in murine splenocytes, whereas its analogue, ACC-22, with an ACCGGT palindrome did not. The binding of AAC-22 to splenocytes did not differ from that of ACC-22. Lipofection of AAC-22 to splenocytes remarkably enhanced IFN production and NK cell activity, whereas that of ACC-22 caused little enhancement. These results strongly suggest that the prerequisite for IFN production is not the binding of AAC-22 to the cell surface receptors, but its penetration into the spleen cells [24].

A 6-mer palindromic ODN (5′-AACGTT-3′) induced IFN from cultured mouse spleen cells when added with cationic liposomes. Accordingly, 32 kinds of 6-mer palindromic ODNs were tested for their ability to induce IFN in the presence of cationic liposomes. The results showed that ODNs with NACGTN and NTCGAN sequences (where N represents any nucleotide) exhibited the strongest activity. ACGCGT and TCGCGA also possessed moderate but significant activity. In contrast, palindromes without CG motif(s) were devoid of the activity. No 6-mer ODNs showed activity when liposomes were absent. A complete palindromic sequence was essential as any single base substitution resulted in diminished activity. Among the palindromic ODNs of different sizes with an ACGT sequence at the center, the tetramer ODN showed no activity, whereas 6-mer and longer ODNs induced an activity that was almost equally high. These results strongly suggest that the minimal essential structure required for IFN induction is a 6-mer palindromic sequence with CG motif(s) [17].

ODNs with certain palindromes stimulate human PBL in vitro

The ability of single-stranded 30-mer ODNs with three different kinds of 6-mer palindromic sequences to stimulate IFN production by human PBL was studied. When

PBL were cultured with oligoDNA with an AACGTT or GACGTC palindrome, IFN activity was detected by bioassay in the culture fluid after 8 h, and the amounts of IFN reached the maximum after 18 h. IFN-α was predominantly produced, and small amounts of IFN-β and IFN-γ were also found. OligoDNA with the ACCGGT palindrome had no effect [23].

We examined the effect of ODNs on highly purified human NK and T cells. MY-1 or synthetic ODNs induced NK cells to produce IFN-γ with increased CD69 expression, and the autocrine IFN-γ enhanced their cytotoxicity. The response of NK cells to ODNs was enhanced when the cells were activated with IL-2, IL-12 or anti-CD16 antibody. T cells did not produce IFN-γ in response to ODNs but did respond independently of IL-2 when they were stimulated with anti-CD3 antibody. In the action of ODNs, the palindrome sequence containing unmethylated CG motif(s) appeared to play an important role in IFN-γ-producing ability of NK cells. The changes of base composition inside or outside the palindrome sequence altered its activity. The homo-oligoG-flanked GACGATCGTC was the most potent IFN-γ inducer for NK cells. The CG palindrome was also important for IFN-γ production in activated NK and T cells, although certain non-palindromes also acted on them.

Among the sequences tested, cell activation- or cell lineage-specific sequences were found; i.e., palindrome ACCGGT and non-palindromic AACGAT were favored by activated NK cells but not by nonactivated NK or activated T cells. These results indicate that ODNs containing the CG palindrome act directly on human NK and activated T cells to induce IFN-γ production. To clarify the cell type targeted by immunostimulatory ODNs to produce IFN-γ, we separated LGL and T cells from NAC. When these two cell fractions were cultured for 24 h, only the large granular lymphocyte fraction produced IFN-γ in the presence of MY-1. Nonadherent cells, which contained 20–30% NK and 70–80% T cells, produced IFN-γ in response to MY-1 when the cell density was increased to 4×10^6 cells/ml, whereas the purified T cell fraction did not produce IFN-γ even when cultured at 1×10^7 cells/ml or for longer periods. We purified $CD56^+$ cells from the LGL fraction and found that they were responsive to MY-1. NK cells produced IFN-γ in response to MY-1. The doses of MY-1 necessary to induce maximum amounts of IFN-γ were between 12.5–50 μg/ml in NK cultures. IFN-γ production in the culture with MY-1 was first observed at 18 h and increased thereafter. The amount of IFN-γ produced without MY-1 after 24 h of culture was below 4 pg/ml and did not increase. These results show that NK cells are responsive in terms of IFN-γ production. To prove that the MY-1-induced IFN-γ production is due to a direct action on NK cells, the effect of monoclonal antibody against IL-12 or TNF-α on the IFN-γ production of NK cells in the stimulation of ODNs was examined. Neither anti-IL-12 nor anti-TNF-α monoclonal antibodies influenced the IFN-γ production by NK cells cultured with or without ODN. The combined addition of monoclonal antibodies against IL-12 and TNF-α also did not inhibit the production of IFN-γ. In addition, monoclonal antibodies to IL-18, IL-15 or IFN-α did not alter the level of IFN-γ production induced by the ODNs [4].

Conclusion

We pointed out in 1992 that a hexamer palindromic sequence with –CpG– motif(s) is essential for NK augmentation and IFN production, with some exceptions [10].

Krieg et al. [8] also noted the importance of the CpG motif as the basic structure required for B cell stimulation, and stated that the CpG dinucleotides flanked by two 5′ purines and two 3′ pyrimidines is optimal. Ballas et al. [1] examined the necessity of palindromic sequences for NK activation and observed that the presence of a hexamer palindrome was irrelevant; for instance, GTCGTT and GACGTT were active, and GACGTC was inactive. They concluded that the unmethylated CpG motif, but not the palindromic sequence, was definitely required, and that the two flanking bases at the 5′ and 3′ ends were a stringent requirement. Boggs et al. [3] tested various sequences of ODNs, and showed that the CpG motif was stimulatory for NK cells only in specific sequence contexts [3]. Monteith et al. [12] tested various ODN sequences for inducing splenomegaly and B cell stimulation; ODNs containing a 5′-AACGTT-3′ palindrome were the most effective. The general formula, Pu-Pu-CG-Py-Py, proposed by Krieg [8] and Klinman et al. [7], also has many exceptions, although the formula has been widely used by many investigators. Therefore we think that at present either the term "immunostimulatory sequences (ISS) of DNA" [13, 14, 18] or "CpG dinucleotides in particular base contexts" [3, 26] is appropriate for indicating immunostimulatory sequences.

References

1. Ballas ZK, Rasmussen WL, Krieg AM (1996) Induction of NK activity in murine and human cells by CpG motifs in oligodeoxynucleotides and bacterial DNA. J Immunol 157:1840
2. Benimetskaya L, Loike JD, Khaled Z, Loike G, Silverstein SC, Cao L, Khoury JE, Cai T-Q, Stein CA (1997) Mac-1 (CD11b/CD18) is an oligodeoxynucleotide-binding protein. Nat Med 3:414
3. Boggs RL, McGraw K, Condon T, Flournoy S, Villiet P, Bennett CF, Monia BP (1997) Characterization and modulation of immune stimulation by modified oligonucleotides. Antisense Nucleic Acid Drug Dev 7:461
4. Iho S, Yamamoto T, Takahashi T, Yamamoto S (1999) Oligodeoxynucleotides containing palindrome sequences with internal 5′-CpG-3′ act directly on human NK and activated T cells to induce IFN-γ production in vitro. J Immunol 163:3642
5. Kataoka T, Yamamoto S, Yamamoto T, Kuramoto E, Kimura Y, Yano O, Tokunaga T (1992) Antitumor activity of synthetic oligonucleotides with sequences from cDNA encoding proteins of *Mycobacterium bovis* BCG. Jpn J Cancer Res 83:244
6. Kimura Y, Sonehara K, Kuramoto E, Makino T, Yamamoto S, Yamamoto T, Kataoka T, Tokunaga T (1994) Binding of oligoguanylate to scavenger receptors is required for oligonucleotides to augment NK cell activity and induce IFN. J Biochem 116:991
7. Klinman DM, Yi A-K, Beaucaga SL, Conover J, Krieg AM (1996) CpG motifs present in bacterial DNA rapidly induce lymphocytes to secrete interleukin 6, interleukin 12, and interferon gamma. Proc Natl Acad Sci USA 93:2879
8. Krieg AM, Yi A-K, Matson S, Waldschmidt TJ, Bishop GA, Teasdale R, Koretzky GA, Klinman DM (1995) CpG motifs in bacterial DNA trigger direct B-cell activation. Nature 374:546
9. Kuramoto E, Toizumi S, Shimada S, Tokunaga T (1989) In situ infiltration of natural killer-like cells induced by intradermal injection of the nucleic acid fraction from BCG. Microbiol Immunol 33:929
10. Kuramoto E, Yano O, Kimura Y, Baba M, Makino T, Yamamoto S, Yamamoto T, Kataoka T, Tokunaga T (1992) Oligonucleotide sequences required for natural killer cell activation. Jpn J Cancer Res 83:1128
11. Mashiba H, Matsunaga K, Tomoda H, Furusawa M, Jimi S, Tokunaga T (1988) In vitro augmentation of natural killer activity of peripheral blood cells from cancer patients by a DNA fraction from *Mycobacterium bovis* BCG. Jpn J Med Sci Biol 41:197
12. Monteith DK, Henry SP, Howard RB, Flournoy S, Levin AA, Bennett CF, Crooke ST (1997) Immune stimulation – a class effect of phosphorothioate oligonucleotides in rodents. Anticancer Drug Des 12:421

13. Roman M, Orozco EM, Goodman JS, Nguyen MD, Sato Y, Raz E (1997) Immunostimulatory DNA sequences function as T helper-1 promoting adjuvants. Nat Med 3:849
14. Sato Y, Roman M, Tighe H, Lee D, Corr M, Nguyen MD, Silverman GJ, Lotz M, Carson DA, Ratz E (1996): Immunostimulatory DNA sequences necessary for effective intradermal gene immunization. Science 273:352
15. Shimada S, Yano O, Inoue H, Kuramoto E, Fukuda T, Yamamoto H, Kataoka T, Tokunaga T (1985) Antitumor activity of the DNA fraction from *Mycobacterium bovis* BCG. II. Effects on various syngeneic mouse tumors. J Natl Cancer Inst 74:681
16. Shimada S, Yano O, Tokunaga T (1986) In vivo augmentation of natural killer cell activity with a deoxyribonucleic acid fraction of BCG. Jpn J Cancer Res 77:808
17. Sonehara K, Saito H, Kuramoto E, Yamamoto S, Yamamoto T, Tokunaga T (1996) Hexamer palindromic oligonucleotides with 5′-CG-3′ motif(s) induce production of interferon. J Interferon Cytokine Res 16:799
18. Tighe H, Corr M, Roman M, Ratz E (1998) Gene vaccination: plasmid DNA is more than just a blueprint. Immunol Today 19:89
19. Tokunaga T, Yamamoto S, Shimada S, Abe H, Fukuda T, Fujisawa Y, Furutani Y, Yano O, Kataoka T, Sudo T, Makiguchi N, Suganuma T (1984) Antitumor activity of deoxyribonucleic acid fraction from *Mycobacterium bovis* BCG. I. Isolation, physicochemical characterization, and antitumor activity. J Natl Cancer Inst 72:955
20. Tokunaga T, Yano O, Kuramoto E, Kimura Y, Yamamoto T, Kataoka T, Yamamoto S (1992) Synthetic oligonucleotides with particular base sequences from the cCNA encoding proteins of *Mycobacterium bovis* BCG induce interferons and activate natural killer cells. Microbiol Immunol 36:55
21. Yamamoto S, Kuramoto E, Shimada S, Tokunaga T (1988) In vitro augmentation of natural killer cell activity and production of interferon-α/β and -γ with deoxyribonucleic acid fraction from *Mycobacterium bovis* BCG. Jpn J Cancer Res 79:866
22. Yamamoto S, Yamamoto T, Kataoka T, Kuramoto E, Yano O, Tokunaga T (1992) Unique palindromic sequences in synthetic oligonucleotides are required to induce IFN and augment IFN-mediated natural killer activity. J Immunol 148:4072
23. Yamamoto T, Yamamoto S, Kataoka T, Komuro K, Kohase M, Tokunaga T (1994) Synthetic oligonucleotides with certain palindromes stimulate interferon production of human peripheral blood lymphocytes in vitro. Jpn J Cancer Res 85:775
24. Yamamoto T, Yamamoto S, Kataoka T, Tokunaga T (1994) Lipofection of synthetic oligodeoxyribonucleotide having a palindromic sequence of AACGTT to murine splenocytes enhances interferon production and natural killer activity. Microbiol Immnol 38:831
25. Yamamoto T, Yamamoto S, Kataoka T, Tokunaga T (1994) Ability of oligonucleotides with certain palindromes to induce interferon production and augment natural killer cell activity is associated with their base length. Antisense Res Dev 4:119
26. Yi A-K, Tuetken R, Redford T, Waldschmidt M, Kirsch J, Krieg AM (1998) CpG motifs in bacterial DNA activate leukocytes though the pH-dependent generation of reactive oxygen species. J Immunol 160:4755

Activation of skin dendritic cells by immunostimulatory DNA

Jonathan C. Vogel, Mark C. Udey

Dermatology Branch, National Cancer Institute, Bethesda, MD 20892, USA

Introduction

Our laboratory is interested in developing methods that allow expression of exogenous genes in skin for therapeutic purposes (skin gene therapy). One approach involves direct introduction of genetic material by intradermal (ID) injection of naked plasmid DNA [15, 28]. Following ID injection of plasmid DNA, the encoded proteins are transiently and predominantly expressed in keratinocytes in a dose-dependent manner. Gene expression in other skin cells [including dendritic cells (DC), fibroblasts and adipocytes] has also been observed after injection of plasmid DNA into skin [16].

Because injection of plasmid DNA results in high level, transient gene expression and skin contains numerous epidermal and dermal DC that play important roles in the initiation of primary responses in naive T cells, genetic immunization via skin is a promising option. DNA vaccines can elicit effective humoral and cellular immune responses against pathogenic organisms when plasmid DNA encoding the appropriate antigens are introduced intramuscularly (IM) or ID [4, 7, 12, 25, 43, 44]. Immune responses induced by DNA immunization are characterized by IL-12-dependent production of interferon (IFN)-γ by helper T cells, and accumulation of antibodies of the IgG2a subclass in sera [7, 29]. Development of IFN-γ-predominant Th1 immune responses results in control of infections caused by intracellular pathogens. In contrast to immunization with plasmid DNA, immunization protocols that utilize protein antigens in conjunction with standard adjuvants preferentially result in Th2 immune responses characterized by production of IL-4, IL-5, IL-10, as well as antibodies of the IgE and IgG1 subclasses. Typically, Th2 immune responses do not lead to clearance of intracellular pathogens.

Genetic vaccination and leishmaniasis

To determine if a protective immune response against *Leishmania* could be elicited in a murine model of leishmaniasis, plasmid DNA encoding a *Leishmania major* cell surface protein (gp63) was injected into susceptible mice. The immunology of

Correspondence to: J.C. Vogel

Table 1. ODN sequences

ODN 1911	5′-TCCAGGACTTTCCTCAGGTT-3′
CpG/ISS-ODN 1826	5′-TCCATGA**CG**TTCCTGA**CG**TT-3′
Consensus CpG/ISS motiff	5′-A/GA/G**CG**C/TC/T-3′

CpG dinucleotides are in bold letters
ISS-ODN, Immunostimulatory sequence oligodeoxynucleotide

L. major infection has been well characterized in inbred strains of mice [23, 30, 31]. Development of Th1 immune responses in C75BL/6 and C3H mice correlates with resistance or protective immunity, while susceptibility to infection in BALB/c mice is associated with a Th2 response [1, 26, 35, 36]. Previously, protein vaccines have not provided protection from *Leishmania* infection in susceptible mice, most likely because they preferentially induce Th2-type immune responses. In contrast to protein vaccines, we and others have demonstrated that ID genetic immunization with plasmid DNA encoding conserved *Leishmania* proteins induces protective Th1 immune responses and can protect susceptible mice from *Leishmania* infection [13, 46, 48].

Immunostimulatory DNA

Although the mechanisms involved in DNA immunization are still being defined, the associated Th1 immune responses are probably due, in large part, to immunostimulatory DNA sequences contained within plasmid DNA [34]. Immunostimulatory sequences (ISS) in plasmid DNA are comprised of central unmethylated CpG dinucleotides flanked by 5′ purine nucleotides and 3′ pyrimidine nucleotides (Table 1), and have the capacity to induce production of a variety of cytokines (including IL-12 and IFN-γ) from immune and inflammatory cells in vitro and in vivo [20, 21, 27, 33]. Synthetic oligodeoxynucleotides (ODN) containing homologous non-methylated CpG dinucleotide sequences are also immunostimulatory and can induce monocyte cytokine secretion, B cell proliferation and IFN-γ production, and activation of natural killer (NK) cells with IFNγ release [2, 21, 33]. Consequently, ODN that contain CpG ISS (CpG/ISS-ODN) can be co-administered with protein and induce Th1 cellular immune responses against that protein, while administration of protein alone (or with an adjuvant such as alum) typically results in Th2-type immune responses with high titers of neutralizing antibodies and poor cellular immunity [6, 10, 22, 33, 41, 47]. In aggregate, these data suggest that CpG/ISS in DNA or CpG/ISS-ODN function as effective adjuvants that promote Th1 immune responses to antigens encoded by plasmids or to co-administered proteins. To determine if the Th1 adjuvant activity of ISS might be useful in the prevention or treatment of an important infectious disease, we tested the ability of ISS to redirect immune responses to *L. major* in susceptible BALB/c mice.

Leishmaniasis vaccine enhancement by CpG/ISS-ODN

ODN containing optimal CpG/ISS were identified by assessing the effects of various ODN on BALB/c splenocyte cytokine production [45]. One CpG/ISS-ODN (1826) was then co-injected ID with the *L. major* lysate as a source of protein antigens to determine if a *Leishmania*-specific Th1 immune response, similar to the one observed earlier for plasmid DNA vaccines, could be induced. At 9 days after ID immunization, draining lymph nodes were removed and lymph node cells were cultured with *Leishmania* antigens. In these in vitro stimulation assays, lymph node cells from mice injected with CpG/ISS-ODN plus *Leishmania* protein produced two- to eightfold more IFN-γ than lymph node cells from mice injected ID with *Leishmania* antigen alone [45]. ID injection of CpG/ISS-ODN plus *Leishmania* antigens also elicited protective immunity in approximately 40% of susceptible mice that were challenged with *Leishmania* parasites 6 weeks after a subsequent boost; a level of protection comparable to that seen following ID DNA vaccination with plasmids encoding *Leishmania* gp63 protein [45, 46]. In contrast, none of the susceptible mice vaccinated with either composition-matched ODN lacking CpG motifs (1911) plus *Leishmania* protein or *Leishmania* protein alone were protected from parasite challenges.

CpG/ISS-ODN as therapeutics for leishmaniasis

Because co-injection of CpG/ISS-ODN and *Leishmania* proteins induced a Th1-type cytokine response and provided partial protection from *Leishmania* infection in susceptible mice, we wanted to determine if CpG/ISS-ODN would have a therapeutic effect when given after susceptible mice had already been infected with *Leishmania*. After inoculation of susceptible mice with *Leishmania*, CpG/ISS-ODN were injected into the site of infection. Prolonged survival was seen in 65–95% of infected susceptible mice treated with CpG/ISS-ODN, while sham-injected mice or mice receiving control ODN developed progressive fatal infections [45]. Interestingly, the similar enhancement of survival was seen when CpG/ISS-ODN were injected into sites remote from the sites of infection, suggesting that ID injection of CpG/ISS-ODN exerted systemic therapeutic effects. The effect of the CpG/ISS-ODN was dose dependent, with a maximal therapeutic effect at approximately 10 μg CpG/ISS-ODN per mouse. These results are consistent with those obtained by Heeg and co-workers [49].

Although we had previously demonstrated that CpG/ISS-ODN could induce IL-12 and IFN-γ production by splenocytes in vitro, we wanted to determine if the anti-*Leishmania* activity of CpG/ISS-ODN was dependent on IL-12 and IFN-γ production in vivo. Susceptible mice that were deficient in either IL-12 or IFN-γ were inoculated with *Leishmania* parasites and then treated with ID injections of CpG/ISS-ODN 4 h later. None of the mice deficient in either IL-12 or IFN-γ survived *Leishmania* challenge, demonstrating that the protective effects of CpG/ISS-ODN are dependent on, and likely mediated through, IL-12 and IFN-γ [45].

While the effectiveness of CpG/ISS-ODN in the *Leishmania* model may be attributable, in part, to activation of NK cells, it is likely that effects of local or systemic administration of CpG/ISS-ODN also involve accessory cells that, in the presence of IL-12, will promote Th1 development. Following ID injection of CpG/ISS-ODN, IL-12 may be produced by accessory cells in selected sites such as the skin or draining lymph nodes or at distant sites. In the skin, DC such as epidermal Langerhans cells (LC) and dermal DC may be crucial targets for CpG/ISS-ODN action.

Activation of skin DC by CpG/ISS-ODN

Skin DC are potent antigen-presenting cells (APC) that are critical for initiating antigen-specific immune responses to antigens or pathogens that are encountered in skin. Following antigen acquisition and activation, skin DC migrate to regional lymph nodes where antigens are presented to naive T cells and immune responses are initiated [40]. To assess the response of skin DC to CpG/ISS-ODN, the biological behavior of LC was modeled in vitro. LC-like DC were expanded in primary cultures of C57BL/6 fetal skin and isolated as tight aggregates [immature fetal skin-derived DC (FSDDC-I)] [17]. Like murine epidermal LC, FSDDC-I spontaneously give rise to cells that resemble mature antigen-presenting interdigitating DC [mature FSDDC (FSDDC-M)] during a several-day subculture period and can be triggered to differentiate into FSDDC-M by inflammatory mediators such as IL-1, TNF-α, and LPS. Because FSDDC recapitulate the transition of epidermal LC into mature interdigitating DC, we assessed the responses of these cells to CpG/ISS-ODN.

We have previously determined that adhesion within the FSDDC aggregates is mediated by E-cadherin and established that this correlates with the ability of LC to adhere to keratinocytes in vitro [17, 42]. Additionally, the ability of inflammatory mediators (IL-1, TNF-α and LPS) to down-regulate E-cadherin-mediated adhesion in FSDDC aggregates and to initiate maturation correlates with activation and the initiation of LC migration from epidermis to regional lymph nodes [18]. Therefore, we assessed the effect of CpG/ISS-ODN on E-cadherin-mediated adhesion using a simple disaggregation assay. FSDDC-I were incubated with CpG/ISS-ODN (6 μg/ml) or LPS (100 ng/ml) for 18 h and observed at various times. Both the CpG/ISS-ODN and LPS caused almost complete loss of adhesion in FSDDC-I aggregates within 18 h, while base composition-matched (non-CpG-containing) control ODN were without effect [19]. Loss of adhesion in the disaggregation assay was dose dependent and was accompanied by a reduction in cell surface E-cadherin expression.

Cytokine- and LPS-induced disaggregation of FSDDC-I is also associated with DC maturation, manifested by increased expression of MHC class II antigen and co-stimulator molecules [18]. We used multicolor flow cytometry to assess the effects of CpG/ISS-ODN on the expression of FSDDC cell surface markers of activation. Single-cell suspensions of EDTA-dissociated FSDDC-I were stained with anti-CD45 monoclonal antibodies (mAb) and mAb reactive with MHC antigens and co-stimulator molecules (CD40, CD80, and CD86), and viable cells (>95% of all cells present) were selected for analysis. Both CpG/ISS-ODN (6 μg/ml) and LPS treatment (100 ng/ml) for 18 h induced dramatically increased expression of MHC class II antigens, CD40, and CD86 and slightly increased expression of CD80 [19]. In contrast, the control non-CpG-ODN did not result in significant changes in cell surface phenotype. Dose-response studies revealed that concentrations of CpG/ISS-ODN of more than 2 μg/ml resulted in FSDDC-I activation and enhanced MHC class II antigen expression. High concentrations (>60 mg/ml) of control ODN lacking CpG/ISS motifs also activated FSDDC-I to some extent.

CpG/ISS-ODN and DC IL-12 production

Whether Th1- or Th2-predominant immune responses ensue after interactions between APC and T cells depends on the cytokines that are produced as well as the co-

Table 2. Cytokine release from skin-derived dendritic cells in vitro

Agonist	*TNF-α*	*IL-6*	*IL-12*
None	ND	46±36	80±80
LPS	757±228	946±453	1643±520
CpG/ISS-ODN 1826	155±114	133±16	16,582±5,742
ODN 1911	ND	62±28	1,266±1,215

Numerical values represent pg/5×10^5 cells per18 h in response to LPS (100 ng/ml) or ODN (6 μg/ml)
ND, Not detectable (<40 pg)

stimulator molecules that are expressed by APC. To address the issue of effects of CpG-ISS DNA on DC cytokine production, we characterized the cytokines produced by FSDDC following CpG/ISS-ODN stimulation. FSDDC-I aggregates were cultured with CpG/ISS-ODN or LPS, and IL-1β, IFN-γ, TNF-α, IL-6, and IL-12 (p40) were assayed in cell-free supernatants by ELISA. As expected, LPS-treated FSDDC released significant amounts of TNF-α, IL-6, and IL-12 into the medium (Table 2). Addition of CpG/ISS-ODN to FSDDC-I also stimulated cytokine production. However, CpG/ISS-ODN induced about fivefold less TNF-α, about sevenfold less IL-6 and, interestingly, about tenfold more IL-12 production. Neither IL-1β, nor IFN-γ was detected in FSDDC supernatants under any of these conditions.

We also assessed IL-12 production at the single-cell level by staining for both cell surface MHC class II expression and intracellular accumulation of IL-12 using an anti-IL-12 p40 mAb and analytical flow cytometry. LPS treatment of FSDDC-I caused an approximately tenfold increase in the level of MHC class II antigen expression by almost all cells during the incubation period with accumulation of intracellular IL-12 p40 in only a minor population (≈3%) of FSDDC (Fig. 1). The effects of CpG/ISS-ODN on MHC class II expression by FSDDC-I were similar to that of LPS, but CpG/ISS-ODN also stimulated a dramatic accumulation of IL-12 p40 in a major subset of FSDDC (14–32%) in a dose-dependent fashion (Fig. 1) [19]. By comparison, treatment of FSDDC-I with control ODN (non-CpG/ISS) induced IL-12 p40 accumulation in only a minor subpopulation (1–2%). These results conclusively demonstrate that the IL-12 produced in response to CpG/ISS-ODN was synthesized by the DC (FSDDC) and not by a minor contaminant in the preparation. Additionally, these data indicate that IL-12 is preferentially induced by CpG/ISS-ODN in the FSDDC that expressed the highest levels of MHC class II antigen (i.e. the most mature DC) in the FSDDC preparations. These effects, as well as effects on other parameters of DC activation, were observed with CpG/ISS-ODN with a phosphorothioate or phosphodiester backbone.

To determine if CpG/ISS-ODN enhanced DC APC activity, FSDDC-I were incubated for 18 h in either LPS (10 ng/ml) or CpG/ISS-ODN (6 μg/ml), washed, and then tested for allo-stimulatory activity in a mixed leukocyte reaction using accessory cell-depleted BALB/c T cells as responders. Treatment of FSDDC with CpG/ISS-ODN resulted in a several-fold increase in the potency of FSDDC APC activity. Although less than the tenfold increase in APC activity induced by LPS, the increased stimulation by CpG/ISS-ODN treated DC was significantly greater than DC incubated with control ODN, which had no APC-augmenting activity.

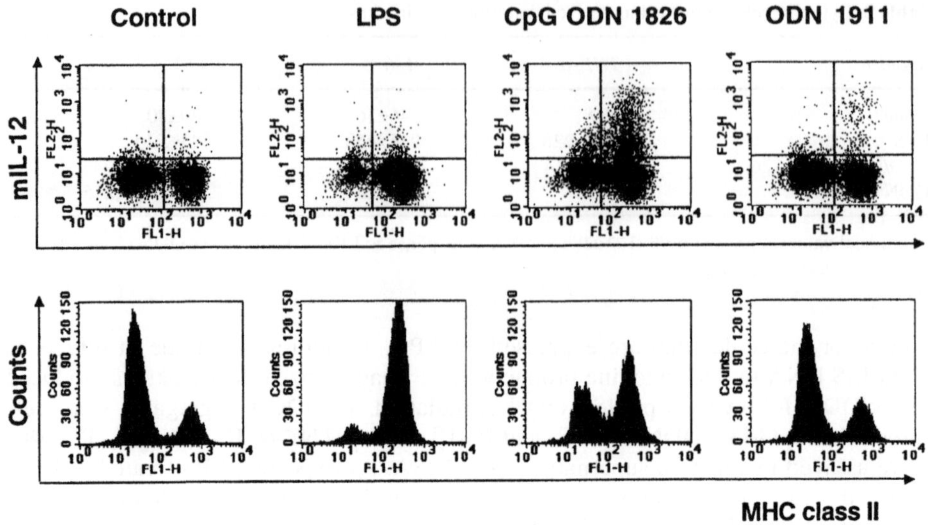

Fig. 1. Activation and induction of IL-12 in dendritic cells treated with CpG/ISS-ODN. Aggregates of skin-derived dendritic cells were treated with LPS (100 ng/ml) or ODN (6 μg/ml) for 18 h [brefelden A (1 μg/ml) was added for the final 4 h]. At the end of the incubation, cells were stained for cell surface MHC class II, fixed, permeabilized, stained for intracytoplasmic IL-12 accumulation and analyzed via flow cytometry

In vivo activation of skin DC by CpG/ISS-ODN

Although FSDDC model various aspects of LC biology in vitro, it was important to determine if CpG/ISS-ODN could activate immature non-lymphoid DC in vivo. Activation of epidermal LC following ID injection of CpG/ISS-ODN could provide a mechanism for the observed protective and therapeutic effect of the CpG/ISS-ODN in the murine *Leishmania* model. Subpopulations of LC become activated by exposure to contact allergens, IL-1, TNF-α, and LPS and are subsequently induced to emigrate from epidermis [9, 11, 24, 32]. Before activated LC exit the epidermis, they express increased levels of cell surface MHC class II and CD86 Antigen and can be distinguished from unstimulated LC and quantitated using multicolor flow cytometry. To assess LC activation, we injected IL-1β, CpG/ISS-ODN, control ODN (non-CpG/ISS), or diluent into the dorsal ear skin of BALB/c mice, and prepared epidermal cell suspensions from the overlying epidermis 12 h later. Cells were stained for simultaneous expression of MHC class II and CD86 antigen, and analyzed by flow cytometry (Table 3). Injection of LPS and CpG/ISS-ODN into murine skin led to increased expression of MHC class II and CD86 antigen by significant subpopulations of LC [19]. The proportion of LC activated by CpG/ISS-ODN in vivo was always less than that activated by IL-1β, but was significantly greater than that due to injection of control ODN (non-CpG/ISS) or PBS. Similar results were obtained in an identical experiment conducted in C57BL/6 mice.

We also assessed intracellular levels of IL-12 in LC from the ears of BALB/c mice injected with LPS (200 ng) or CpG/ISS-ODN (50 μg) using methodology analogous to that used to evaluate IL-12 intracellular production by FSDDC. Activated

Table 3. Activation of Langerhans cells by CpG/ISS-ODN in situ

LC phenotype	Intradermal injection		
	Sham	CpG/ISS-ODN 1826	ODN 1911
MHC class II^{high}	9.0±5.2	29.6±13.5	10.4±4.7
$CD86^{high}$	4.4±2.1	28.6±2.6	5.1±1.6
MHC II^{high} $CD86^{high}$	2.6±1.1	19.4±7.6	3.2±0.3

Epidermal cell suspensions were prepared from mouse ear skin that was injected with PBS or ODN (50 μg) 12 h earlier, stained for simultaneous expression of MHC class II and CD86 and analyzed by flow cytometry. The values reported represent percentages of Langerhans cells (LD) expressing levels of the indicated antigens that exceeded those on LC from the skin of uninjected mice

epidermal LC that expressed increased levels of MHC class II could be clearly resolved from MHC class II-negative epidermal cells. Intracellular levels of IL-12 in LC activated by LPS were compared with IL-12 levels in LC stimulated with CpG/ISS-ODN. We found that in three experiments, a small subpopulation of LC activated by CpG/ISS-ODN in vivo (4.3%±1.6%), contained detectable levels of intracellular IL-12, while LPS-activated LC did not [19]. This data demonstrates that CpG/ISS-ODN can selectively induce IL-12 production by cutaneous DC in vivo as well as in vitro.

Conclusion

DNA vaccines, such as those used to protect susceptible mice from *Leishmania* infection, are efficacious because of ISS containing a core CpG dinucleotide flanked by the appropriate consensus nucleotides [20, 21, 27, 33]. ODN containing these CpG/ISS are effective adjuvants that elicit Th1-predominant immune responses when combined with protein vaccines [6, 10, 22, 33, 41, 47]. Previous studies have demonstrated that CpG/ISS-ODN can activate B cells [21, 34], NK cells [2, 8], macrophages [5, 14, 22, 38, 39] and T cells [3]. We (and others [37]) now demonstrate that CpG/ISS-ODN are also capable of stimulating DC and LC. These results provide a framework for understanding how Th1-predominant immune responses are elicited by genetic vaccination via skin.

A model consistent with our data suggests that ID introduction of CpG/ISS activates DC in skin. Activation of epidermal LC is associated with attenuation of E-cadherin-mediated adhesion to epidermal keratinocytes [17, 42] and enhanced expression of MHC class II and co-stimulator molecules. LC that have acquired antigen synthesized endogenously or by other skin cells (e.g., keratinocytes or fibroblasts) are mobilized and carry antigen from skin to regional lymph nodes. In lymph nodes, these cells localize in T cell-dependent areas as mature interdigitating DC [4, 7, 24] capable of initiating Th1 responses in naive T cells. Elaboration of IL-12 in this microenvironment will promote development of Th1 as compared with Th2 immunity. ID injected CpG/ISS-ODN may also have important immunostimulatory effects on cells (DC as well as non-DC) in tissues other than the skin. Determining the relative contributions of the various immune cells that are activated by immunostimulatory DNA to the immune responses that ultimately ensue is one of several major challenges for the future.

Acknowledgements We would like to gratefully acknowledge Drs. Patricia Walker, Thilo Jakob, and Arthur Krieg whose efforts and contributions made the above studies possible.

References

1. Afonso LCC, Scharton TM, Vieira LW, Wysocka M, Trinchieri G, Scott P (1994) The adjuvant effect of interleukin-12 in a vaccine against Leishmania major. Science 263:235
2. Ballas ZK, Rasmussen WL, Krieg AM (1996) Induction of NK activity in murine and human cells by CpG motifs in oligodeoxynucleotides and bacterial DNA. J Immunol 157:1840
3. Bendigs S, Salzer U, Lipford GB, Wagner H, Heeg K (1999) CpG-oligodeoxynucleotides co-stimulate primary T cells in the absence of antigen-presenting cells. Eur J Immunol 29:1209
4. Casares S, Inaba K, Brumeanu T-D, Steinman RM, Bona CA (1997) Antigen presentation by dendritic cells after immunization with DNA encoding a major histocompatibility complex class II-restricted viral epitope. J Exp Med 186:1481
5. Chace JH, Hooker NA, Mildenstein KL, Krieg AM, Cowdery JS (1997) Bacterial DNA-induced NK cell IFN-γ production is dependent on macrophage secretion of IL-12. Clin Immunol Immunopathol 84:185c
6. Chu RS, Targoni OS, Krieg AM, Lehmann PV, Harding CV (1997) CpG oligodeoxynucleotides act as adjuvants that switch on T helper 1 (Th1) immunity. J Exp Med 186:1623
7. Condon C, Watkins SC, Celluzzi CM, Thompson K, Falo LD Jr (1996) DNA-based immunization by in vivo transfection of dendritic cells. Nat Medicine 2:1122
8. Cowdery JS, Chace JH, Yi A-K, Krieg AM (1996) Bacterial DNA induces NK cells to produce IFN-gamma in vivo and increases the toxicity of lipopolysaccharides. J Immunol 156:4570
9. Cumberbatch M, Fielding I, Kimber I (1994) Modulation of epidermal Langerhans cell frequency by tumor necrosis factor-α. Immunology 81:395
10. Davis HL, Weeranta R, Waldschmidt TJ, Tygrett L, Schorr J, Krieg AM (1998) CpG DNA is a potent enhancer of specific immunity in mice immunized with recombinant hepatitis B surface antigen. J Immunol 160:870
11. Enk AH, Angeloni VL, Udey MC, Katz SI (1993) An essential role for Langerhans cell-derived IL-1ß in the initiation of primary immune responses in skin. J Immunol 150:3698
12. Fynan EF, Webster RG, Fuller DH, Haynes JR, Santoro JC, Robinson HL (1993) DNA Vaccines: Protective immunizations by parenteral, mucosal, and gene-gun inoculations. Proc Natl Acad Sci USA 90:11478
13. Gurunathan S, Sacks DL, Brown DR, Reiner SL, Charest H, Glaichenhaus N, Seder RA (1997) Vaccination with DNA encoding the immunodominant LACK parasite antigen confers protective immunity to mice infected with *Leishmania major*. J Exp Med 186:1137
14. Halpern MD, Kurlander RJ, Pisetsky DS (1996) Bacterial DNA induces murine interferon-gamma production by stimulation of interleukin-12 and tumor necrosis factor-α. Cell Immunol 167:72
15. Hengge UR, Chan EF, Foster RA, Walker PS, Vogel JC (1995) Cytokine gene expression in epidermis with biological effects following injection of naked DNA. Nat Genet 10:161
16. Hengge UR, Walker PS, Vogel JC (1996) Expression of naked DNA in human, pig, and mouse skin. J Clin Invest 97:2911
17. Jakob T, Saitoh A, Udey MC (1997) E-cadherin-mediated adhesion involving Langerhans cell-like dendritic cells expanded from murine fetal skin. J Immunol 159:2693
18. Jakob T, Udey MC (1998) Regulation of E-cadherin-mediated adhesion in Langerhans cell-like dendritic cells by inflammatory mediators that mobilize Langerhans cells in vivo. J Immunol 160:4067
19. Jakob T, Walker PS, Krieg AM, Udey MC, Vogel JC (1998) Activation of cutaneous dendritic cells by CpG-containing oligodeoxynucleotides: a role for dendritic cells in the augmentation of Th1 responses by immunostimulatory DNA. J Immunol 161:3042
20. Klinman DM, Yi A-K, Beaucage SL, Conover J, Krieg AM (1996) CpG motifs present in bacterial DNA rapidly induce lymphocytes to secrete interleukin 6, interleukin 12, and interferon gamma. Proc Natl Acad Sci USA 93:2879
21. Krieg AM, Yi AK, Matson S, Waldschmidt TJ, Bishop GA, Teasdale R, Koretzky GA, Klinman DM (1995) CpG motifs in bacterial DNA trigger direct B-cell activation. Nature 374:546
22. Lipford GB, Bauer M, Blank C, Reiter R, Wagner H, Heeg K (1997) CpG-containing synthetic oligonucleotides promote B and cytotoxic T cell responses to protein antigen: a new class of vaccine adjuvant. Eur J Immunol 94:2340

23. Locksley RM, Scott P (1991) Helper T-cell subsets in mouse leishmaniasis: induction, expansion and effector function. Immunol Today 12:A58
24. Macatonia SE, Knight SC, Edwards AJ, Griffiths S, Fryer P (1987) Localization of antigen on lymph node dendritic cells after exposure to the contact sensitizer fluorescein isothiocyanate: functional and morphologic studies. J Exp Med 166:16545
25. McClements WL, Armstrong ME, Keys RD, Liu MA (1996) Immunization with DNA vaccines encoding glycoprotein D or glycoprotein B, alone or in combination, induces protective immunity in animal models of herpes simplex virus-2 disease. Proc Natl Acad Sci USA 93:11414
26. Nabors GS, Afonso LCC, Farrell JP, Scott P (1995) Switch from a type 2 to a type 1 T helper cell response and cure of established *Leishmania major* infection in mice is induced by combined therapy with interleukin 12 and Pentostam. Proc Natl Acad Sci USA 92:3142
27. Pisetsky DS (1996) Immune activation by bacterial DNA: a new genetic code. Immunity 5:303
28. Raz E, Carson DA, Parker SE, Parr TB, Abai AM, Aichinger G, Gromkowski SH, Singh M, Lew D, Yankauckas MA, Baird SM, Rhodes GH (1994) Intradermal gene immunization: the possible role of DNA uptake in the induction of cellular immunity to viruses. Proc Natl Acad Sci USA 91:9519
29. Raz E, Tighe H, Sato Y, Corr M, Dudler JA, Roman M, Swain SL, Spiegelberg HL, Carson DA (1996) Preferential induction of a Th1 immune response and inhibition of specific IgE antibody formation by plasmid DNA immunization. Proc Natl Acad Sci USA 93:5141
30. Reed SG, Scott P (1993) T-cell and cytokine responses in leishmaniasis. Curr Opin Immunol 5:524
31. Reiner SL, Locksley RM (1995) The regulation of immunity to *Leishmania major*. Annu Rev Immunol 13: 151
32. Roake JA, Rao AS, Morris PJ, Larsen CP, Hankins DF, Austyn JM (1995) Dendritic cell loss from nonlymphoid tissues after systemic administration of lipopolysaccharide, tumor necrosis factor and interleukin-1. J Exp Med 181:2237
33. Roman M, Martin-Orozco G, Goodman JS, Nguyen M-D, Sato Y, Ronaghy A, Kornbluth RS, Richman DD, Carson DA, Raz E (1997) Immunostimulatory DNA sequences function as T helper-1-promoting adjuvants. Nat Medicine 3:849
34. Sato Y, Roman M, Tighe H, Lee D, Corr M, Nguyen M-D, Silverman GJ, Lotz M, Carson DA, Raz E (1996) Immunostimulatory DNA sequences necessary for effective intradermal gene immunization. Science 273:352
35. Scharton-Kersten T, Afonso LCC, Wysocka M, Trinchieri G, Scott P (1995) IL-12 is required for natural killer cell activation and subsequent T helper 1 cell development in experimental leishmaniasis. J Immunol 154:53230
36. Scharton-Kersten T, Scott P (1995) The role of the innate immune response in Th1 cell development following *Leishmania major* infection. J Leukoc Biol 57:515
37. Sparwasser T, Koch E, Vabulas RM, Heeg K, Lipford GB, Ellwart JW, Wagner H (1998) Bacterial DNA and immunostimulatory CpG oligonucleotides trigger maturation and activation of murine dendritic cells. Eur J Immunol 28:2045
38. Sparwasser T, Miethke T, Lipford G, Erdmann A, Hacker H, Heeg K, Wagner H (1997) Macrophages sense pathogens via DNA motifs: induction of tumor necrosis factor-mediated shock. Eur J Immunol 27:1671
39. Stacey KJ, Sweet MJ, Hume DA (1996) Macrophages ingest and are activated by bacterial DNA. J Immunol 157:2116
40. Steinman RM (1991) The dendritic cell system and its role in immunogenicity. Annu Rev Immunol 9:271
41. Sun S, Kishimoto H, Sprent J (1998) DNA as an adjuvant: capacity of insect DNA and synthetic oligodeoxynucleotides to augment T cell responses to specific antigen. J Exp Med 187:1145
42. Tang A, Amagai M, Granger LG, Stanley JR, Udey MC (1993) Adhesion of epidermal Langerhans cells to keratinocytes mediated by E-cadherin. Nature 361:82
43. Tang D, DeVit M, Johnston SA (1992) Genetic immunization is a simple method for eliciting an immune response. Nature 356:152
44. Ulmer JB, Donnelly JJ, Parker SE, Rhodes GH, Felgner PL, Dwarki VJ, Gromkowski SH, Deck RR, DeWitt CM, Friedman A, Hawe LA, Leander KR, Martinez D, Perry HC, Shiver JW, Montgomery DL, Liu MA (1993) Heterologous protection against influenza by injection of DNA encoding a viral protein. Science 259:1745
45. Walker PS, Scharton-Kersten T, Krieg AM, Love-Homan L, Rowton ED, Udey MC, Vogel JC (1999) Immunostimulatory oligonucleotides promote protective immunity and provide systemic therapy for leishmaniasis via IL-12- and IFN-γ-dependent mechanisms. Proc Natl Acad Sci USA 96:6970

46. Walker PS, Scharton-Kersten T, Rowton ED, Hengge U, Bouloc A, Udey MC, Vogel JC (1998) Genetic immunization with glycoprotein 63 cDNA results in a helper T cell type 1 immune response and protection in a murine model of leishmaniasis. Hum Gene Ther 9:1899
47. Weiner GJ, Liu H-M, Wooldridge JE, Dahle CE, Krieg AM (1997) Immunostimulatory oligodeoxynucleotides containing the CpG motif are effective as immune adjuvants in tumor antigen immunization. Proc Natl Acad Sci USA 94:10833
48. Xu D, Liew FY (1995) Protection against leishmaniasis by injection of DNA encoding a major surface glycoprotein, gp63, of *L. major*. Immunology 84: 173
49. Zimmermann S, Egeter O, Hausmann S, Lipford GB, Rocken M, Wagner H, Heeg K (1998) CpG oligodeoxynucleotides trigger protective and curative Th1 responses in lethal murine leishmaniasis. J Immunol 160:3627

Rescue of B cells from apoptosis by immune stimulatory CpG DNA

Arthur M. Krieg[1], Ae-Kyung Yi[2]

[1] Department of Veterans Affairs Medical Center, Iowa City, IA 52246, USA, Department of Internal Medicine, University of Iowa College of Medicine, 540 EMRB, Iowa City, IA 52242, USA, CpG ImmunoPharmaceuticals, Wellesley, MA 02481, USA
[2] Department of Internal Medicine, University of Iowa College of Medicine, 540 EMRB, Iowa City, IA 52242, USA

Regulation of apoptosis

All higher multicellular organisms use programmed cell death, or apoptosis, as a way to regulate cell numbers. Apoptosis is used to rid the organism of unneeded cells during development as well as to eliminate infected or damaged cells that could pose a threat to organismal integrity. The immune system also uses apoptosis as a means to regulate cell numbers. For example, at the end of an immune response large numbers of antigen-specific lymphocytes have been generated against an infectious agent. The absence of antigens is a sign to the immune system that the infection has been overcome, and is typically followed by the loss via apoptosis of 90% or more of these newly generated lymphocytes. Apoptosis also plays an extremely important role during the generation of the primary immune repertoire. The immune system typically "uses" antigen-receptor signaling of immature lymphocytes as a sign that these lymphocytes may have a level of reactivity with self-antigens that could lead to the development of autoimmune disease. Such autoreactive lymphocytes are instead purged from the emerging repertoire through apoptosis.

Thus, cell death via apoptosis plays an extremely important role in maintaining the size and composition of lymphocyte populations. In this chapter, we primarily focus on the regulation of B cell apoptosis. Depending upon their stage of maturation, cross-linking of the B cell antigen receptor (BCR) may result in activation or apoptosis. Mature B lymphocytes proliferate and secrete immunoglobulin (Ig) in response to BCR cross-linking [1]. In contrast, self-reactive immature B lymphocytes are eliminated by apoptosis in the bone marrow and in the germinal centers of peripheral lymphoid organs [2, 3]. Antigen-receptor cross-linking on these immature B lymphocytes triggers apoptosis, which is thought to be an important mechanism in the maintenance of immune tolerance. Because a breakdown in this process is thought to lead to the development of autoimmune diseases, such as systemic lupus erythematosus, there has been a great deal of interest in the mechanisms responsible for its regulation. In different experimental models, the relative roles of apoptosis versus receptor editing may differ [4, 5].

Correspondence to: A.M. Krieg

Several B cell lines have been found to be useful models for studying the induction of apoptosis by BCR cross-linking. For example, the WEHI-231 murine B cell lymphoma has some phenotypic characteristics of immature B cells and undergoes rapid growth arrest and apoptosis in response to cross-linking of the BCR by anti-IgM [6]. The phenotype of WEHI-231 is membrane IgM^+, IgD^-, Fc receptor-low, and MHC class II-low [7]. BCR cross-linking in WEHI-231 cells induces rapid growth arrest in the G_0/G_1 stage of the cell cycle with chromatin fragmentation and death by apoptosis [6, 8]. These characteristics have made the WEHI-231 cell line a popular model system for investigating BCR-induced apoptosis and the regulation of immune tolerance. Strong mitogenic stimuli such as LPS and ligation of the CD40 ligand can rescue WEHI-231 cells from apoptosis induced by BCR cross-linking [6, 9].

Aside from BCR cross-linking, a wide range of signals have been found to induce the apoptotic pathways. Some of the second messenger pathways that have been shown to induce apoptosis include exposure to ceramides or activation of sphingomyelinase, inhibition of calcium homeostasis, activation of protein kinase C, the generation of reactive oxygen species (ROS), glucocorticoids, and a wide variety of chemotherapeutic agents that interfere with cellular metabolism. This wide variety of biochemical signals is thought to induce apoptosis through certain final common pathways which involve caspaces. In general, apoptosis can be prevented by increased expression or activity of certain protective genes such as BCL_2 and BCL_X [9, 10].

CpG DNA prevents B cell apoptosis triggered by BCR cross-linking

As detailed in the other chapters of this volume, oligodeoxynucleotides (ODN) containing CpG motifs are extraordinarily powerful B cell mitogens and immune activators. In addition to driving more than 95% of B cells into the cell cycle, CpG DNA induces B cells to produce high levels of IL-6 and to secrete Ig [11, 12]. These B cell stimulatory effects are further enhanced by the release of IFN-γ from NK cells activated by CpG DNA [13, 14]. The stimulatory effects of CpG DNA on mature B cells are dramatically enhanced by BCR cross-linking, indicating that this may be a mechanism that preferentially activates B cells that have bound their specific antigen [11]. Thus, CpG DNA is not only a B cell mitogen, but also a costimulatory factor for B cell activation.

These studies suggested the possibility that like other B cell mitogens and costimulatory signals, CpG DNA may protect WEHI-231 cells from the apoptosis induced by BCR cross-linking. We found this to be the case. CpG DNA not only protects WEHI-231 cells from the growth arrest triggered by BCR cross-linking, but also rescues the cells against apoptosis as measured by the failure of BCR cross-linking to induce the formation of hypodiploid nuclei, which is an indicator of apoptotic cell death [15]. Studies using panels of different CpG ODN demonstrated that a variety of CpG motifs could protect WEHI-231 B cells. As used herein, a "CpG motif" refers to a CpG dinucleotide and the two bases on its 5′ and 3′ sides. ODN need contain only a single CpG motif to protect against apoptosis. Protective motifs include AACGTT, GTCGCT, GTCGAT, and GACGTT [15]. Thus, although the CpG motif has sometimes been described as purine-purine CG pyrimidine-pyrimidine, there is actually more flexibility than is implied by this simple formula. However, the CpG motif has to be unmethylated, since methylation at the 5 position of the cytosine abolished apoptosis protection.

If the CpG DNA acted quite early on the signaling pathways induced by BCR cross-linking, then the protective effects of CpG DNA should only be seen when it is added very early after BCR ligation. In fact, the addition of CpG to BCR-cross-linked WEHI-231 cells can be delayed as long as 3 h with no loss of protection and for at least 9 h with partial protection [15].

The mechanism of this anti-apoptotic effect of CpG DNA has been of great interest. BCR ligation in WEHI-231 cells leads to an initial increase in expression of the proto-oncogene *c-myc* followed by a decline below basal levels [15]. BCR ligation also results in decreased mRNA levels for the protooncogene *myn* as well as the apoptosis-regulating genes bcl_2, $bcl\text{-}x_L$, and *bax* [15, 16]. BCL_2 protein levels do not change, but the levels of the anti-apoptotic protein BCL_{XL} are greatly reduced by 12 h after BCR ligation. These alterations in gene expression presumably result from changes in transcription factor activity. One such transcription factor is NF-κB, which appears to have an important role in the regulation of apoptosis in WEHI-231 cells. BCR cross-linking leads to decreased activity of the p50/c-Rel heterodimer with an increase in the NF-κB p50/p50 homodimer within approximately 3–8 h [17]. The RNA level for *egr*-1, an immediate early gene encoding a transcriptional activator, also falls after BCR ligation [18].

CpG DNA reverses all of these changes in gene expression, and even induces increased levels of mRNA for *myc*, $bcl\text{-}x_L$, and *egr*-1 [15, 18]. In fact, CpG DNA is even more effective than LPS in protecting WEHI-231 cells from BCR-induced apoptosis. CpG DNA causes a sustained activation of the p50/c-Rel heterdimer of NF-κB in WEHI-231 cells. BCR cross-linking normally causes a decrease in p50/c-Rel levels with an increase in the p50/p50 homodimer. Since the homodimer is a putative transcriptional repressor, this may lead to decreased expression of genes whose expression is dependent upon NF-κB, such as *c-myc*. Considering the anti-apoptotic function of *c-myc*, this decrease in NF-κB function would result in increased apoptosis. Indeed, chemical inhibitors of IκB degradation, which prevent NF-κB activation, promote WEHI-231 apoptosis and prevent the ability of CpG DNA to maintain *c-myc* mRNA levels [17]. A role for *egr*-1 induction in the anti-apoptotic activity of CpG ODN has been suggested by the loss of CpG protection in cells treated with antisense ODN against *egr*-1 [18]. However, the antisense ODN used to inhibit *egr*-1 expression in this study contained two poly-G sequences (four Gs in a row) which were not present in the control ODN. Such poly-G ODN have been shown to have nonspecific anti-proliferative effects, suggesting that a poly-G mechanism rather than an "antisense" mechanism may have accounted for the growth inhibition induced by this antisense ODN [19, 20]. Further studies will be required to determine the possible role of *egr*-1 in mediating the anti-apoptotic effects of CpG DNA.

The mitochondrial membrane potential (ψm) is reduced at the onset of apoptosis by the opening of permeability transition pores in the mitochondrial membrane, which is thought to be a point of no return in the cascade of signaling events leading to apoptosis [21]. Of interest, ψm is reduced not only during induced apoptosis, but also during the spontaneous apoptosis of primary splenic B cells [16]. CpG DNA effectively prevented this spontaneous loss of ψm.

The anti-apoptotic effects of CpG DNA on WEHI-231 cells are not limited to BCR ligation. CpG DNA also protects against apoptosis induced by ceramides, sphingomyelinase, induction of intracellular calcium flux with thapsigargin, UV light, TGF-β, anthracycline and vinca chemotherapeutics, oxidative stress induced by menadione, and by the protein phosphatase inhibitor okadaic acid [22]. CpG

DNA was not able to reverse the induction of apoptosis by the protein synthesis inhibitor cyclohexamide, but did reduce the extent of apoptosis induced by the combination of cyclohexamide and BCR ligation. Protein kinase C activity did not seem to be required for the anti-apoptotic effects of CpG DNA since these were not effected by PKC inhibition. These results indicate that CpG DNA inhibits apoptosis at a relatively distal point in the signaling pathways. Overexpression of BCL_{XL} expression has also been shown to protect against apoptosis induction through diverse signaling pathways, providing a possible mechanism for the CpG effect.

Prevention of spontaneous B cell apoptosis by CpG DNA

Mature resting T and B cells differ from immature cells in the constitutive production of pro-apoptotic proteins, which appear to be held in check by labile apoptosis inhibitors. Treatment of mature lymphocytes with inhibitors of protein synthesis or protein kinase C activity leads to accelerated spontaneous apoptosis [23, 24]. In vivo, physiologic homeostatic signals, possibly mediated in part through the BCR, maintain the viability of these mature lymphocytes. However, upon purification, mature resting splenic T and B cells undergo spontaneous apoptosis in culture, with typically about 25% of B cells undergoing apoptosis by 16 h, and 50% at 40 h (apoptotic cells defined by hypodiploid nuclei on DNA staining) [25, 26].

To determine whether CpG DNA also prevent this spontaneous apoptotic process, purified B cells were studied in the presence or absence of CpG DNA. These studies confirmed that addition of CpG ODN could almost completely prevent spontaneous B cell apoptosis, but ODN containing GpC motifs or methylated CpG motifs could not [26]. In addition, CpG ODN drove B cells into the G_1 and S phases of the cell cycle. CpG ODN also partially protected B cells against cyclohexamide-induced apoptosis, even in the absence of cell cycle entry. These protective effects were associated with marked increases in mRNA expression of *egr*-1, *c-jun*, *c-myc*, and $bcl\text{-}x_L$ [26].

An important clue to the mechanism of the anti-apoptotic effect of CpG DNA is provided by the finding that an inhibitor of endosomal acidification, chloroquine, abolishes the protective effect of CpG DNA but does not diminish the ability of LPS or anti-CD40 to protect against apoptosis [16]. We hypothesize that CpG DNA is taken up by B cells through an endosomal process, and that CpG-induced signal transduction depends on the acidification and/or maturation of these vesicles [27].

Biologic consequences of the anti-apoptotic effects of CpG DNA

The anti-apoptotic effects of CpG DNA may be thought of in the context of the role of this DNA as a "danger signal" in alerting the immune system to the presence of infectious pathogens. The B cell response to antigen is normally quite limited by the amount of antigen and costimulatory signals. CpG DNA provides an additional costimulatory signal and maintains the viability of antigen-specific B cells that may otherwise undergo apoptosis. This would tend to enhance the magnitude of antigen-specific immune responses as well as prolonging their duration.

This theoretical prediction is confirmed by experimental studies in which CpG DNA has proven to be an exceptionally strong vaccine adjuvant [28–35]. The adjuvant effects of CpG DNA for inducing antibody production are also seen with thymus-independent antigens in vitro [36].

For reasons that are not entirely clear, vaccination of neonates tends to be quite inefficient. This may be partially due to the tendency of the immature immune system to become tolerant to neoantigens instead of immune. Whatever the case, CpG DNA has proven to be an extremely effective adjuvant at driving antigen-specific immune responses in neonatal mice, even for driving antibody production against thymus-independent antigens [36–38].

Like T and B cells, primary human dendritic cells also tend to die in culture in the absence of growth factors or other stimuli. Although this process has not been shown to be due to apoptosis, it is noteworthy that CpG DNA is a survival factor for human as well as mouse dendritic cells, not only maintaining their viability, but also stimulating their antigen-presentation function [39–41].

Because of the potent anti-apoptotic effects of CpG DNA and its ability to drive such a high percentage of B cells into the cell cycle, it might be expected that exposure to CpG DNA would be a trigger for autoimmune disease. Autoimmune diseases have certainly been suggested to be triggered by infectious agents, and circumstantial evidence supports the hypothesis that CpG DNA could trigger autoimmunity [42]. However, animal studies demonstrate that administration of CpG DNA not only fails to induce lupus but actually reduces its severity in genetically disposed mice [43–45]. These studies provide convincing evidence that CpG DNA as a single agent, does not trigger systemic autoimmunity in these disease models. On the other hand, when CpG DNA is administered together with a central nervous system antigen or a molecular mimic of a self-antigen, potent adjuvant activity can lead to induction of autoimmune disease [46, 47].

Another theoretical possibility is that CpG DNA could prevent the apoptosis of malignant B cells, thus increasing the risk of lymphoma development. However, CpG DNA does not promote lymphoma development in a transgenic mouse model of Burkat's lymphoma, but actually can prevent tumor development in this model [48].

Conclusions

CpG DNA is extremely effective at protecting primary B cells or B cell lines against apoptosis induced by multiple different stimuli. These protective effects are mediated through a chloroquine-sensitive pathway and are associated with increased activity of NF-κB and increased expression of the anti-apoptotic factor, BCL_{XL}. This anti-apoptotic property of CpG DNA is yet another manifestation of its important role in regulating lymphocyte homeostasis. It seems likely that the anti-apoptotic effects of CpG DNA contribute to its remarkable efficacy as a vaccine adjuvant.

Acknowledgements The authors thank Vickie Akers for secretarial assistance. Financial support was provided through a Career Development Award from the Department of Veterans Affairs and grants from the National Institutes of Health, Cystic Fibrosis Foundation, and CpG ImmunoPharmaceuticals, Inc.

References

1. DeFranco AL (1987) Molecular aspects of B-lymphocyte activation. Annu Rev Cell Biol 3:143
2. Nossal GJ, Pike BL, Battye FL (1979) Mechanisms of clonal abortion tolerogenesis. II. Clonal behavior of immature B cells following exposure to anti-mu chain antibody. Immunology 37:203
3. Liu YJ, Joshua DE, Williams GT, Smith CA, Gordon J, MacLennan IC (1989) Mechanism of antigen-driven selection in germinal centers. Nature 342:929

4. Monroe JG (1996) Tolerance sensitivity of immature-stage B cells: can developmentally regulated B cell antigen receptor (BCR) signal transduction play a role? J Immunol 156:2657
5. Melamed D, Nemazee D (1997) Sel-antigen does not accelerate immature B cell apoptosis, but stimulates receptor editing as a consequence of developmental arrest. Proc Natl Acad Sci USA 94:9267
6. Jakway JP, Unsinger WR, Gold MR, Mishell RI, DeFranco AL (1986) Growth regulation of the B lymphoma cell line WEHI-231 by anti-immunoglobulin, lipopolysaccharide, and other bacterial products. J Immunol 137:2225
7. Hibner U, Benhamou LE, Haury M, Cazenave P-A, Sarthou P (1993) Signaling of programmed cell death induction in WEHI-231 B lymphoma cells. Eur J Immunol 23:2821
8. Scott DW, Tuttle J, Livnat D, Haynes W, Cogswell J, Keng P (1985) Lymphoma models for B-cell activation and tolerance. II. Growth inhibitions by anti-mu of WEHI-231 and the selection of properties of resistants. Cell Immunol 93:124
9. Tsubata T, Wu J, Honjo T (1993) B-cell apoptosis induced by antigen receptor crosslinking is blocked by a T-cell signal through CD40. Nature 364:645
10. Wang Z, Karras JG, Howard RG, Rothstein TL (1995) Induction of *bcl-x* by CD40 engagement rescues sIg-induced apoptosis in murine B cells. J Immunol 155:3722
11. Krieg AK, Yi A-K, Matson S, Waldschmidt TJ, Bishop GA, Teasdale R, Koretzky G, Klinman D (1995) CpG motifs in bacterial DNA trigger direct B-cell activation. Nature 374:546
12. Klinman D, Yi A-K, Beaucage SL, Conover J, Krieg AM (1996) CpG motifs expressed by bacterial DNA rapidly induce lymphocytes to secrete IL-6, IL-12 and IFN. Proc Natl Acad Sci USA 93:2879
13. Yi A-K, Chace JH, Cowdery JS, Krieg AM (1996) IFN-γ promotes IL-6 and IgM secretion in response to CpG motifs in bacterial DNA and oligodeoxynucleotides. J Immunol 156:558
14. Cowdery JS, Chace JH, Yi A-K, Krieg AM (1996) Bacterial DNA induces NK cells to produce interferon-γ *in vivo* and increases the toxicity of lipopolysaccharides. J Immunol 156:4570
15. Yi A-K, Hornbeck P, Lafrenz DE, Krieg AM (1996) CpG DNA rescue of murine B lymphoma cells from anti-IgM induced growth arrest and programmed cell death is associated with increased expression of *c-myc* and bcl_{xL}. J Immunol 157:4918
16. Yi A-K, Peckham DW, Ashman RF, Krieg AM (1999) CpG DNA rescues B cells from apoptosis by activating NF-κB and preventing mitochondrial membrane potential disruption via a chloroquine-sensitive pathway. Int Immunol 11:2015
17. Yi A-K, Krieg AM (1998) CpG DNA rescue from anti-IgM induced WEHI-231 B lymphoma apoptosis via modulation of IκBα and IκBβ and sustained activation of nuclear factor-κB/c-Rel. J Immunol 160:1240
18. Han S-S, Chung S-T, Robertson DA, Chelvarajan RL, Bondada S (1999) CpG oligodeoxynucleotides rescue BKS-2 immature B cell lymphoma from anti-IgM-mediated growth inhibition by up-regulation of egr-1. Int Immunol 11:871
19. Yaswen P, Stampfer MR, Ghosh K, Cohen JS (1993) Effects of sequence of thioated oligonucleotides on cultured human mammary epithelial cells. Antisense Res Dev 3:67
20. Burgess TL, Fisher EF, Ross SL, Bready JV, Qian Y-X, Bayewitch LA, Cohen AM, Herrera CJ, Hu SS-F, Kramer FB, Lott FD, Martin FH, Pierce GF, Simone L, Farrell CL (1995) The antiproliferative activity of c-myb and *c-myc* antisense oligonucleotides in smooth muscle cells is caused by a nonantisense mechanism. Proc Natl Acad Sci USA 92:4051
21. Zamzani N, Marchetti P, Castedo M, Zanin C, Vayssiere J-L, Petit PX, Kroemer G (1995) Reduction in mitochondrial potential constitutes an early irreversible step of programmed lymphocyte death *in vivo*. J Exp Med 181:1661
22. MacFarlane DE, Manzel L, Krieg AM (1997) Unmethylated CpG-containing oligodeoxynucleotides inhibit apoptosis in WEHI 231 B lymphocytes induced by several agents: evidence for blockade of apoptosis at a distal signalling step. Immunology 91:586
23. Illera VA, Perandones E, Stunz LL, Mower DA Jr, Ashman RF (1993) Apoptosis in splenic B lymphocytes: regulation by protein kinase C and IL-4. J Immunol 151:2965
24. Perandones CE, Illera VA, Peckham D, Stunz LL, Ashman RF (1993) Regulation of apoptosis in vitro in mature murine spleen T cells. J Immunol 151:3521
25. Mower DA Jr, Peckham DW, Illera VA, Fishbaugh JK, Stunz LL, Ashman RF (1994) Decreased membrane phospholipid packing and decreased cell size precede DNA cleavage in mature mouse B cell apoptosis. J Immunol 152:4832
26. Yi A-K, Chang M, Peckham DW, Krieg AM, Ashman RF (1998) CpG oligodeoxyribonucleotides rescue mature spleen B cells from spontaneous apoptosis and promote cell cycle entry. J Immunol 160:5898

27. Yi A-K, Tuetken R, Redford T, Kirsch J, Krieg AM (1998) CpG motifs in bacterial DNA activates leukocytes through the pH-dependent generation of reactive oxygen species. J Immunol 160:4755
28. Roman M, Martin-Orozco E, Goodman JS, Nguyen M-D, Sato Y, Ronaghy A, Kornbluth RS, Richman DD, Carson DA, Raz E (1997) Immunostimulatory DNA sequences function as T helper-1-promoting adjuvants. Nat Med 3:849
29. Lipford GB, Sparwasser T, Bauer M, Zimmermann S, Koch E-S, Heeg K, Wagner H (1997) Immunostimulatory DNA: sequence-dependent production of potentially harmful or useful cytokines. Eur J Immunol 27:3420
30. Chu RS, Targoni OS, Krieg AM, Lehmann PV, Harding CV (1997) CpG oligodeoxynucleotides act as adjuvants that switch on Th1 immunity. J Exp Med 186:1623
31. Davis HL, Weeranta R, Waldschmidt TJ, Tygrett L, Schorr J, Krieg AM (1998) CpG DNA is a potent adjuvant in mice immunized with recombinant hepatitis B surface antigen. J Immunol 160:870
32. Weiner GJ, Liu H-M, Wooldridge JE, Dahle CE, Krieg AM (1997) Immunostimulatory oligodeoxynucleotides containing the CpG motif are effective as immune adjuvants in tumor antigen immunization. Proc Natl Acad Sci USA 94:10833
33. Moldoveanu Z, Love-Homan L, Huang WQ, Krieg AM (1998) CpG DNA, a novel adjuvant for systemic and mucosal immunization with influenza virus. Vaccine 16:1216
34. Jones TR, Obaldia N III, Gramzinski RA, Charoenvit Y, Kolodny N, Davis HL, Krieg AM, Hoffman SL (1999) Synthetic oligodeoxynucleotides containing CpG motifs enhance immunogenicity of a peptide malaria vaccine in Aotus monkeys. Vaccine 17:3065
35. Davis HL, Suparto I, Weeratna R, Juminarto, Iskandriati D, Krieg AM, Heriyanto, Sajuthi D (2000) CpG DNA overcomes hypo-responsiveness to hepatitis B vaccine in orangutans. Vaccine 18:1920
36. Chelvarajan RL, Raithatha R, Venkataraman C, Kaul R, Han S-S, Robertson DA, Bondada S (1999) CpG oligodeoxynucleotides overcome the unresponsiveness of neonatal B cells to stimulation with the thymus-independent stimuli anti-IgM and TNP-Ficoll. Eur J Immunol 29:2808
37. Brazolot Millan CL, Weeratna R, Krieg AM, Siegrist CA, Davis HL (1998) CpG DNA can induce strong Th1 humoral and cell-mediated immune responses against hepatitis B surface antigen in young mice. Proc Natl Acad Sci USA 95:15553
38. Kovarik J, Bozzotti P, Love-Homan L, Pihlgren M, Davis HL, Lambert P-H, Krieg AM, Siegrist C-A (1999) CpG oligodeoxynucleotides can circumvent the Th2 polarization of neonatal responses to vaccines but may fail to fully redirect Th2 responses established by neonatal priming. J Immunol 162:1611
39. Hartmann G, Weiner G, Krieg AM (1999) CpG DNA as a signal for growth, activation and maturation of human dendritic cells. Proc Natl Acad Sci USA 96:9305
40. Jakob T, Walker PS, Krieg AM, Udey MC, Vogel JC (1998) Activation of cutaneous dendritic cells by CpG-containing oligodeoxynucleotides: a role for dendritic cells in the augmentation of Th1 responses by immunostimulatory DNA. J Immunol 161:3042
41. Sparwasser T, Koch E-S, Vabulas RM, Heeg K, Lipford GB, Ellwart J, Wagner H (1998) Bacterial DNA and immunostimulatory CpG oligonucleotides trigger maturation and activation of murine dendritic cells. Eur J Immunol 28:2045
42. Krieg AM (1995) CpG DNA: a pathogenic factor in systemic lupus erythematosus? J Clin Immunol 15:284
43. Gilkeson GS, Conover J, Halpern M, Pisetsky DS, Feagin A, Klinman DM (1998) Effects of bacterial DNA on cytokine production by (NZB/NZW)F1 mice. J Immunol 161:3890
44. Gilkeson GS, Ruiz P, Pippen AMM, Alexander AL, Lefkowith JB, Pisetsky DS (1996) Modulation of renal disease in autoimmune NZB/NZW mice by immunization with bacterial DNA. J Exp Med 183:1389
45. Mor G, Singla M, Steinberg AD, Hoffman SL, Okuda K, Klinman DM (1997) Do DNA vaccines induce autoimmune disease? Hum Gene Ther 8:293
46. Bachmaier K, Neu N, Maza LM de la, Pal S, Hessel A, Penninger JM (1999) Chlamydia infections and heart disease linked through antigenic mimicry. Science 283:1335
47. Segal BM, Klinman DM, Shevach EM (1997) Microbial products induce autoimmune disease by an IL-12-dependent pathway. J Immunol 158:5087
48. Smith JB, Wickstron E (1998) Antisense *c-myc* and immunostimulatory oligonucleotide inhibition of tumorigenesis in a murine B-cell lymphoma transplant model. J Natl Cancer Inst 90:1146

The response of human B lymphocytes to oligodeoxynucleotides

Hua Liang, Peter E. Lipsky

Department of Internal Medicine, University of Texas Southwestern Medical Center at Dallas, 5323 Harry Hines Blvd., Dallas, TX 75235-8884, USA

Introduction

Until recently, DNA has generally been viewed as having limited immunogenic potential. Although antibody production could be induced by certain DNA structures, including denatured DNA, Z-DNA, A-DNA, and triple helical DNA [1], it was difficult to induce antibody by immunization with native right-handed helical DNA. Therefore, DNA was generally considered to be poorly immunostimulatory.

However, certain forms of DNA can be immunostimulatory. In 1984, Tokunaga and his colleagues [2, 3] found that the DNA component from *Mycobacterium bovis* strain Bacille Calmette-Guerin (BCG) inhibited growth of various syngeneic mouse and guinea pig tumors. This nucleic acid-rich fraction purified from BCG (MY-1) also augmented NK cell activity and stimulated IFN-α/β and -γ production by murine spleen cells and human peripheral blood mononuclear cells (PBMCs) [4, 5]. After cloning different BCG genes and testing the stimulatory activity of synthesized oligodeoxynucleotides (ODNs) identical to specific regions of the mycobacterial genome, Tokunaga and his colleagues identified palindromic single-stranded immunostimulatory DNA sequences (ISS), including the following CpG containing hexamers: 5′-GACGTC-3′, 5′-AGCGCT-3′, and 5′-AACGTT-3′ [6, 7]. They concluded that bacterial DNA containing ISS activated the immune system.

In the past few years, the immunostimulatory activities of DNA have been investigated intensively. Studies in mice demonstrated that DNA from various microorganisms and invertebrates, including bacteria, insects, yeasts, nematodes, and molluscs, induced polyclonal B cell activation. In contrast, mammalian and plant DNA did not stimulate B cell responses [8, 9]. The stimulatory activity of microbial DNA could be attributed to an ISS, the CpG motif, in which an unmethylated CpG dinucleotide was flanked by two 5′ purines and two 3′ pyrimidines. An additional 5′ thymidine appended to the CpG motif could enhance the stimulatory activity [9].

In 1996, Raz et al. [10] found that mice immunized intradermally with expression vectors encoding β-galactosidase (β-Gal) and containing a bacterial ampicillin resistance gene (ampR) developed high titers of β-Gal-specific antibodies [10]. In con-

Correspondence to: P.E. Lipsky

trast, mice immunized with a similar expression vector containing the kanamycin resistance gene (kanR) produced a weak antibody response to β-Gal [10, 11]. Comparison of the sequences of the ampR and kanR genes indicated that two repeats of the CpG motif were present in the ampR gene, whereas none was present in kanR gene. Subcloning the CpG motif to the sites flanking the kanR gene in the vector conferred the ability to induce strong humoral and cellular responses [11]. These results confirmed that DNA and plasmids containing CpG motifs can activate the immune system.

Certain phosphorothioate oligodeoxynucleotides (sODNs) also stimulated murine B cells. One of the most stimulatory sODNs is complementary to a portion of the rev region of the HIV genome. This antisense compound induced marked proliferation and immunoglobulin production by murine B cells in vitro. Moreover, mice developed massive splenomegaly and polyclonal hypergammaglobulinemia within 2 days after intravenous injection of this sODN [12]. B cell stimulation by the antisense sODNs did not appear to result from inhibition of specific genes, but rather from direct stimulation of B cells. Therefore, certain sODNs can activate murine B cells.

Some of the immunostimulatory activity of DNA, plasmids and sODNs can be accounted for the CpG motif, one of the ISS. However, murine B cell activation could also be induced by sODNs containing no CpG at all [13, 14]. Therefore, there might be other ISS besides the CpG motif.

ISS demonstrate a variety of influences on the immune system. They directly activate murine B cells, macrophages/monocytes, and dendritic cells both in vivo and in vitro. Activated myeloid cells produce a variety of cytokines, including IL-12, that subsequently stimulate NK cells to secrete IFN-γ and enhance their lytic activity [8, 9, 12–19]. Moreover, because of the ability to induce production of IL-12 and IFN-γ, ISS stimulate a selective Th1 response both in vivo and in vitro [10, 20–22].

The stimulatory effects of ISS on murine B cells include induction of increased expression of activation markers, proliferation, differentiation and cytokine production [8, 9, 12–14, 23]. ISS also prevent murine B cells from undergoing apoptosis [24–26]. It should be noted, however, that many of the effects on murine B cells were assessed in mixed cell culture, and therefore, many of the effects could be indirectly mediated by stimulation of contaminating cells.

Because of the variety of activities on the immune system leading to antibody production and Th1 responses, ISS could be important adjuvants for conventional protein vaccination and necessary components for DNA vaccination against a variety of targets [11, 22, 27–31]. It has been demonstrated that mice immunized with recombinant hepatitis B surface antigen (HBsAg) and a CpG containing sODN had titers of HBsAb that were five times higher than those of mice immunized with HBsAg and alum. In addition, CpG containing sODNs also induced strong Th1 and cytotoxic T lymphocyte (CTL) responses, whereas immunization with antigens in alum induced Th2 responses and no CTL [27]. It was also shown that the addition of either *Escherichia coli* DNA or CpG containing sODNs to inactivated influenza virus or protein antigens promoted production of influenza-specific antibodies and CTLs in mice [21, 22, 28]. Moreover, mice immunized with a tumor-specific antigen and CpG containing sODN produced higher titers of tumor antigen-specific IgG2a antibody and exhibited more prolonged survival than mice immunized with tumor antigen and complete Freund's adjuvant. The degree of tumor protection induced by CpG containing sODN was greater than that by complete Freund's adjuvant, but with less local inflammation [29]. Furthermore, combination of CpG containing sODNs and antitumor monoclonal antibodies (mAb) enhanced the efficacy of mAb therapy of murine B cell lymphoma 38C13 [30]. Therefore, ISS may be effective adjuvants for DNA or protein vaccination designed to induce Th1 or CTL responses.

Because of the ability to induce a Th1-biased response, ISS may be important for treating allergy, asthma, and chronic parasitic infection [32–36]. It has been reported that coadministration of sODNs containing a CpG motif with antigen inhibited production of Th2 cytokines, IgE, airway eosinophilia and bronchial hyperactivity in a murine model of asthma. In addition, CpG containing sODNs prevented allergen-induced airway inflammation in a presensitized mouse [34, 35]. Moreover, CpG containing sODNs triggered protective and curative Th1 responses in a murine model of *Leishmania major* infection [36]. These results suggested that ISS might be a good treatment for allergy, asthma, and chronic parasitic infection.

Taken together, ISS may have important roles in vaccination, tumor resistance and modification of Th2-mediated responses in humans. However, little information is available on the potential immunostimulatory effects of ISS in humans. Because human and murine lymphocytes may behave differently in immune responses, results obtained from mouse models cannot be extrapolated to man directly. Therefore, investigation of the ability of ISS to induce activation of human lymphocytes is necessary to determine the potential impact of these materials on human immune responsiveness as well as their potential role as immune modulators.

Human B cell activation induced by ODNs

The first evidence for the possible immunostimulatory activity of DNA in man came from studies on the binding of sera from normal human subjects to a variety of mammalian and nonmammalian DNA. It was found that sera from normal subjects contained antibodies that bound DNA from two bacterial species, *Micrococcus lysodeikticus* and *Staphylococcus epidermidis*. These antibodies had high affinity and specificity for bacterial and nonmammalian DNA, which suggested that they bound to structural epitopes unique to these DNA [37–40]. It was also shown that sera from normal subjects contained antibodies that bound to DNA from BK polyomavirus [41]. It should be noted that the nonmammalian DNA studied contained numerous ISS [8, 9, 42–44]. Despite finding anti-DNA antibodies in the sera of normal human subjects, these studies did not examine the direct effect of nonmammalian DNA or specific ISS on human B cell function. Evidence has been presented that antisense sODNs complementary to parts of the HBV genome could stimulate proliferation of B lymphocytes from chronic hepatitis patients [45]. Furthermore, it has been demonstrated that 27-mer and 21-mer antisense sODNs to the rev region of the HIV genome increased proliferation and Ig production by PBMCs from normal subjects [46, 47]. Taken together, these reports suggest that ISS can induce lymphocyte proliferation and antibody production from patients and normal human subjects. However, whether ISS can directly activate normal human B cells and the mechanism of the human B cell activation remain to be completely delineated.

A series of experiments was carried out to determine whether bacterial DNA and various oligodeoxynucleotides, including phosphorothioates (sODNs) and phosphodiesters (ODNs), could activate human B cells directly [48]. These studies employed highly purified human peripheral blood B cells so that a direct stimulatory activity on human B cells could be assessed. As shown in Fig. 1, three sODNs (HSVas,

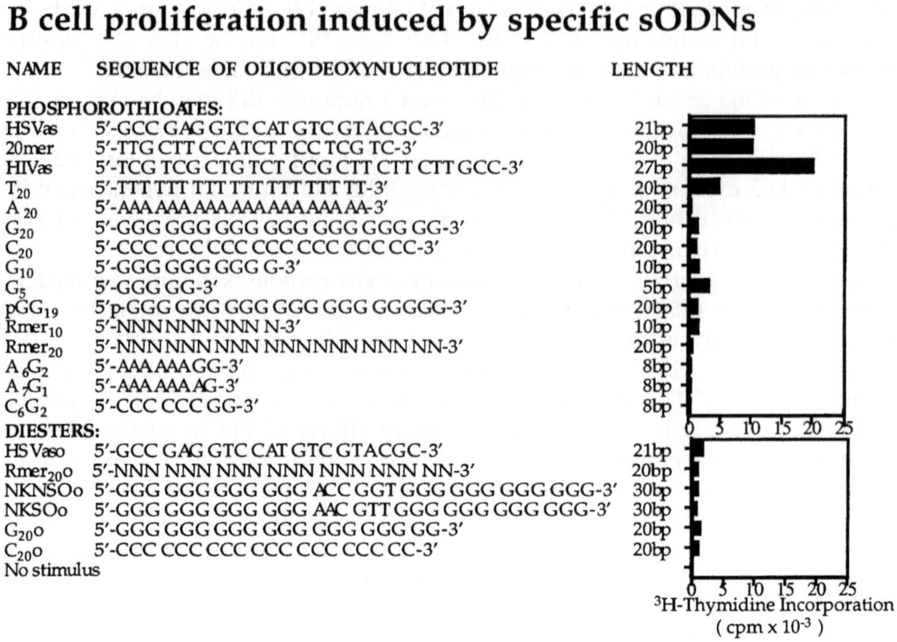

Fig. 1. B cell proliferation induced by specific's ODNs. Highly purified human peripheral blood B cells (50×10^3/well) were cultured with various concentrations of sODNs, ODNs, or DNA (1 μg/ml to 50 μg/ml) for 4 days and proliferation was assessed by [^{3}H]thymidine incorporation. The data indicate the results with the optimal stimulatory concentrations, usually 5 μg/ml (except 1 μg/ml for HIVas and 25 μg/ml for R-mer10). Data with HSVaso were obtained by incubation of B cells with 5 μg/ml HSVaso and then adding 5 μg/ml of HSVaso to culture daily. A single addition of HSVaso induced no response. The data are the mean of triplicate cultures with a SEM of less than 10% and are representative of three separate experiments, each carried out with B cells from a different donor. HSVas is a 21-bp antisense sODN complementary to a translation initiation region of HSV; HIVas is a 27-bp antisense sODN complementary to the rev region of HIV [12]; NKSOo is a 30-bp antisense sODN that has been shown to induce IFN-γ production and enhance NK cell lytic activity [6]; NKNSO is the control sODN for NKSOo [6] (*ODN* oligodeoxnucleotide; *sODN* phosphorothioate oligonucleotide)

20-mer, and HIVas) consistently induced significant human B cell proliferation. Of note, neither *E. coli* DNA nor calf thymus DNA was stimulatory. Other sODNs (poly G, poly C, poly T, randomers) and ODNs induced minimal, but nonetheless detectable responses that were statistically different from [^{3}H]thymidine incorporation manifested by B cells cultured alone. Poly A and three 8-mer sODNs did not stimulate B cells at all. Moreover, the diester form of the herpes simplex virus (HSV) antisense (HSVaso) was also much less stimulatory than its phosphorothioate counterpart (HSVas) within this concentration range, even when added to culture repetitively (mean maximum response to HSVaso was 615±22 cpm vs 3113±93 cpm for HSVas). Although modest, the response induced by the diester form of HSVas (HSVaso) was significantly greater than tritiated thymidine incorporation of control B cells (99±7, $P<0.01$) [48]. These results indicated that certain sODNs stimulated human B cell proliferation and they were more efficient than their phosphodiester counterparts.

sODNs that induced maximal human B cell proliferation also increased the expression of activation markers by highly purified B cells. Thus, the most stimulatory

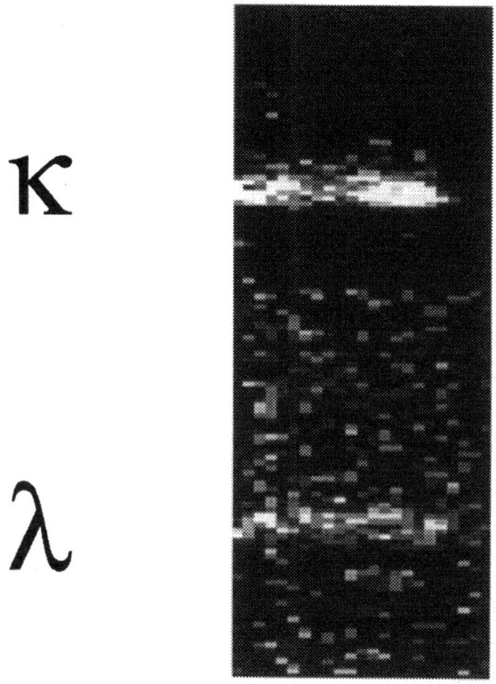

Fig. 2. Polyclonal activation of human B cells induced by HIVas. B cells (25×10^3/well) were cultured with IL-2 and HIVas for 8 days, after which RNA was harvested and analyzed for the content of light chain variable gene products by reverse transcriptase-PCR using V_κ- or V_λ-specific primers. The data are representative of two separate experiments, each using B cells from an individual donor

sODNs activated more than 80% of B cells to express activation markers, including CD69, CD86 and CD25. In contrast, sODNs that stimulated minimal proliferation also induced minimal or no increased expression of activation markers ([48] and unpublished data). The finding that sODNs induced activation marker expression by more than 80% of B cells implies that the response of human B cells to sODNs is polyclonal.

Moreover, the sODNs that induced maximal proliferation also stimulated production of IgM, IgG and IgA from purified B cells in the absence of exogenous cytokines or T cells. The other sODNs and DNA induced little or no Ig production. The most stimulatory sODNs also induced low affinity anti-DNA antibody production [48]. Taken together, these results clearly indicate that ISS can directly trigger activation, proliferation and differentiation of highly purified human B cells.

Certain cytokines and T cells can augment human B cell activation induced by ISS. Thus, IL-2 and IL-6, but not IL-4 and IL-10, enhanced human B cell responses to the most stimulatory sODNs, but B cell activation was not dependent on IL-2 or IL-6 ([48] and unpublished data). In addition, purified human T cells also enhanced the responses of human B cells to the most stimulatory sODNs [48], although T cells did not bind sODNs and did not proliferate when cultured with immunostimulatory sODNs ([48] and unpublished data). These results indicated that certain cytokines and intact T cells enhanced B cell responses to ISS, but they were not required for the stimulatory activity of sODNs.

The nature of B cell responses to sODNs is polyclonal. This was confirmed by documenting that B cells expressed mRNA for all six major V_H families [48] and for both κ and λ light chain variable genes (Fig. 2) when activated by the most stimulatory sODNs. However, the large number of B cells induced to express activation markers compared to the modest degree of proliferation implied that many B cells were initially activated, but few underwent clonal expansion in response to sODNs. Additional experiments directly analyzing cell cycle entry and progression confirmed that active sODNs stimulated a few cells to enter cell cycle and these cells underwent multiple rounds of proliferation. Of note, many of the originally activated B cells underwent apoptosis rather than clonal expansion after stimulation by sODNs.

Taken together, ISS induced polyclonal activation of human B cells in vitro in the absence of T cells and other cells capable of facilitating B cell activation. Many B cells were initially activated, but only a small number of activated B cells proliferated and differentiated into Ig-secreting cells, whereas others were induced to undergo programmed cell death.

Mechanism of human B cell activation induced by ODNs

ODNs activate human B cells by cross-linking surface Ig

To examine whether sODNs activate human B cells by engaging surface receptors or whether cellular entry of sODNs is necessary for the stimulatory activities, the most stimulatory sODNs were covalently coupled to CNBr-activated Sepharose 4B beads and the ability of the immobilized sODNs to induce human B cell activation was tested. The results showed that Sepharose-bound sODNs stimulated B cells as effectively as their soluble counterparts [48). Additional experiments documented that the stimulatory activity did not result from soluble sODNs released from the beads. These results indicate that ISS activate human B cells by engaging sODN-binding surface receptors.

Examination of binding of fluorescein isothiocyanate-labeled-(FITC) sODNs indicated that binding was rapid, saturable, specific and initially temperature independent, suggesting that the binding is likely to be receptor mediated. Most sODNs tested appeared to bind to the same receptor(s) in that cross-competition of binding was evident. Analysis of B cell subsets binding sODN-FITC (Fig. 3, Table 1) showed that a greater percentage of IgM^+ cells than IgM^- cells bind HIVas (Fig. 3A). Similar results were obtained with IgD (Fig. 3B), CD20 (Fig. 3E), and CD44 (Fig. 3F). Comparable percentages of $CD5^+$ and $CD5^-$ cells bound HIVas (Fig. 3C). Similar results were obtained with CD38 (Fig. 3D). These results indicate that HIVas binds preferentially to B cells expressing IgM, IgD and CD44, implying that IgM, IgD, and CD44 may be the candidate proteins for sODNs receptor(s).

It was possible that the most stimulatory sODNs triggered human B cell activation by directly binding surface IgM. A number of findings support this conclusion. HIVas was found to bind to FlowMetrix beads coated with IgM but not bovine serum albumin. Moreover, HIVas was found to bind to B cells and cap at 37°C. Colocalization of surface IgM into these HIVas caps was found, strongly implying that HIVas may bind and cross-link surface IgM. These data indicate that the most stimulatory sODNs directly bind to and crosslink surface IgM, thereby inducing polyclonal activation of human B cells.

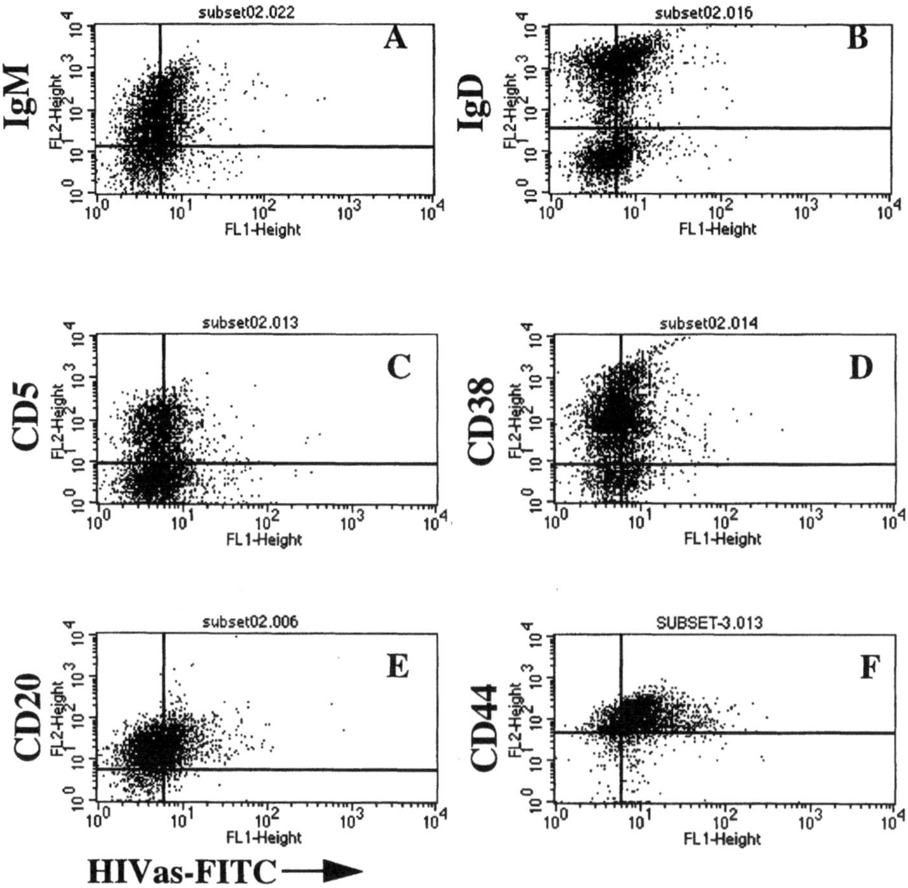

Fig. 3. HIVas binds preferentially to B cells expressing IgM, IgD, and CD44. B cells (2×10^5/sample) were incubated with or without HIVas-FITC (2 μg/sample) at 37 C for 30 min, after washing to remove unbound HIVas-FITC, B cells were stained with mAb against IgM (**A**), IgD (**B**), CD5 (**C**), CD38 (**D**),CD20 (**E**), CD44 (**F**), or their isotype-matched controls and analyzed by flow cytometry. FL1 represents HIVas-FITC and FL2 represents mAb against cell surface markers. The results of one of three experiments, each using B cells from a different donor, with similar findings are shown

The nature of ODNs

The nature of ISS has not been completely delineated. To identify the stimulatory sequences necessary for human B cell activation, one of the most stimulatory sODN, HIVas, was examined in detail. Three 15-mer sODNs containing the sequences corresponding to the 5′, central, and 3′ regions of HIVas were synthesized and tested. The 5′ 15-mer of HIVas stimulated comparable DNA synthesis as the full-length 27-mer, whereas the central and 3′ 15-mers were less stimulatory [48]. Comparison of the sequences indicated that TCGTCG was present only in the 5′ 15-mer of HIVas, but not in the others. To determine whether TCG is a stimulatory motif, the activity of additional 15-mer sODNs was tested. Of these compounds, $(TCG)_5$ in-

Table 1. HIVas binds preferentially to B cells expressing IgM, IgD, and CD44

B cell subpopulation	% of cells in the subpopulation	% of cells in the subpopulation binding HIVas
IgM^+	73	43
IgM^-	27	22
IgD^+	66	56
IgD^-	34	33
$CD5^+$	44	39
$CD5^-$	56	35
$CD38^+$	82	42
$CD38^-$	18	40
$CD44^+$	89	80
$CD44^-$	11	59
$CD20^+$	93	36
$CD20^-$	7	17

duced equal or greater B cell activation to HIVas, whereas a 5′ TCG doublet followed by a 3′ G nonamer failed to stimulate B cells. Additional sODNs, in which the TCG repeat was altered to ACG, TCC or TGG, had no stimulatory activity [48]. Therefore, a TCG repeat is a stimulatory motif for human B cells. The minimal length of ISS appears to be nine base pairs, since sODNs containing three TCG repeats were stimulatory, but a tandem TCG had minimal stimulatory activity. In addition to TCG repeats, repeats of the entire CpG motif that stimulated murine B cell also activated human B cells [48]. However, these motifs are not necessary for human B cell activation, since sODNs containing no CpG also induce maximal human B cell activation. The combined results of examining the stimulatory activity of 70 ODNs and sODNs did not indicate that a unique sequence accounted for the stimulatory activity of sODNs.

Several methods have been utilized to determine whether secondary or tertiary structure rather than a specific sequence might be involved in human B cell activation. The results indicate that the stimulatory activity of sODNs does not correlate with their ability to form hairpins or double-stranded molecules. In addition, the aberrant mobility of some sODNs on native polyacrylamide gel does not correlate with their stimulatory activity. However, HIVas induces capping of human B cell surface IgM, implying that HIVas can cross-link surface IgM. Therefore, it is possible that HIVas molecules interact with each other to form a complex which cross-links surface IgM and activates B cells. In this regard, it is possible that other stimulatory sODNs may be capable of facilitating the cross-linking of surface IgM and thereby activating human B cells. Taken together, these results suggested that structure rather than primary sequence might be an important determinant of the stimulatory capacity of sODNs, but the structures that could be necessary for stimulating B cells remain unknown.

Differences between human and murine B cells in the responsiveness to ODNs

Human B cell activation induced by ISS may be governed by different principles than those observed in the mouse (Table 2). First, the responses of human and mu-

Table 2. Differences between human and murine B cells in responsiveness to immunostimulatory DNA sequences

	Murine B cells	Human B cells
Stimulation by bacterial DNA	*E. coli*	None
Activation motifs	CpG motif (necessary)	CpG motif (not necessary)
Cellular entry of stimulus	Necessary	Not necessary, activation is receptor mediated
Activation character	Prevent apoptosis	Induce apoptosis
Mechanism of stimulation	IgM production requires IL-6	IgM production is independent of IL-6

rine B cells to bacterial DNA may be different. It has been demonstrated that *E. coli* DNA stimulated murine B cells both in vivo and in vitro [8, 9, 42–44]. In contrast, *E. coli* DNA did not activate human B cells [48]. However, sera from normal subjects contained antibodies that bound DNA from two bacterial species, *M. lysodeikticus* and *S. epidermidis*, suggesting that DNA from these bacteria might induce human B cell activation. It is not known, however, whether DNA from these microorganisms can directly stimulate human B cells. In summary, human and murine B cells appear to respond differently to bacterial DNA, at least that derived from *E. coli*.

Secondly, the basic activation motif appears to be different in man and mouse. The CpG motif has been shown to be sufficient and necessary for inducing murine B cell activation [9]. In contrast, for stimulation of human B cells, the CpG motif is sufficient, but not necessary. In addition, $(CpG)_n$, which is a potent stimulator of murine B cells, does not appear to be capable of inducing maximal human B cell activation, although it did stimulate human B cells minimally [48]. Of note, TCG repeats activate human B cells comparably to CpG motifs [48], but this sequence has not been tested in the murine system. Of importance, sODNs containing no CpG dinucleotides are also capable of activating human B cells. It should be noted that sODNs containing no CpG motifs also have been found to activate murine spleen mononuclear cells [13, 14], suggesting that the difference between mouse and human in this regard may be more relative than absolute. Lastly, methylation of cytosine in CpG dinucleotides totally abolished the stimulatory activity of ISS for murine B cells, suggesting that unmethylated CpG was necessary for murine B cells activation induced by ISS [9]. In contrast, for human B cells, methylation of cytosines in HSVas did not abolish the stimulatory activity of this ISS, suggesting that the methylation status of cytosine is not important in the stimulatory activity of sODNs for human B cells. Taken together, the basic activation motifs may be different in man and mouse.

Thirdly, the mechanism of B cell activation appears to be different between mice and humans. It has been suggested that ISS did not activate murine B cells by engaging surface receptor and cellular uptake of ISS seemed to be required [9]. In contrast, immobilized sODNs induced maximal activation of human B cells [48], suggesting that cell entry of sODNs is not necessary for human B cell activation. In addition, the most stimulatory sODNs activated human B cells by engaging sIgM. Therefore, the mechanism of B cell activation appears to be different between mice and humans.

Fourthly, the character of B cell activation seems to be different in man and mouse. It has been reported that ISS rescued murine B cells from apoptosis [24–26]. In contrast, the most stimulatory sODNs induced apoptosis of human B cells. Whether this represents a species difference or is related to a comparison of the responsiveness of human peripheral blood B cells to murine splenic B cells remains to be determined.

Finally, the cellular mechanism of B cell activation induced by ISS seems to be different between mice and humans. It has been shown that ISS induced marked IL-6 secretion from murine B cells and that IL-6 was necessary for IgM production induced by ISS [23, 49, 50]. In contrast, limited IL-6 secretion was detected in the supernatant of human B cells cultured with the most stimulatory sODNs and neutralizing antibodies to IL-6 inhibited the IgM production of human B cells only minimally or not at all. These results suggest that IL-6 does not play a role in human B cell activation induced by ISS. Therefore, the cellular mechanism of B cell activation induced by ISS seems to be different between mice and humans.

Taken together, human and murine B cells appear to be different in the responsiveness to ISS, implying that results derived from studies of murine B cells can not be directly extrapolated to human B cell responses.

The adjuvant effect of human monocytes

The study of binding of sODNs by PBMCs showed that the most stimulatory sODNs bound to nearly all the monocytes and most NK cells in addition to B cells, but they did not bind to T cells. Moreover, highly purified human monocytes enhanced B cell Ig production induced by the stimulatory sODNs, but not B cell proliferation. These results suggested that in addition to a direct stimulatory effect on human B cells, sODNs may also exert an adjuvant effect or a costimulatory effect on human B cells by activating human monocytes. Of note, this adjuvant effect on monocytes resulted in enhanced production of Ig but not increased proliferation.

Conclusions

ISS induce T cell-independent polyclonal activation of human B cell by engaging surface Ig. Manifestations of ISS-induced human B cell activation include expression of activation markers, proliferation, and Ig production as well as anti-DNA antibody production. IL-2, IL-6 and intact T cells enhanced B cell responses to ISS, but were not required for B cell activation. Human monocytes enhanced B cell responses induced by ISS, particularly Ig secretion. The chemical nature of sODNs capable of stimulating human B cells has not been completely delineated. Further studies will be necessary and important for developing novel therapeutic and preventive agents in humans using ISS.

Acknowledgements The authors would like to thank Dr. David S. Pisetsky for providing the oligonucleotide reagents and for many helpful discussions. The work described in this review was supported by NIH grant 2-P01-AI31229-8.

References

1. Stollar BD (1986) Antibodies to DNA. CRC Crit Rev Biochem 20:1
2. Tokunaga T, Yamamoto H, Shimada S, Abe H, Fukuda T, Fujisawa Y, Furutani Y, Yano O, Kataoka T, Sudo T, Makiguchi N, Suganuma T (1984) Antitumor activity of deoxyribonucleic acid fraction from *Mycobacterium bovis* BCG. I. Isolation, physicochemical characterization, and antitumor activity. J Natl Cancer Inst 72:955
3. Shimada S, Yano O, Inoue H, Kuramoto E, Fukuda T, Yamamoto H, Kataoka, T, Tokunaga T (1985) Antitumor activity of the DNA fraction from *Mycobacterium bovis* BCG. II. Effects on various syngeneic mouse tumors. J Natl Cancer Inst 74:681
4. Shimada S, Yano O, Tokunaga T (1986) In vivo augmentation of natural killer cell activity with a deoxyribonucleic acid fraction of BCG. Jpn J Cancer Res 77:808
5. Yamamoto S, Kuremoto E, Shimada S, Tokunaga T (1988) In vitro augmentation of natural killer cell activity and production of interferon α/β and -γ with deoxyribonucleic acid fraction from *Mycobacterium bovis* BCG. Jpn J Cancer Res 79:866
6. Yamamoto S, Yamamoto T, Kataoka T, Kuramoto E, Yana O, Tokunaga T (1992) Unique palindromic sequences in synthetic oligonucleotides are required to induce IFN and augment IFN-mediated natural killer activity. J Immunol 148:4072
7. Yamamoto T, Yamamoto S, Kataoka T, Komuro K, Kohase M, Tokunaga T (1994) Synthetic oligonucleotides with certain palindromes stimulate interferon production of human peripheral blood lymphocytes in vitro. Jpn J Cancer Res 85:775
8. Sun S, Beard C, Jaenisch R, Jones P, Sprent J (1997) Mitogenicity of DNA from different organisms for murine B cells. J Immunol 159:3119
9. Krieg AM, Yi A, Matson S, Waldschmidt TJ, Bishop GA, Teasdale R, Koretzky GA Klinman DM (1995) CpG motifs in bacterial DNA trigger direct B cell activation. Nature 371:546
10. Raz E, Tighe H, Sato Y, Corr M, Daudler JA, Roman M, Swain S, Spiegelberg HL, Carson DA (1996) Preferential induction of a Th1 immune response and inhibition of specific IgE antibody formation by plasmid DNA immunization. Proc Natl Acad Sci USA 93:5141
11. Sato Y, Roman M, Tighe H.m Lee D, Corr M, Nguyen M, Silverman GJ, Lotz M, Carson DA, Raz E (1996) Immunostimulatory DNA sequences necessary for effective intradermal gene immunization. Science 273:352
12. Branda RF, Moore AL, Mathews L, McCormarck JJ, Zon G (1993) Immune stimulation by an antisense oligomer complementary to the rev gene of HIV-1. Biochem Pharmacol 45:2037
13. Branda RF, Moore AL, Lafayette AR, Mathews L, Hong R, Zon G, Brown T, McCormack JJ (1996) Amplification of antibody production by phosphorothioate oligodeoxynucleotides. J Lab Clin Med 128:329
14. Monteith DK, Henry SP, Howard RB, Flournoy S, Levin AA, Bennett CF, Crooke ST (1997) Immune stimulation – a class effect of phosphorothioate oligodeoxynucleotides in rodents. Anticancer Drug Des 12:421
15. Stacey KJ, Sweet MJ, Hume DA (1996) Macrophages ingest and are activated by bacterial DNA. J Immunol 157:2116
16. Sparwasser T, Miethke T, Lipford G, Erdmann A, Hacker H, Heeg K, Wagner H (1997) Macrophages sense pathogen via DNA motifs: induction of tumor necrosis factor-α-mediated shock. Eur J Immunol 27:1671
17. Sparwasser T, Koch E, Vabulas RM, Heeg K, Lipford GB, Ellwart JW, Wagner H (1998) Bacterial DNA and immunostimulatory CpG oligonucleotides trigger maturation and activation of murine dendritic cells. Eur J Immunol 28:2045
18. Ballas ZK, Rasmussn WL, Krieg AM (1996) Induction of NK activity in murine and human cells by CpG motifs in oligodeoxynucleotides and bacterial DNA. J Immunol 157:1840
19. Chace JH, Hooker NA, Mildenstein KL, Krieg AM, Cowdery JS (1997) Bacterial DNA-induced NK cell IFN-gamma production is dependent on macrophage secretion of IL-12. Clin Immunol Immunopathol 84:185
20. Carson DA, Raz E (1997) Oligonucleotide adjuvants for T helper 1 (Th1)-specific vaccination. J Exp Med 186:1621
21. Chu RS, Targoni OS, Krieg AM, Lehmann PV, Harding CV (1997) CpG oligodeoxynucleotides act as adjuvants that switch on T helper (Th1) immunity. J Exp Med 186:1623

22. Roman M, Martin-Orozco E, Goodman JS, Nguyen M, Sato Y, Ronaghy A, Kornbluth RS, Richman DD, Carson DA, Raz E (1997) Immunostimulatory DNA sequences function as T helper-1-promoting adjuvants. Nat Med 3:849
23. Klinman DM, Yi A, Beaucage SL, Conover J, Krieg AM (1996) CpG motifs present in bacterial DNA rapidly induce lymphocytes to secret interleukin 6, interleukin-12, and interferon-γ. Proc Natl Acad Sci USA 93:2879
24. Yi A, Krieg AM (1998) CpG DNA rescue from anti-IgM-induced WEHI-231 B lymphoma apoptosis via modulation of IκBα and IκBβ and sustained activation of nuclear factor-κB/c-Rel. J Immunol 160:1240
25. Yi A, Chang M, Peckham DW, Krieg AM, Ashman RF (1998) CpG oligodeoxynucleotides rescue mature spleen B cells from spontaneous apoptosis and promote cell cycle entry. J Immunol 160:5898
26. Wang Z, Karras JG, Colarusso TP, Foote LC, Rothstein TL (1997) Unmethylated CpG motifs protect murine B lymphocytes against FAS-mediated apoptosis. Cell Immunol 180:162
27. Davis HL, Weeranta R, Waldschmidt TJ, Tygreett L, Schorr J, Krieg AM (1998) CpG DNA is a potent enhancer of specific immunity in mice immunized with recombinant hepatitis B surface antigen. J Immunol 160:870
28. Moldoveanu Z, Love-Homan L, Huang WQ, Krieg AM (1998) CpG DNA, a novel immune enhancer for systemic and mucosal immunization with influenza virus. Vaccine 16:1216
29. Weiner GJ, Liu H, Wooldridge JE, Dahle CE, Krieg AM (1997) Immunostimulatory oligodeoxynucleotides containing the CpG motifs are effective as immune adjuvants in tumor antigen immunization. Proc Natl Acad Sci USA 94:10833
30. Wooldridge JE, Ballas Z, Krieg AM, Weiner GJ (1997) Immunostimulatory oligodeoxynucleotides containing CpG motifs enhance the efficacy of monoclonal antibody therapy of lymphoma. Blood 89:2994
31. Lipford GB, Bauer M, Blank C, Reiter R, Wagner H, Heeg K (1997a) CpG-containing synthetic oligonucleotides promote B and cytotoxic T cell responses to protein antigen: a new class of vaccine adjuvants. J Exp Med 27:2340
32. Vogel G (1997) New clues to asthma therapies. Science 276:1643
33. Goodman JS, Van Uden JH, Kobayashi H, Broide D, Raz E (1998) DNA immunotherapeutics: new potential treatment modalities for allergic disease. Int Arch Allergy Immunol 116:177
34. Broide D, Schwarze J, Tighe H, Gifford T, Nguyen M, Malek S, Van Uden J, Martin-Orozco E, Gelfand EW, Raz E (1998) Immunostimulatory DNA sequences inhibit IL-5, eosinophilic inflammation, and airway hyperresponsiveness in mice. J Immunol 161:7054
35. Kline JN, Waldschmidt TJ, Businga TR, Lemish JE, Weinstock JV, Thorne PS, Krieg AM (1998) Cutting edge: modulation of airway inflammation by CpG oligodeoxynucleotides in a murine model of asthma. J Immunol 160:2555
36. Zimmermann S, Egeter O, Hausmann S, Lipford GB, Rocken M, Wagner H, Heeg K (1998) CpG oligodeoxynucleotides trigger protective and curative Th1 responses in lethal murine leishmaniasis. J Immunol 27(12):3420
37. Karounos DG, Grudier JP, Pisetsky DS (1988) Spontaneous expression of antibodies to DNA of various species origin in sera of normal subjects and patients with systemic lupus erythematosis. J Immunol 140:451
38. Robertson CR, Gilkeson GS, Ward MM, Pisetsky DS (1992) Patterns of heavy and light chains utilization in the antibody response to single-stranded bacterial DNA in normal human subjects and patients with systemic lupus erythematosis. Clin Immunol Immunopathol 62:25
39. Bunyard MP, Pisetsky DS (1994) Characterization of antibodies to bacterial double-stranded DNA in the sera of normal human subjects. Int Arch Allergy Immunol 105:122
40. Wu Z, Drayton D, Pisetsky DS (1997) Specificity and immunochemical properties of antibodies to bacterial DNA in sera of normal human subjects and patients with systemic lupus erythematosis (SLE). Clin Exp Immunol 109:27
41. Fredriksen K, Skogsholm T, Flaegstad T, Traavik T, Rekvig OP (1993) Antibodies to ds DNA are produced during primary BK virus infection in man, indicating that anti-dsDNA antibodies may be related to virus replication in vivo. Scand J Immunol 38:401
42. Klinman DM, Yamshchikov G, Ishigatsubo Y (1996a) Contribution of CpG motifs to the immunogenicity of DNA vaccines. J Immunol 158:3635
43. Krieg AM (1996) An innate immune defense mechanism based on the recognition of CpG motifs in microbial DNA. J Lab Clin Med 128:128

44. Pisetsky DS (1996) Immune activation by bacterial DNA: a new genetic code. Immunity 5:303
45. Chen C, Zhou Y, Yao Z, Zhang Y, Feng Z (1996) Stimulation of human lymphocyte proliferation and CD40 Ag expression by phosphorothioate oligodeoxynucleotides complementary to hepatitis B virus genome. J Viral Hepat 3:167
46. Branda RF, Moore AL, Mathews L, McCormack JJ, Zon G (1993) Stimulation of peripheral blood mononuclear cells (PBMCs) from chronic lymphatic leukemia (CLL) patients by an antisense phosphorothioate oligomer to the rev gene of HIV. Proc Am Assoc Cancer Res 34:455
47. Branda RF, Moore AL, Hong R, McCormack JJ, Zon G, Cunningham-Rundles C (1996) Cell proliferation and differentiation in common variable immunodeficiency patients produced by an antisense oligomer to the rev gene of HIV-1. Clin Immunol Immunopathoogy 79:115
48. Liang H, Nishioka Y, Reich CF, Pisetsky DS, Lipsky PE (1996) Activation of human B cells by phosphorothioate oligodeoxynucleotides. J Clin Invest 98:1119
49. Yi A, Chace JH, Cowdery JH, Krieg AM (1996) IFN-γ promotes IL-6 and IgM secretion in response to CpG motifs in bacterial DNA and oligodeoxynucleotides. J Immunol 156:558
50. Yi A, Klinman DM, Martin TL, Matson S, Krieg AM (1996) Rapid immune activation by CpG motifs in bacterial DNA: systemic induction of IL-6 transcription through an antioxidant-sensitive pathway. J Immunol 157:5494

Multiple effects of immunostimulatory DNA on T cells and the role of type I interferons

Siquan Sun[1], Xiaohong Zhang[2], David Tough[3], Jonathan Sprent[2]

[1] R.W. Johnson Pharmaceutical Research Institute, 3210 Merryfield Row, La Jolla, CA 92121, USA
[2] Department of Immunology, IMM4, The Scripps Research Institute, 10550 North Torrey Pines Road, La Jolla, CA 92037, USA
[3] The Edward Jenner Institute for Vaccine Research, Compton, Newbury, Berkshire RG20 7NN, UK

Introduction

It is now well established that DNA from non-vertebrates contains immunostimulatory sequences (ISS) which are able to stimulate a variety of lymphohemopoietic cells, notably antigen-presenting cells (APCs) and B cells [1, 6, 7, 9, 11–14, 17, 23–25]. This property of DNA applies to bacteria, yeast, insects and molluscs and is under the control of unmethylated CpG motifs in conjunction with appropriate flanking sequences. A similar capacity to stimulate APCs and B cells applies to synthetic oligodeoxynucleotides (ODNs) containing unmethylated CpG motifs [1, 7, 11, 16, 17]. In this article we summarize our recent evidence on the capacity of CpG DNA and ODNs to influence various facets of T cell function in vivo. To begin, we discuss the capacity of CpG DNA and other products of microorganisms to cause bystander proliferation of T cells.

Bystander stimulation of memory $CD8^+$ cells and the role of IFN-I

Stemming from initial studies on bromodeoxyuridine (BrdU) incorporation by T cells during viral infections [18], evidence has been obtained that proliferation of memory-phenotype $CD8^+$ cells in vivo is driven in part by a T cell receptor (TCR) -independent bystander reaction [18]. This reaction can be elicited by injecting mice with lipopolysaccharide (LPS) [19], polyI:C [18], CpG DNA (insect DNA) or CpG ODNs (S. Sun and J. Sprent, unpublished data). A single injection of these agents in saline causes a transient burst of proliferation at the level of memory-phenotype ($CD44^{hi}$) $CD8^+$ cells; proliferation of $CD44^{hi}$ $CD4^+$ cells and naive-phenotype ($CD44^{lo/int}$) $CD8^+$ and $CD4^+$ cells is largely unaffected.

In the case of polyI:C injection, bystander proliferation of $CD44^{hi}$ $CD8^+$ cells does not appear to require TCR ligation. The evidence here came from adoptive transfer studies with β2 microglobulin ($\beta2m^{-/-}$) hosts [18]. Thus, when $\beta2m^{-/-}$ $CD8^+$ cells (raised from stem cells in $\beta2m^+$ chimeras) were transferred to $\beta2m^{-/-}$ hosts, pro-

Correspondence to: J. Sprent

liferation of CD44^{hi} CD8$^+$ cells after polyI:C injection was the same as in β2m$^+$ hosts. Since expression of MHC class I molecules (the ligands for CD8$^+$ cells) is very low in β2m$^{-/-}$ mice, it is unlikely that the CD8$^+$ T cell response elicited by polyI:C involves TCR/MHC class I interaction (although TCR/MHC class II interaction has yet to be excluded).

For polyI:C, LPS and CpG DNA/ODNs, in vivo proliferation of CD44^{hi} CD8$^+$ cells is apparent in IFN-γ$^{-/-}$ mice but is greatly reduced in mice lacking receptors for type I interferons (IFN-I) ([18, 19] and unpublished data). For these compounds, T cell proliferation thus appears to be largely under the control of IFN-I (IFN-α/β). Indeed, similar proliferation of CD44^{hi} CD8$^+$ cells can be elicited by injecting mice with purified IFN-I [18]. However, bystander T cell proliferation is not under the sole control of IFN-I. Thus, selective proliferation of CD44^{hi} CD8$^+$ cells is also seen after injection of several other cytokines, including IFN-γ, IL-12 and IL-18 (D. Tough and J. Sprent). Here, proliferation is unimpaired in IFN-IR$^{-/-}$ mice but greatly reduced in IFN-γ$^{-/-}$ mice, implying that proliferation is controlled by IFN-γ rather than IFN-I.

Mechanism of bystander proliferation and the role of IL-15

For all of the above agents and cytokines, proliferation of CD44^{hi} CD8$^+$ cells occurs only under in vivo conditions and does not apply to purified T cells cultured in vitro ([26] and unpublished data of the authors). Hence, under in vivo conditions these compounds appear to act on T cells by an indirect mechanism. The simplest idea is that the above agents and cytokines act on other cells and cause these cells to synthesize effector cytokines which are then directly stimulatory for T cells.

In considering this scenario, we reasoned that, to explain the selective proliferation of CD44^{hi} CD8$^+$ cells, the receptors for the putative effector cytokine would have to be expressed selectively on this subset of T cells. In fact, screening T cell subsets for cytokine receptors showed that expression of one receptor, IL-2Rβ (CD122), was much higher on CD44^{hi} CD8$^+$ cells than on CD44^{hi} CD4$^+$ cells (or CD44$^{lo/int}$ CD8$^+$ and CD4$^+$ cells); this skewed expression did not apply to IL-2Rα or IL-2Rγ [26].

Since only two known cytokines, IL-2 and IL-15, bind to IL-2Rβ, these cytokines emerged as likely candidates for controlling bystander T cell proliferation in vivo. *A priori*, IL-15 seemed more promising than IL-2 because, unlike IL-2, IL-15 is synthesized by a wide variety of cell types, including macrophages and other APCs [26]. Indeed, for polyI:C, LPS, CpG DNA/ODNs, IFN-I and IFN-γ, all of these agents induced strong production of IL-15 mRNA by peritoneal macrophages in vitro ([26] and unpublished data). The key finding, however, was that unlike these agents, IL-15 (human recombinant IL-15) caused selective proliferation of CD44^{hi} CD8$^+$ cells when added to purified T cells in vitro [26]; in contrast, IL-2 acted on both CD44^{hi} CD8$^+$ cells and CD44^{hi} CD4$^+$ cells. The capacity of IL-15 to cause selective proliferation of CD44^{hi} CD8$^+$ cells also applied when IL-15 was injected in vivo [26].

Proof that IL-15 is the main effector cytokine driving bystander T cell proliferation in vivo will have to await studies on IL-15$^{-/-}$ mice. Although we have yet to examine these mice, in the interim we have established that, at least for polyI:C, bystander proliferation is minimal in IL-2Rβ$^{-/-}$ mice, indicating a crucial role for IL-2Rβ (X. Zhang and J. Sprent, unpublished data).

Partial activation of naïve T cells

As mentioned above, the capacity of CpG DNA/ODNs, LPS etc. to cause bystander T cell proliferation in vivo is highly selective for CD44^{hi} CD8^{+} cells. For these cells, T cell proliferation is not apparent before day 2 post injection and lasts for only 1–2 days. To our surprise, however, studies with both LPS and CpG DNA/ODNs showed that injection of these compounds in vivo caused strong up-regulation of CD69 on naive (CD44$^{lo/int}$) T cells, including both CD4^{+} and CD8^{+} cells, as well as on B cells and APCs; the capacity of CpG DNA (insect DNA) to induce CD69 up-regulation on T cells is illustrated in Fig. 1. Significantly, as for bystander proliferation of CD44^{hi} CD8^{+} cells, up-regulation of CD69 on naive CD8^{+} and CD4^{+} cells after injection of the above agents was almost undetectable in IFN-IR$^{-/-}$ mice [16]. Moreover, both after in vivo injection and when added to lymphoid cells in vitro, IFN-I caused strong up-regulation of CD69 on naive (and memory) T cells as well as on B cells and APCs; data on purified naive CD8^{+} cells are shown in Fig. 2. This effect of IFN-I did not require the presence of APCs. By contrast, the capacity of CpG DNA/ODNs to cause CD69 up-regulation on T cells was heavily dependent on the presence of APCs. Here, it was notable that when CpG DNA/ODNs were added to purified normal versus IFN-IR$^{-/-}$ T cells, the capacity of normal APCs to promote CD69 up-regulation on T cells applied only to normal and not IFN-IR$^{-/-}$ T cells [16].

Based on these findings, the capacity of CpG DNA/ODNs to cause CD69 up-regulation on naive T cells does not seem to involve a direct effect on T cells but is mediated through production of IFN-I by other cells, e.g., APCs. As mentioned earlier, IFN-I-induced up-regulation of CD69 on naive T cells is not followed by cell division, indicating that IFN-I induces partial rather than full activation of the cells. It should be noted that CD69 up-regulation elicited directly by IFN-I (and indirectly by CpG DNA/ODNs) is accompanied by other signs of partial activation of T cells, e.g., up-regulation of B7-2, Ly-6C and MHC class I [16]; IL-2Rα (CD25) is not up-regulated, implying that the form of partial T cell activation induced by IFN-I does not involve triggering via the TCR.

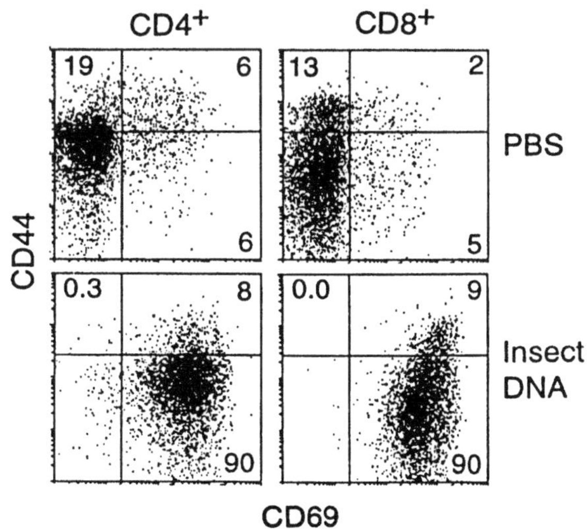

Fig. 1. CD69 up-regulation on T cells in response to *D. melanogaster* DNA in vivo. B6 mice were injected with *D. melanogaster* DNA (100 µg/mouse); 18 h later, draining lymph node cells were triple-stained for CD4 or CD8 and also for CD44 and CD69 expression. Adapted from Sun et al. [16]

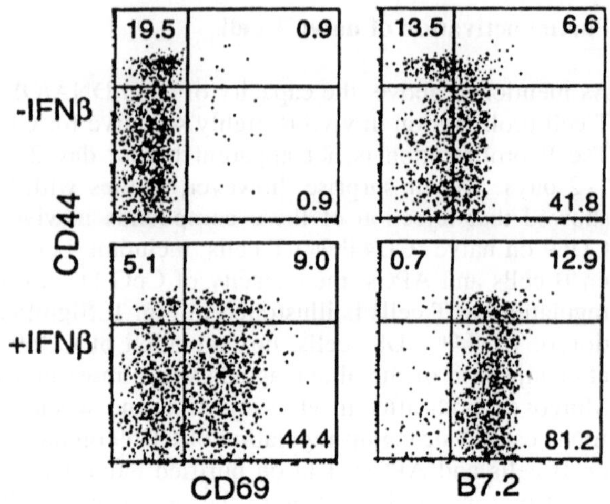

Fig. 2. Upregulation of CD69 and B7-2 on purified CD8+ cells in response to IFN-β in vitro. Purified CD8+ cells (2×10^6 cells/well) were cultured with or without IFN-β (10,000 units/ml) overnight; cells were then triple-stained for CD8, CD44, and CD69 or B7-2. The data shown are for gated CD8+ cells

Adjuvant function of CpG DNA/ODNs

It is well established that immune responses to purified proteins and peptides are generally poor unless accompanied by some form of adjuvant [20]. How adjuvants augment immune responses is still unclear, but a clue is provided by the finding that immune responses to certain antigens, e.g., aggregated human γ-globulin (dHGG) and heterologous erythrocytes, do not require adjuvants [21]. By binding to cells via Fc receptors (dHGG) or by being sufficiently large to induce phagocytosis (erythrocytes), these antigens cause direct activation of APCs, thereby making the MHC/peptide complexes on APCs more immunogenic for T cells; this improvement of immunogenicity correlates with up-regulation of co-stimulatory molecules. Hence the simplest explanation for the role of adjuvants is that these compounds, e.g., complete Freund's adjuvant (CFA), operate by activating APCs, thereby causing increased expression of co-stimulatory molecules such as B7 (B7-1, B7-2) and perhaps also by inducing synthesis of stimulatory cytokines, e.g., IL-1 and IL-6.

Since CFA contains mycobacteria, i.e. a source of many different compounds with the capacity to stimulate APCs, the question arises as to which of these compounds account for the marked adjuvanticity of CFA. With its capacity to cause direct activation of APCs, the CpG DNA of mycobacteria is an obvious possibility. To assess this idea we have examined the capacity of CpG DNA (insect DNA) and CpG ODNs to act as an adjuvant for the responses of CD4+ T cells to fowl (chicken) γ-globulin (FγG).

These studies, as well as studies by others [3, 4, 8, 10, 22], showed that CpG DNA and ODNs do indeed act as a powerful adjuvant, both for T proliferative responses and production of T-dependent antibody [15]. Thus, coinjecting mice with FγG plus either insect DNA or CpG ODNs (but not non-CpG ODNs) gave far stronger production of IgG anti-FγG antibodies than injection of FγG in saline; similar findings applied for priming CD4+ cells for secondary proliferative responses to FγG in vivo. For antibody production, the adjuvant effect of CpG DNA and ODNs was largely restricted to the production of IgG2a and IgG2b, i.e., to Th1 antibodies.

In the case of insect DNA, adjuvant function required that the DNA be suspended in incomplete Freund's adjuvant (IFA, mineral oil), presumably because soluble DNA is subject to rapid enzymatic degradation in vivo. For ODNs, suspension in mineral oil was unnecessary because the ODNs contained a phosphorothioate "backbone", thus retarding enzymatic degradation.

It is of interest that, at least for T proliferative responses, the adjuvant function of insect DNA and CpG ODNs in IFA was stronger than CFA [15]. Hence, the adjuvanticity of CFA could be largely a reflection of the presence of CpG DNA in the mycobacterial component of CFA. Whether other components in CFA contribute to adjuvant function is unknown, and difficult to assess.

Precise information on how CpG DNA/ODNs exert adjuvant function is still unclear. Our initial idea was that these compounds function by inducing the production of IFN-I. However, although IFN-I does indeed act as an adjuvant (see below), preliminary work has shown that insect DNA can provide adjuvant function in IFN-IR$^{-/-}$ mice. The alternative possibility is that CpG DNA/ODNs operate by causing direct activation of APCs. Conclusive evidence on this question, however, is still lacking.

Adjuvant function of IFN-1

Initial evidence on the role of IFN-1 as an adjuvant stemmed from studies with polyI:C, a powerful inducer of IFN-I production in vivo. Using a TCR transgenic model, the proliferative response of $CD8^+$ cells to peptide antigens in vivo was found to be considerably enhanced when mice were coinjected with polyI:C [18]. In addition, the progeny of the proliferating $CD8^+$ cells survived for prolonged periods, suggesting that IFN-I induced by polyI:C may serve not only to augment the primary T proliferative response but cause the responding T cells to differentiate into long-lived memory cells.

Although cytokine production after polyI:C injection is not restricted to IFN-I, more recent studies have shown that the adjuvant properties of polyI:C can be mimicked by injection of purified IFN-I (unpublished data of the authors). Whether other cytokines such as IFN-γ and IL-12 also share this property is currently under investigation.

In vitro effects of IFN-I on T cell function

Elucidating how IFN-I and other cytokines exert an adjuvant effect under in vivo conditions is clearly difficult. For this reason we have been examining the capacity of IFN-I to affect T cell function under defined conditions in vitro. As discussed below the unexpected finding is that, depending upon the conditions used, IFN-I can either inhibit or enhance T cell function.

In clinical situations, IFN-I is commonly used as an anti-proliferative agent to treat certain forms of cancer. Hence, the observation that IFN-I can inhibit proliferative responses of murine T cells is not surprising. In this respect we have found that proliferative responses of purified T cells to a combination of cross-linked anti-TCR and anti-CD28 mAbs in culture is considerably reduced by addition of IFN-I (unpublished data of the authors); this property is not shared by IFN-γ. Interestingly, the inhibitory effect of IFN-I on T cell responses in vitro applies selectively to proliferation. Thus, there is no reduction in the production of cytokines. It would seem likely, therefore, that IFN-I operates at the level of cell cycle control, perhaps by promoting synthesis of cell cycle inhibitors [5].

Although the inhibitory function of IFN-I on TCR/CD28-induced T proliferative responses is conspicuous, discordant results can occur when T cells are supplemented with APCs (unpublished data of the authors). Here, the precise type of APC used is crucial. For responses of TCR transgenic CD8+ T cells to peptide antigens, we routinely use transfected Drosophila cells as APCs, i.e., Drosophila cells transfected with MHC class I, B7 and ICAM-I molecules [2, 14]. With these APCs (which are almost as potent as dendritic cells), addition of IFN-I is strongly inhibitory for T proliferative responses, i.e., as for T cell responses elicited by TCR/CD28 ligation in the absence of APCs. When viable splenic APCs are substituted for Drosophila APCs, however, addition of IFN-I can have the opposite effect and lead to an augmented T proliferative response. This adjuvant effect of IFN-I is not seen until day 3 of culture (day 2 responses are inhibited) and can be countered by increasing the concentration of IFN-I to a high level; the adjuvant effect of IFN-I does not apply to IFN-γ.

The capacity of IFN-I to augment T proliferative responses driven by viable APCs in vitro correlates with the adjuvant activity of IFN-I for T cell responses in vivo (see above). In both situations IFN-I presumably acts by enhancing APC function. The mechanisms involved, however, have yet to be resolved. As discussed earlier, the simplest idea is that IFN-I functions by increasing the expression of co-stimulatory molecules on APCs and/or by causing these cells to synthesize stimulatory cytokines. Alternatively, IFN-I could act by simply augmenting APC survival. These and other possibilities are currently under investigation.

Summary and conclusions

In addition to stimulating antigen-specific immune responses, infectious agents cause nonspecific activation of the innate immune system, notably up-regulation of co-stimulatory/adhesion molecules on APCs and cytokine production. In recent years it has become apparent that stimulation of the immune system by microorganisms is a property of a number of different cellular components, including DNA. As discussed earlier and elsewhere in this volume, the DNA of infectious agents – and indeed of all non-vertebrates tested – differs from mammalian DNA in being enriched for unmethylated CpG motifs. With appropriate flanking sequences, CpG DNA and synthetic CpG ODNs cause strong activation of APCs and other cells.

In this article we have focussed on the capacity of CpG DNA/ODNs to alter T cell function. Whether these compounds act directly on T cells or function indirectly by activating other cells, especially APCs, is controversial [7, 8, 13, 14]. In contrast to other workers [8], we have yet to find definitive evidence that CpG DNA/ODNs can provide a co-stimulatory signal for purified T cells subjected to TCR ligation ([14] and unpublished data of authors). For this reason we lean to the notion that CpG DNA/ODNs modulate T cell function by inducing activation of APC rather than by acting directly on T cells.

When injected in vivo in the absence of specific antigen, CpG DNA/ODNs have two striking effects on T cells, namely (1) induction of overt activation (proliferation) of memory-phenotype CD8+ cells, and (2) partial activation of all T cells, including naïve-phenotype T cells. Both actions of CpG DNA/ODNs are heavily dependent on the production of IFN-I by APC.

For memory-phenotype ($CD44^{hi}$) $CD8^+$ cells, neither CpG DNA nor IFN-I can cause proliferation of purified APC-depleted T cells in vitro. Hence, under in vivo conditions, CpG DNA-induced proliferation of $CD44^{hi}$ $CD8^+$ cells is probably mediated through the production of a secondary cytokine, i.e., by a cytokine that is directly stimulatory for $CD44^{hi}$ $CD8^+$ cells. Based on the available evidence, it is highly likely that the effector cytokine is IL-15. With this assumption, our current model is that proliferation of $CD44^{hi}$ $CD8^+$ cells induced by injection of CpG DNA/ODNs reflects production of IFN-I which, in turn, leads to synthesis of IL-15. Which particular cell types produce these two cytokines is unclear, although APCs are probably of prime importance.

In addition to inducing proliferation of memory-phenotype $CD8^+$ cells via IL-15, the IFN-I induced by CpG DNA/ODNs can also induce partial activation of naive T cells. This form of activation leads to up-regulation of CD69 and other molecules but does not cause entry into cell cycle.

It is of interest that the partial activation of naive T cells induced by IFN-I is associated with decreased T proliferative responses. Thus, proliferation of purified naïve T cells elicited by combined TCR/CD28 ligation in vitro is greatly reduced by addition of IFN-I. This inhibitory effect of IFN-I does not influence cytokine production and probably reflects production of cell cycle inhibitors.

Surprisingly, except at high doses, IFN-I fails to exert an anti-proliferative effect when T proliferative responses are driven by viable APCs. Indeed, in this situation, IFN-I enhances antigen-specific T proliferative responses, both in vivo and in vitro. This adjuvant effect of IFN-I is presumably a reflection of APC activation, but direct evidence on this issue is still lacking.

In this article we have emphasized that contact with CpG DNA/ODNs has multiple effects on T cell function in vivo. Many of these effects seem to be related to the production of certain cytokines by APCs, notably IFN-I and IL-15. It should be stressed, however, that CpG DNA/ODNs probably lead to the production of many other cytokines. Hence, our current models of how CpG DNA/ODNs influence T cell function are undoubtedly oversimplified.

Acknowledgements We thank Ms. Barbara Marchand for typing the manuscript. This work was supported by grants CA38355, CA25803, AI32068 and AG01743 from the United States Public Health Service. Publication no. 12626-IMM from the Scripps Research Institute.

References

1. Ballas ZK, Rasmussen WL, Krieg AM (1996) Induction of NK activity in murine and human cells by CpG motifs in oligodeoxynucleotides and bacterial DNA. J Immunol 157:1840
2. Cai Z, Brunmark A, Jackson MR, Loh D, Peterson PA, Sprent J (1996) Transfected Drosophila cells as a probe for defining the minimal requirements for stimulating unprimed $CD8^+$ T cells. Proc Natl Acad Sci USA 93:14736
3. Chu RS, Targoni OS, Krieg AM, Lehman PV, Harding CV (1997) CpG oligodeoxynucleotides act as adjuvants that switch on T helper 1 (Th1) immunity. J Exp Med 186:1623
4. Davis HL, Weeranta R, Walsschmidt TJ, Tygrett L, Schorr J, Krieg AM (1998) CpG DNA is a potent enhancer of specific immunity in mice immunized with recombinant hepatitis B surface antigen. J Immunol 160:870
5. Grander D, Sangfelt O, Erickson S (1997) How does interferon exert its cell growth inhibitory effect? Eur J Haematol 59:129

6. Hacker H, Mischak H, Miethke T, Liptay S, Schmid R, Sparwasser T, Heeg K, Lipford GB, Wagner H (1998) CpG-DNA-specific activation of antigen-presenting cells requires stress kinase activity and is preceded by non-specific endocytosis and endosomal maturation. EMBO J 17:6230
7. Krieg AM, Yi AK, Matson S, Waldschmidt TJ, Bishop GA, Teasdale R, Koretzky GA, Klinman DM (1995) CpG motifs in bacterial DNA trigger direct B-cell activation. Nature 374:546
8. Lipford GB, Bauer M, Blank C, Reiter R, Wagner H, Heeg K (1997) CpG-containing synthetic oligonucleotides promote B and cytotoxic T cell responses to protein antigen: a new class of vaccine adjuvants. Eur J Immunol 27:2340
9. Messina JP, Gilkeson GS, Pisetsky DS (1991) Stimulation of in vitro murine lymphocyte proliferation by bacterial DNA. J Immunol 147:1759
10. Roman M, Martin-Orozco E, Goodman JS, Nguyen M-D, Sato Y, Ronaghy A, Kornbluth RS, Richman DD, Carson DA, Raz E (1997) Immunostimulatory DNA sequences function as T helper-1-promoting adjuvants. Nat Med 3:849
11. Sparwasser T, Koch ES, Vabulas RM, Heeg K, Lipford GB, Ellwart JW, Wagner H (1998) Bacterial DNA and immunostimulatory CpG oligonucleotides trigger maturation and activation of murine dendritic cells. Eur J Immunol 28:2045
12. Stacey KJ, Sweet MJ, Hume DA (1996) Macrophages ingest and are activated by bacterial DNA. J Immunol 157:2116
13. Sun S, Beard C, Jaenisch R, Jones P, Sprent J (1997) Mitogenicity of DNA from different organisms for murine B cells. J Immunol 159:3119
14. Sun S, Cai Z, Langlade-Demoyen P, Kosaka H, Brunmark A, Jackson MR, Peterson PA, Sprent J (1996) Dual function of Drosophila cells as APC for naive CD8+ T cells: implications for tumor immunotherapy. Immunity 4:555
15. Sun S, Kishimoto H, Sprent J (1998) DNA as an adjuvant: capacity of insect DNA and synthetic oligodeoxynucleotides to augment T cell responses to specific antigen. J Exp Med 187:1145
16. Sun S, Zhang X, Tough DF, Sprent J (1998) Type I interferon-mediated stimulation of T cells by CpG DNA. J Exp Med 188:2335
17. Tokunaga T, Yano O, Kuramoto E, Kimura Y, Yamamoto T, Kataoka T, Yamamoto S (1992) Synthetic oligonucleotides with particular base sequences from the cDNA encoding proteins of *Mycobacterium bovis* BCG induce interferons and activate natural killer cells. Microbiol Immunol 36:55
18. Tough DF, Borrow P, Sprent J (1996) Induction of bystander T cell proliferation by viruses and type I interferon in vivo. Science 272:1947
19. Tough DF, Sun S, Sprent J (1997) T cell stimulation in vivo by lipopolysaccharide (LPS). J Exp Med 185:2089
20. Warren HS, Vogel FR, Chedid LA (1986) Current status of immunological adjuvants. Annu Rev Immunol 4:369
21. Weigle WO (1973) Immunological unresponsiveness. Adv Immunol 16:61
22. Weiner GJ, Liu HM, Wooldridge JE, Dahle CE, Krieg AM (1997) Immunostimulatory oligodeoxynucleotides containing the CpG motif are effective as immune adjuvants in tumor antigen immunization. Proc Natl Acad Sci USA 94:10833
23. Yamamoto S, Yamamoto T, Shimada S, Kuramoto E, Yano O, Kataoka T, Tokunaga T (1992) DNA from bacteria, but not from vertebrates, induces interferons, activates natural killer cells and inhibits tumor growth. Microbiol Immunol 36:983
24. Yi AK, Krieg AM (1998) CpG DNA rescue from anti-IgM-induced WEHI-231 B lymphoma apoptosis via modulation of IKBa and IKBb and sustained activation of nuclear factor-K B/c-Rel. J Immunol 160:1240
25. Yi AK, Tuetken R, Redford T, Waldschmidt M, Kirsch J, Krieg AM (1998) CpG motifs in bacterial DNA activate leukocytes through the pH-dependent generation of reactive oxygen species. J Immunol 160:4755
26. Zhang X, Sun S, Hwang I, Tough DF, Sprent J (1998) Potent and selective stimulation of memory-phenotype CD8+ T cells in vivo by IL-15. Immunity 8:591

Pre-priming: a novel approach to DNA-based vaccination and immunomodulation

Hiroko Kobayashi[1], Anthony A. Horner[2], Elena Martin-Orozco[2], Eyal Raz[2]

[1] Department of Medicine II, Fukushima Medical University, School of Medicine, Hikarigaoka, Fukushima, 960-1295, Japan
[2] The Sam and Rose Stein Institute for Research on Aging, Department of Medicine, University of California, San Diego, 9500 Gilman Drive, La Jolla CA 92093-06631, USA

Introduction

The increasing prevalence of allergic diseases, a rise in microbial resistance, and new and emerging pathogens represent major health threats as we enter the new millennium. Traditional protein-based immunotherapy and anti-allergy medications have proven effective in the treatment of the majority of allergic patients. Vaccination has proven to be a potent modality for the prevention of many infectious diseases and a number of effective antimicrobial therapies exist for the treatment of others. However, there are serious deficiencies in our ability to prevent and treat allergic and infectious diseases and new and better therapeutic modalities continue to be needed. Recently, gene vaccination has gained attention as a potential approach for the development of vaccines that prevent and treat both allergic and infectious diseases [7, 14, 25, 29, 32, 38]. It has been shown that gene vaccination induces long-lasting and potent Th1-biased immune responses, which include cytotoxic T lymphocyte (CTL) activity [7, 25, 29, 38]. In contrast, immunization with the same antigen as a protein induces a Th2-biased immune response without CTL activity [29, 31, 38]. The immune response elicited with gene vaccines is well suited for the induction of protection against allergic pathology and the prevention of infection. Furthermore, plasmid immunization has proven effective in the prevention of allergic responses and infection in animal models [7, 14, 25, 32]. However, there is limited evidence that gene vaccination can reverse allergic hypersensitivity and no evidence that gene vaccination can modify the course of an ongoing infection [29].

While testing the efficacy of various plasmid vectors, we and others have shown that cryptic CpG motifs or immunostimulatory DNA sequences, within the plasmid backbone are likely to play an important role in mediating the immune response induced by gene vaccines [17, 31, 33]. Therefore, it has been proposed that vaccination plasmids contain two functional domains: (1) a transcription domain which is responsible for antigen expression, and (2) an adjuvant domain which contains immunostimulatory DNA sequences [38]. A number of investigators have shown that the Th1-biased immune response elicited by gene vaccination can in fact be mimicked by im-

Correspondence to: H. Kobayashi

munization with native protein and immunostimulatory sequence oligodeoxynucleotide (ISS-ODN) [6, 13, 19, 31, 33]. Furthermore, co-immunization with ISS-ODN and protein antigens has proven effective in the induction of protective immune responses in animal models of allergic and infectious disease [16, 28]. In addition, when delivered independently of antigen, ISS-ODN has been shown to modify ongoing immune responses, and has proven effective in preventing allergic pathology and attenuating infection [3, 9, 37]. The data presented in this review provides insight into the adjuvant and immunomodulatory capacity of ISS-ODN, and offers a novel paradigm for understanding its ability to both prevent and treat allergic and infectious diseases.

ISS-ODN activates the innate immune system for an extended period of time

Early reports on the immunological activity of ISS-ODN focused on its ability to induce NK cell activation, B cell proliferation, and the production of type-1 cytokines such as IL-12, type 1 IFNs, and IFN-γ from antigen-presenting cells (APCs), B cells, and NK cells in an antigen-independent manner [1, 11, 18, 20, 22, 40, 41]. In addition to these effects, ISS-ODN has more recently been shown to increase the expression of various co-stimulatory molecules on APCs and B cells (Fig. 1A, B) [15, 23, 35]. Up-regulation of MHC class I and II expression serves to enhance antigen presentation to T cells [23]. Increased expression of B7 improves the efficacy of T cell priming by APCs and promotes productive immunological cross talk between T and B cells [21, 23]. CD40 engagement by CD40 ligand (CD40L) leads to IL-12 production by APCs, which in turn provides an important signal for Th1 differentiation [2, 23, 26, 27, 30]. In addition, CD40-CD40L interactions play an important role in B cell isotype switching, and promote B cell proliferation [2, 23]. Increased ICAM-1 expression leads to stabilization of cell-cell interactions via binding to its ligand LFA-1 [8, 23]. Interestingly, while ISS-ODN induced an innate cytokine response and increased co-stimulatory molecule expression by APCs and B cells, ISS-ODN did not appear to activate T cells directly [19, 23].

Our own experience is that when splenocytes are incubated with ISS-ODN, cytokine levels in supernatants and cell surface expression of co-stimulatory molecules are maximal after 72 and 48 h, respectively [23]. These results suggested that ISS-ODN might have a prolonged effect on the innate immune system. To better understand the time course of ISS-ODN activation of the innate immune system, we conducted *in vivo* experiments. Our results demonstrate that ISS-ODN induced increased cytokine production in injected mice for about 2 weeks (Table 1) [19]. Increased expression of co-stimulatory molecules on the surface of immunocytes of ISS-ODN-injected mice lasted for about the same period (Fig. 2) [23].

Fig. 1A, B. ISS-ODN effect on BMDM and B cell expression of co-stimulatory molecules in vitro. Purified BMDM (2×10^5/ml; **A**) or splenic B cells (2×10^6/ml; **B**) were incubated with ISS-ODN: 5'-TGACTGTG*AACGTTCG*AGATGA-3' (1 μg/ml), M-ODN: 5'-TGACTGTG*AACCTTAG*AGATGA-3' (1 μg/ml), LPS (5 μg/ml), or were left unstimulated. After 48 h cells were stained and subjected to flow cytometry. On the *x-axis* a log scale of fluorescence intensity for each surface molecule is presented, and the *y-axis* represents the number of Mac3+ (BMDM) or B220+ (B cells) cells found at that fluorescence intensity. For each histogram, the surface molecule-specific antibody (*black line*) is compared to the appropriate isotype control (*gray line*). The *number in the right upper corner* of each graph is the mean fluorescence intensity ratio given as: (surface molecule-specific mean fluorescence intensity)/(isotype control mean fluorescence intensity) [23] (*BMDM* bone marrow-derived macrophages, *ISS-ODN* immunostimulatory sequence oligodeoxynucleotide, *M-ODN* mutated ODN)

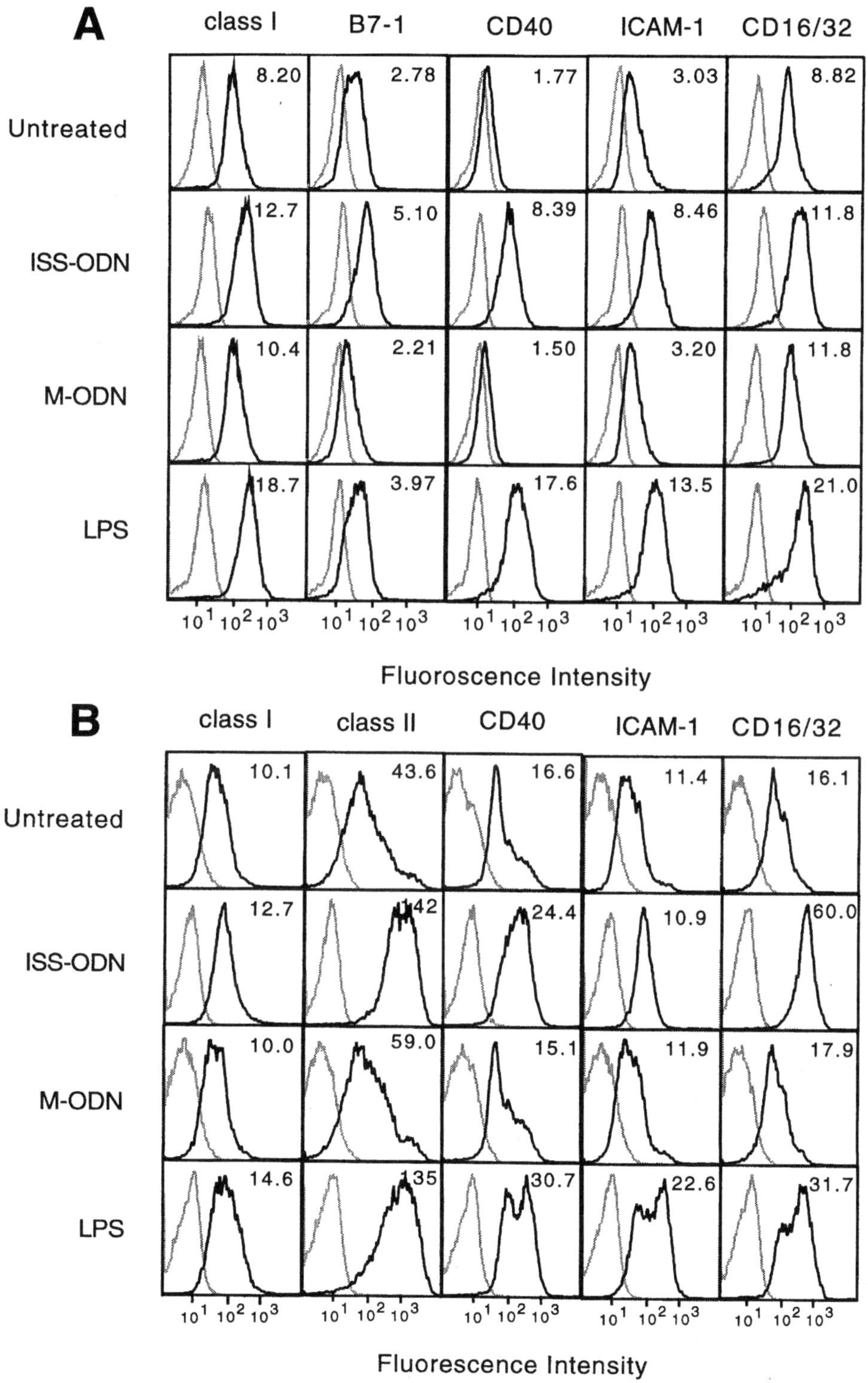
A
class I
B7-1
CD40
ICAM-1
CD16/32
Untreated
ISS-ODN
M-ODN
LPS
8.20
2.78
1.77
3.03
8.82
12.7
5.10
8.39
8.46
11.8
10.4
2.21
1.50
3.20
11.8
18.7
3.97
17.6
13.5
21.0
Fluoroscence Intensity
B
class I
class II
CD40
ICAM-1
CD16/32
Untreated
ISS-ODN
M-ODN
LPS
10.1
43.6
16.6
11.4
16.1
12.7
142
24.4
10.9
60.0
10.0
59.0
15.1
11.9
17.9
14.6
135
30.7
22.6
31.7
Fluorescence Intensity

Table 1. In vivo cytokine production induced by ISS-ODN

ISS-ODN	IL-12 (pg/ml)	IFN-γ (pg/ml)
	<42	<14
Day (1)	4028±1878	343±83
Day (3)	2356±464	312±101
Day (7)	2034±288	174±36
Day (14)	763±255	35±71
LPS Day 7	<42	<14

At serial time points after mice were injected i.d. with ISS-ODN (50 μg) or LPS (10 μg), serum was obtained and cytokine levels were analysed by ELISA. Results represent the mean ± SE for 3 mice in each time point. Injection of M-ODN did not result in any detectable IL-12 or IFN-γ production [19]

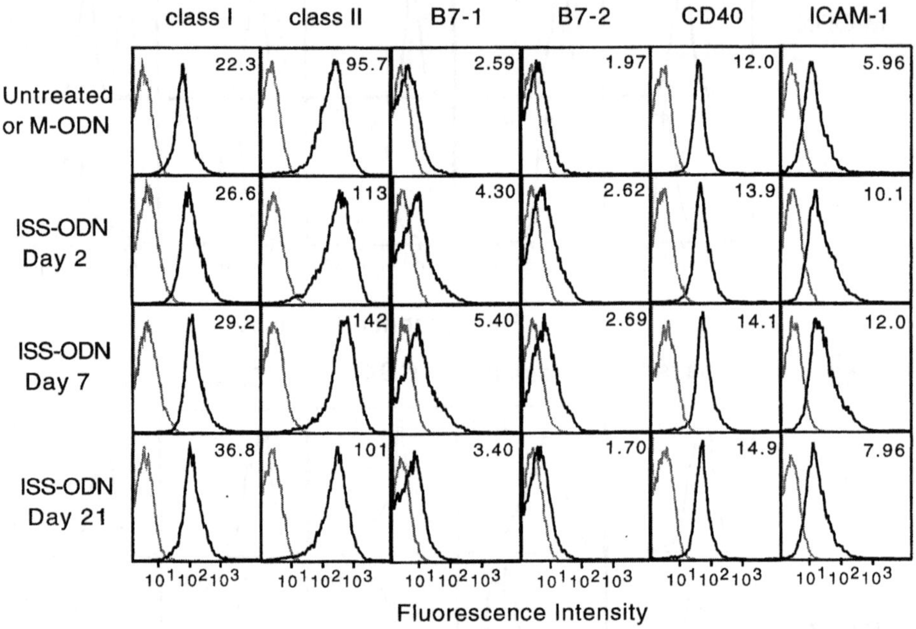

Fig. 2. ISS-ODN effect on in vivo B cell co-stimulatory molecules expression. Mice were injected i.p. with ISS-ODN: 5'-TGACTGTG*AACGTTCG*AGATGA-3' (100 μg), M-ODN: 5'-TGACTGTG*AACCTTAG*AGATGA-3' (100 μg) or saline. Mice were killed on day 2, 7, or 21 after injection, splenocytes were harvested and stained for flow cytometry. On the *x-axis* a log scale of fluorescence intensity for each surface molecule is presented, and the *y-axis* represents the number of B220+ cells found at that fluorescence intensity. For each histogram, the surface molecule specific antibody (*black line*) is compared to the appropriate isotype control (*gray line*). The mean fluorescence intensity ratio is shown in the right upper corner

Fig. 3A, B. ISS-ODN effect on APC function. APCs and TCR-OVA TG T cells were harvested from (DO11.10) mice. APCs were harvested on day 14 after i.d. injections of ISS-ODN (50 μg), M-ODN (50 μg), or saline on days 0 and 7. T cells were obtained from naive TCR-OVA TG littermates. APCs and TCR-OVA TG T cells were cultured in supplemented RPMI at a final concentration of 5×10^6 cells/ml (1:1 ratio) with various concentrations of OVA for 4 days. Results represent mean values ± SD for four mice per group and are representative of three similar and independent experiments [23]. **A** T cell proliferation.

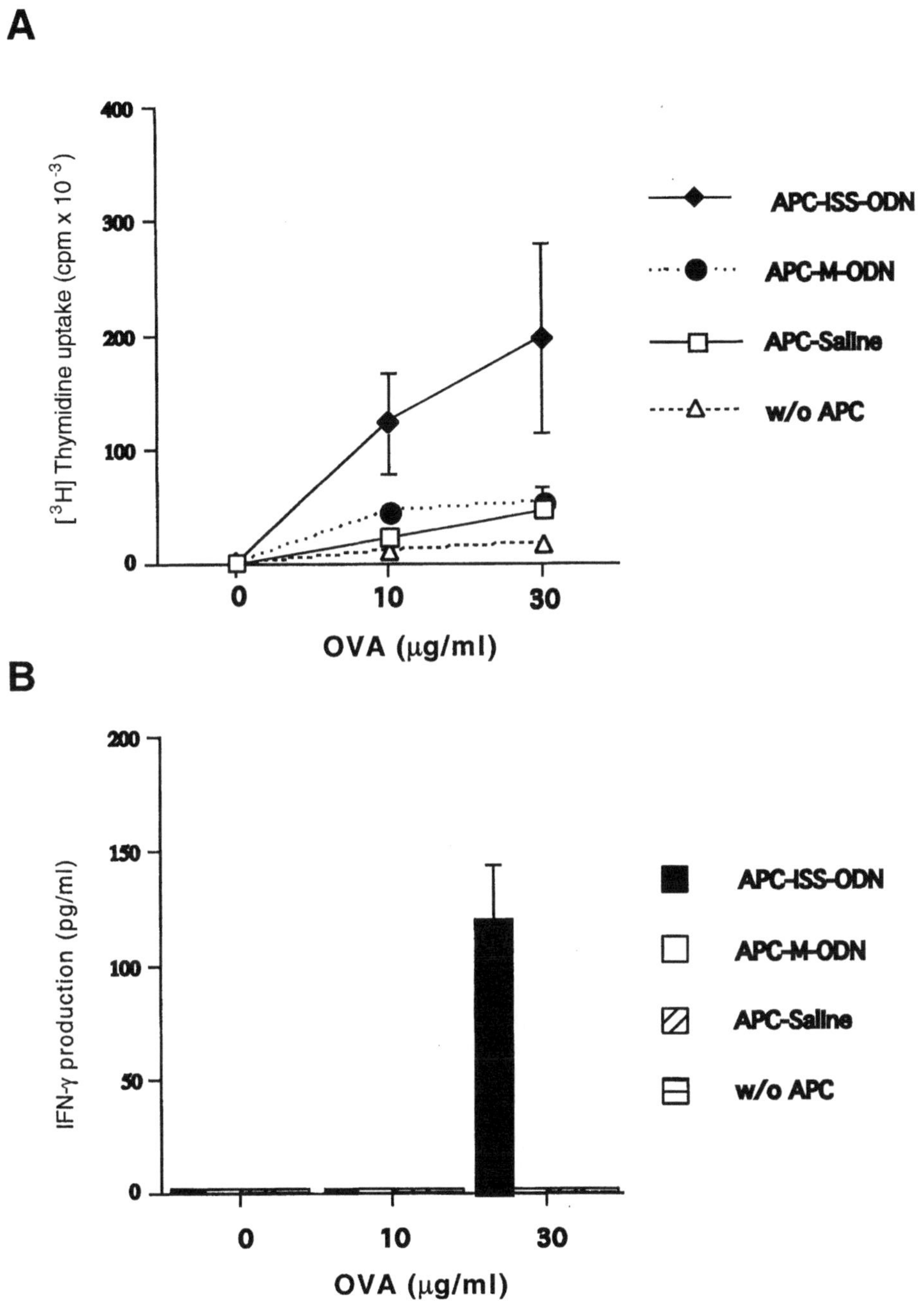

Cells were harvested and [^{3}H]thymidine incorporation was determined after an 18-h incubation with [^{3}H]thymidine (1 μCi/well). APCs obtained from ISS-ODN-injected mice induced four fold more OVA-specific T cell proliferation than APCs obtained from mice injected with saline or M-ODN. **B** OVA-specific cytokine response. Only APCs obtained from TCR-OVA TG mice injected with ISS-ODN induced OVA-specific IFN-γ production from naive T cells. Levels of IL-5 and IL-4 were below detectable limits in this system (*APC* antigen-presenting all, *TCR* T cell receptor, *OVA* ovalbumin, *TG* transgenic, *w/o* without)

Innate activation of APCs by ISS-ODN plays a central role in its mediation of Th1-biased adaptive immune responses

The functionality of APC activation by ISS-ODN on T cell responses has been confirmed in experiments utilizing T cell receptor-ovalbumin (TCR-OVA) transgenic (TG) mice (DO.11.10 mice) [23]. Splenic APC were harvested on day 14 from TCR-OVA TG mice injected with ISS-ODN, mutated ODN (M-ODN), or saline on days 0 and 7. Unstimulated T cells were obtained from naive TCR-OVA TG littermates. APCs and T cells were then cultured with OVA. APCs from ISS-ODN-injected mice induced four-fold more T cell proliferation than splenic APCs obtained from mice injected with M-ODN or saline (Fig. 3A). Furthermore, incubation of APCs from ISS-ODN-injected mice with naive TCR-OVA TG T cells and OVA resulted in antigen-specific IFN-γ production (Fig. 3B), indicating the differentiation of naive Th cells toward a Th1 phenotype [23]. Therefore, it appears that ISS-ODN functions as a Th1 adjuvant in large part via the induction of an innate immune response involving APCs. These results further demonstrate that APC exposure to ISS-ODN enhances their ability to induce T cell responses for at least 7 days.

ISS-ODN pre-priming Th1 biases immune responses for a prolonged period of time

Given that ISS-ODN can activate the innate immune system for up to 2 weeks, we hypothesized that injection of mice with ISS-ODN would Th1 bias adaptive immune responses for an extended period (ISS-ODN pre-priming). The data presented here demonstrate that ISS-ODN provides a 14-day window of Th1 adjuvant activity for antigens injected into the same site [19]. Mice were injected i.d. with ISS-ODN from 14 to 1 day prior to β-galactosidase (β-gal), or with β-gal only. When compared to mice i.d. immunized with ß-gal alone, mice receiving i.d. ISS-ODN up to 14 days prior to β-gal had a significant increase ($P<0.05$). in their serum IgG2a response (Fig. 4). Furthermore, the IgG2a response was improved over ISS-ODN/β-gal co-immunization if ISS-ODN was given 3–7 days before antigen ($P<0.05$ for day –7 ISS-ODN delivery versus ISS-ODN/β-gal co-immunization). In contrast to the relatively IFN-γ-dependent IgG2a response, which increased, the relatively IL-4-dependent IgG1 response was not affected by ISS-ODN pre-priming or by co-delivery with β-gal (unpublished data and [4, 19]).

ISS-ODN has previously been reported to induce a Th1 cytokine profile and a CTL response to soluble protein antigens [6, 13, 16, 28, 31, 33]. Therefore, the ISS-ODN pre-priming effect on cellular immunity was investigated [19]. As shown in Fig. 5A, antigen-specific IFN-γ production was significantly increased in mice pre-primed with ISS-ODN up to 14 days before β-gal immunization compared to mice immunized with antigen alone ($P<0.05$). Furthermore, mice pre-primed with ISS-ODN 3–7 days before β-gal immunization demonstrated a 100% increase in their IFN-γ response compared to mice co-immunized with ISS-ODN and β-gal ($P<0.05$). However, ISS-ODN pre-primed and co-immunized mice did not develop antigen-specific IL-4 or IL-5 responses (unpublished data and [19]). Further studies evaluated the CTL response of ISS-ODN-pre-primed mice [19]. These results again demonstrate a prolonged window of ISS-ODN adjuvant activity. Administration of

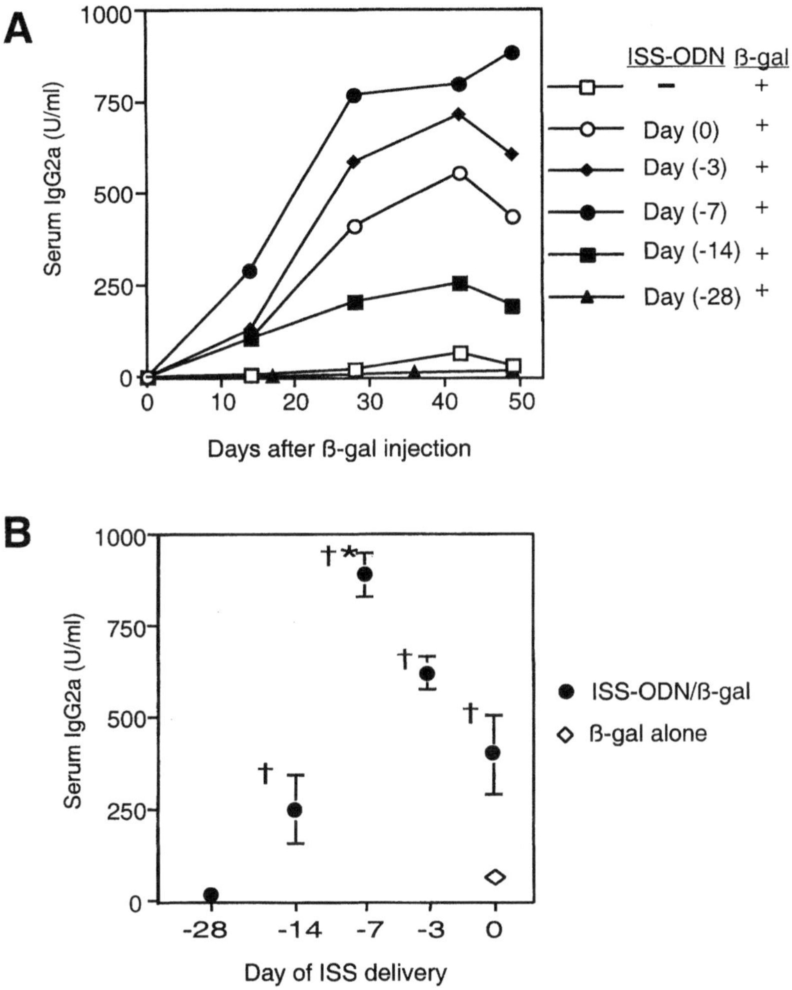

Fig. 4A, B. ISS-ODN pre-priming effect on humoral immunity. Mice received a single i.d. injection with ISS (50 μg) either 3, 7, 14, or 28 days before or with β-gal (10 μg) immunization via the same route (day 0). Control mice received β-gal immunization without ISS-ODN. Serial bleeds were perormed after β-gal immunization and serum anti-β-gal IgG2a levels were analyzed by ELISA. Results represent mean values ± SE for four mice per group and are representative of three similar and independent experiments [23]. **A** Time course of IgG2a production. **B** Serum IgG2a at 7 weeks post immunization. Mice receiving ISS-ODN up to 14 days prior to β-gal injection demonstrated an elevated IgG2a response when compared to mice immunized with β-gal alone († $P \leq 0.05$). Mice receiving ISS-ODN 7 days before β-gal immunization had a significantly increased IgG2a response when compared to mice co-administered ISS with β-gal (* $p<0.05$). ISS-ODN delivery prior to, or with, β-gal did not significantly increase the IgG1 response (data not shown) (*β-gal* β-galactosidase)

ISS-ODN up to 14 days before β-gal delivery led to a significantly improved CTL response over β-gal vaccination without adjuvant ($P<0.05$, Fig. 5B). Although ISS-ODN pre-priming 3–7 days prior to antigen did not lead to statistically significant increases in CTL activity when compared to ISS-ODN/β-gal co-immunization, again there was a trend toward improved responses if ISS-ODN pre-priming

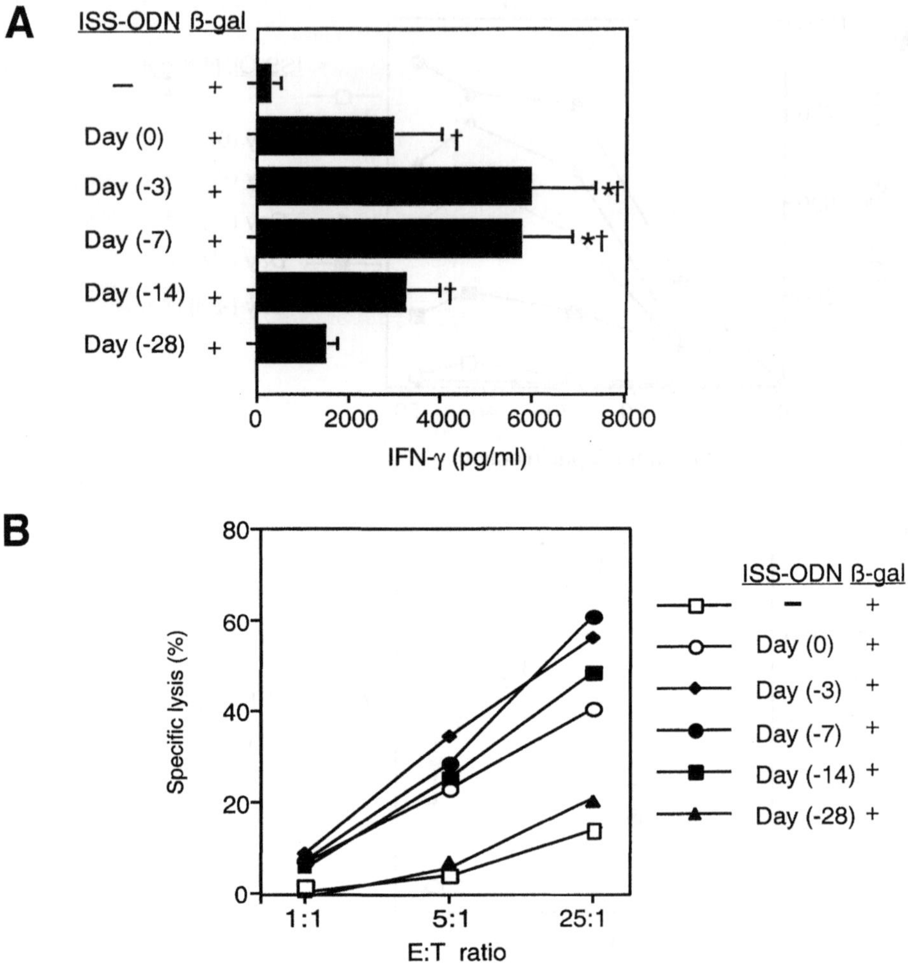

Fig. 5A, B. ISS-ODN pre-priming effect on cellular immune responses. Mice received a single i.d. injection with ISS-ODN (50 μg) either 3, 7, 14, or 28 days before or with β-gal (10 μg) immunization via the same route (day 0). Control mice received β-gal immunization without ISS-ODN. Mice were killed during week 8 for determination of splenocyte cytokine and CTL responses. Results represent the mean ± SE for four mice in each group and similar results were obtained in two other independent experiments [19]. **A** IFN-γ response. Mice receiving ISS-ODN up to 14 days prior to β-gal demonstrated an improved IFN-γ response when compared to mice immunized with β-gal alone († $P \leq 0.05$). Delivery of ISS-ODN from 3 to 7 days before β-gal led to an increased IFN-γ response when compared to mice receiving ISS-ODN/β-gal co-immunization (* $p \leq 0.05$). **B** CTL response. Mice receiving ISS-ODN up to 14 days prior to β-gal demonstrated a significantly improved CTL response when compared to mice immunized with β-gal alone ($P \leq 0.05$)

occurred on these days. Interestingly, when ISS-ODN was injected 1 week prior to or simultaneously with β-gal but at two different sites, the pre-priming effect was not seen, even when the injected dose of ISS-ODN was increased five-fold (unpublished data and [19]). This observation demonstrates that the ISS-ODN-pre-priming effect is local and not systemic.

Discussion

The data presented demonstrate that i.d. delivery of ISS-ODN, up to 2 weeks prior to i.d. β-gal administration and into the same site, results in improved antigen-specific immune responses when compared to i.d. vaccination with β-gal alone [19]. Anti-β-gal IgG2a (Th1 isotype), IFN-γ release by β-gal-specific T cells, and CTL activity against β-gal peptide-pulsed target cells, are all higher in mice pre-primed (up to 14 days) with ISS-ODN compared to mice immunized with β-gal alone. This pre-priming effect does not occur if the interval between ISS-ODN and β-gal delivery is extended to 28 days or if ISS-ODN and antigen are injected into different sites (unpublished data). These results further demonstrate that in addition to providing an extended window of local adjuvant activity, i.d. ISS-ODN delivery 3–7 days prior to i.d. β-gal delivery leads to significantly stronger immune responses then i.d. β-gal/ISS-ODN co-immunization. We have previously demonstrated that ISS-ODN is an effective mucosal adjuvant [13]. In an accompanying review we present data demonstrating that the ISS-ODN pre-priming effect also occurs with intranasal (i.n.) delivery (the review by Horner et al. discusses this ISS-ODN pre-priming effect on mucosal immune responses).

A previous epidemiological study conducted on approximately 1,000 Japanese school children demonstrated a correlation between exposure to *Mycobacterium tuberculosis* (MTB) and a Th1-biased serum cytokine profile in study subjects. In addition, PPD converters demonstrated significantly lower serum IgE levels compared to PPD negative school children [34]. Similar observations have been made in an experimental murine system [10]. In this respect, exposure to MTB may be considered to pre-prime the host toward Th1 immunity. Moreover, a recent study demonstrated that infection of dendritic cells with MTB resulted in the release of TNF-γ and IL-12 as well as the up-regulation of MHC class I, ICAM-1, CD40, and B7 co-stimulatory molecules [12]. This activation profile is very similar to the pattern induced by ISS-ODN [23]. As ISS-ODN DNA was initially identified and isolated from MTB DNA [20, 24, 39, 41], it is conceivable that this DNA adjuvant plays a role in biasing the immune profile of MTB-exposed hosts toward a Th1 phenotype, as does synthetic ISS-ODN in mice.

In this review, as well as in recent papers by other investigators data have been presented which suggest that in gene-vaccinated animals ISS-ODN within the plasmid DNA backbone generate a type 1 cytokine milieu and induce the expression of co-stimulatory molecules on APCs and B cells [11, 15, 17–19, 23, 31, 33, 35, 36, 40, 41]. This innate activation of the innate immune system would be expected to foster a Th1 response to the antigen encoded in the vaccination plasmid. Thus, gene vaccination plasmids provide both a source of adjuvant and antigen [5, 17, 31, 33, 38]. In the light of current findings, these two activities are probably not simultaneous. The local induction of cytokines by ISS-ODN is rapid and probably precedes the expression of sufficient amounts of antigen to elicit an effective immune response. A similar argument can be made for the up-regulation of co-stimulatory ligands. Thus, in gene vaccination, the pre-priming effects mediated by immunostimulatory sequences in the pDNA are likely to contribute to the Th1-biased immune response to the encoded antigen.

ISS-ODN can not only be used as an adjuvant in the traditional sense, but also as an immunomodifying therapeutic agent. For example, ISS-ODN might be i.d. injected or applied i.n. for the treatment of allergic rhinitis or inhaled to treat asthma. Due to the prolonged secretion of type 1 cytokines after ISS-ODN delivery, this immunological strategy would be expected to provide relatively prolonged immunological protection against continuous exposure to inhaled allergens in a Th2-sensitized host. Instead of amplifying the pre-existing Th2-biased immune response and increasing allergic inflammation of the nasal mucosa and bronchial surface with allergen exposure, the numerous type-1 cytokines released after ISS-ODN delivery would be expected to inhibit these responses. This theoretical approach to the treatment of allergic respiratory disease has already proven to be extremely effective in a murine model of asthma [3, 37]. A similar approach has been used successfully in the prevention and treatment of *Francisella tularensis* and *Listeria monocytogenes* infections [9], indicating that ISS-ODN-pre-priming also induces protective immunity to microbial pathogens. Further research is needed to establish the clinical utility of the ISS-ODN pre-priming effect for the prevention and treatment of infectious and allergic diseases. However, the data generated to date suggest that ISS-ODN can function as both a vaccine adjuvant and as an immunomodulatory therapeutic agent.

Acknowledgement This work was supported in part by NIH grants AI40682 and AI01490 and by Dynavax Technologies Corporation.

References

1. Ballas ZK, Rasmusen WL, Krieg AM (1996) Induction of NK activity in murine and human cells by CpG motifs in oligodeoxynucleotides and bacterial DNA. J Immunol 157: 1840
2. Banchereau J, Bazan F, Blanchard D, Briere F, Galizzi JP, Van Kooten C, Liu YJ, Rousset F, Saeland S (1994) The CD40 antigen and its ligand. Ann Rev Immunol 12: 881
3. Broide D, Schwarze J, Tighe H, Gifford T, Nguyen M-D, Malek S, Van Uden J, Martin-Orozco E, Gelfand EW, Raz E (1998) Immunostimulatory DNA sequences inhibit IL-5, eosinophilic inflammation, and airway hyperresponsiveness in mice. J Immunol 161: 7054
4. Coffman RL, Mosmann TR (1988) Isotype regulation by helper T cells and lymphokines. Monogr Allergy 24: 96
5. Cohen AD, Boyer JD, Weiner DB (1998) Modulating the immune response to genetic immunization. FASEB J 15: 1611
6. Davis HL, Weeranta R, Waldschmidt TJ, Tygrett L, Schorr J, Krieg AM (1998) CpG DNA is a potent enhancer of specific immunity in mice immunized with recombinant hepatitis B surface antigen. J Immunol 160: 870
7. Donnelly J, Ulmer JB, Shiver JW, Liu MA (1997) DNA vaccines. Annu Rev Immunol 15: 617
8. Dustin ML, Springer TA (1989) T cell crosslinking transiently stimulates adhesiveness through LFA-1. Nature 341: 619
9. Elkins K, Rhinehart-Jones TR, Stibitz S, Conover JS, Klinman DM (1999) Bacterial DNA containing CpG motifs stimulates lymphocyte-dependent protection of mice against lethal infection with intracellular bacteria. J Immunol 162: 2291
10. Erb KJ, Holloway JW, Sobeck A, Moll H, Le Gros G (1998) Infection of mice with *Mycobacterium bovis*-Bacillus Calmette-Guerin (BCG) suppresses allergen-induced airway eosinophilia. J Exp Med 187: 561
11. Halpern MD, Kurlander RJ, Pisetsky DS (1996) Bacterial DNA induces murine interferon-gamma production by stimulation of interleukin-12 and tumor necrosis factor-alpha. Cell Immunol 167: 72
12. Henderson RA, Watkins SC, Flynn JL (1997) Activation of human dendritic cells following infection with *Mycobacterium tuberculosis*. J Immunol 159: 635
13. Horner AA, Ronaghy A, Cheng PM, Nguyen MD, Cho HJ, Broide D, Raz E (1998) Immunostimulatory DNA is a potent mucosal adjuvant. Cell Immunol 190: 77
14. Hsu CH, Chua KY, Tao MH, Lai YL, Wu HD, Huang SK, Hsieh KH (1996) Immunoprophylaxis of allergen-induced immunoglobulin E synthesis and airway hyperresponsiveness in vivo by genetic immunization. Nat Med 2: 540

15. Jakob T, Walker PS, Krieg AM, Udey MC, Vogel JC (1998) Activation of cutaneous dendritic cells by CpG-containing oligodeoxynucleotides: a role for dendritic cells in the augmentation of Th1 responses by immunostimulatory DNA. J Immunol 161: 3042
16. Kline JN, Waldschmidt TJ, Businga J, Lemish JE, Weinstock JV, Thorne PS, Krieg AM (1998) Modulation of airway inflammation by CpG oligodeoxynucleotides in a murine model of asthma. J Immunol 160: 25
17. Klinman DM, Yamshchikov G, Ishigatsubo Y (1997) Contribution of CpG motifs to the immunogenicity of DNA vaccines. J Immunol 158: 3635
18. Klinmann DM, Yi AK, Beaucage SL, Conover J, Krieg AM (1996) CpG motifs present in bacterial DNA rapidly induce lymphocytes to secrete interleukin 6, interleukin 12, and interferon gamma. Proc Natl Acad Sci USA 93: 2879
19. Kobayashi H, Horner AA, Takabayashi K, Nguyen M-D, Huang E, Cinman N, Raz E (1999) Immunostimulatory DNA prepriming: a novel approach for prolonged Th1-biased immunity. Cell Immunol 198: (in press)
20. Krieg AM, Yi A., Matson S, Waldschmidt TJ, Bishop GA, Teasdale R, Koretzky GA, Klinman DM (1995) CpG motifs in bacterial DNA trigger direct B-cell activation. Nature 374: 546
21. Lenschow DJ, Walunas TL, Bluestone JA (1996) CD28/B7 system of T cell costimulation. Annu Rev Immunol 14: 233
22. Liang H, Nishioka Y, Reich CF, Pisetsky DS, Lipsky PE (1996) Activation of human B cells by phosphorothioate oligodeoxynucleotides. J Clin Invest 98: 1119
23. Martin-Orozco E, Kobayashi H, Van Uden J, Nguyen M-D, Kornbluth RS, Ras E (1999) Enhancement of antigen-presenting cell surface molecules involved in cognate interactions by immunostimulatory DNA sequences. Int Immunol 11: 1111
24. Mashiba H, Matsunaga K, Tomoda H, Furusawa M, Jimi S, Tokunaga T (1988) In vitro augmentation of natural killer activity of peripheral blood cells from cancer patients by a DNA fraction from *Mycobacterium bovis* BCG. Jap J Med Sci and Biol 41: 197
25. McDonnell WM, Squires HR Jr (1996) DNA vaccines. N Engl J Med 334: 42
26. McDyer JF, Goletz TJ, Thomas E, June CH, Seder RA (1998) CD40 ligand/CD40 stimulation regulates the production of IFN from human peripheral blood mononuclear cells in an IL-12- and or CD28-dependent manner. J Immunol 160: 1701
27. Medzhitov R, Janeway CA Jr (1997) Innate immunity: the virtues of a nonclonal system of recognition. Cell 91: 295
28. Oxenius A, Martinic MM, Hengartner H, Klenerman P (1999) CpG-containing oligonucleotides are efficient adjuvants for induction of protective antiviral immune responses with T-cell peptide vaccines. J Virol 73: 4120–4126
29. Raz E (1998) Immune deviation of the allergic response by DNA vaccination. In: Marone G, Austen KF, Holgate ST, Kay AB, Lichtenstein LM (eds) Asthma and allergic diseases: physiology, immunopharmacology, and treatment. Academic Press, San Diego, CA, pp 417
30. Reise SC, Hieny S, Scharton-Kersten T, Jankovic D, Charest H, Germain RN, Sher A (1997) *In vivo* microbial stimulation induces rapid CD40 ligand-independent production of IL-12 by dendritic cells and their redistribution to T cell areas. J Exp Med 186: 1819
31. Roman M, Martin-Orozco E, Goodman JS, Nguyen M-D, Sato Y, Ronaghy A, Kornbluth RS, Richman DD, Carson DA, Raz E (1997) Immunostimulatory DNA sequences function as T helper-1-promoting adjuvants. Nat Medicine 3: 849
32. Roy K, Mao HQ, Huang SK, Leong KW (1999) Oral gene delivery with chitosan-DNA nanoparticles generates immunologic protection in a murine model of peanut allergy. Nat Med 5: 387
33. Sato Y, Roman M, Tighe H, Lee D, Corr M, Nguyen M-N, Silverman GJ, Lotz M, Carson DA, Raz E (1996) Immunostimulatory DNA sequences necessary for effective intradermal gene immunization. Science 273: 352
34. Shirakawa T, Enomoto T, Shimazu S, Hopkin JM (1997) The inverse association between tuberculin responses and atopic disorder. Science 275: 77
35. Sparwasser T, Koch ES, Vabulas RM, Heeg K, Lipford GB, Ellwart JW, Wagner H (1998) Bacterial DNA and immunostimulatory CpG oligonucleotides trigger maturation and activation of murine dendritic cells. Eur J Immunol 28: 2045
36. Sun S, Zhang X, Tough DF, Sprent J (1998) Type I interferon-mediated stimulation of T cells by CpG DNA. J Exp Med 188: 2335
37. Sur S, Wild JS, Choudhury BK, Sur N, Alam R, Klinman DM (1999) Long term prevention of allergic lung inflammation in a mouse model of asthma by CpG oligodeoxynucleotides. J Immunol 162: 6284

38. Tighe H, Corr M, Roman M, Raz E (1998) Gene vaccination: plasmid DNA is more than just a blue print. Immunol Today 19: 89
39. Tokunaga T, Yamamoto H, Shimada H, Abe H, Fukuda T, Fujisawa Y, Furutani Y, Yano O, Kataoka T, Sudo T, Makiguchi N, Saganuma T (1984) Antitumor activity of deoxyribonucleic acid fraction from *Mycobacterium bovis* BCG. Isolation, physicochemical characterization, and antitumor activity. J Natl Cancer Inst 72: 955
40. Tokunaga T, Yano O, Kuramoto E, Kimura Y, Yamamoto T, Kataoka T, Yamamoto S (1992) Synthetic oligonucleotides with particular base sequences from the cDNA encoding proteins of *Mycobacterium bovis* BCG induce interferons and activate natural killer cells. Microbiol Immunol 36: 55
41. Yamamoto S, Kuramoto E, Shimada S, Tokunaga T (1988) In vitro augmentation of natural killer cell activity and protection of interferon-alpha/beta and gamma with deoxyribonucleic acid fraction from *Mycobacterium bovis* BCG. Jpn J Cancer Res 79: 866

Signal transduction induced by immunostimulatory CpG DNA

Arthur M. Krieg[1–3]

[1] Department of Veterans Affairs Medical Center, Iowa City, IA 52246, USA
[2] Department of Internal Medicine, University of Iowa College of Medicine, 540 EMRB, Iowa City, IA 52242, USA
[3] CpG ImmunoPharmaceuticals, Wellesley, MA 02481, USA

Abstract. The immune recognition of unmethylated CpG motifs appears to be an example of the ability of the immune system to detect molecular patterns which are characteristic of microbes, but are not present in vertebrates. This detection is accomplished by the means of pattern recognition receptors (PRR). Unlike some other examples of PRR, immune recognition of CpG DNA appears to require cell uptake and to be accomplished through an intracellular PRR system. This then results in the activation of mitogen-activated protein kinases, culminating in the phosphorylation of transcription factors and the activation of transcription and translation. The rapid activation of these pathways by CpG DNA leads to the induction of protective immune responses.

Introduction

Since the initial demonstration in 1984 that bacterial DNA possesses immune stimulatory and anti-tumor activity [50], an important question has been the structure within the DNA which is responsible for these effects, and the mechanism through which the effects are mediated. By 1991, it was realized that bacterial DNA induced murine B cell proliferation and immunoglobulin secretion, but vertebrate DNA did not [35]. By the following year, Yamamoto and et al. [53] concluded that the immune stimulatory effects of bacterial DNA could be reproduced with synthetic oligodeoxynucleotides (ODN), if these ODN contained certain self-complementary palindromes. Not all palindrome-containing ODN were immune stimulatory; the palindromes had to contain at least one CpG dinucleotide, but the methylation status of the CpG was reported to have no effect on the immune stimulatory properties of the DNA [28]. It was hypothesized that the stimulatory effects of bacterial DNA compared to vertebrate DNA might be explained by an increased frequency of these palindromes [28]. Of note, the following year it was reported that polymers of dC.dG were B cell mitogens, and that this mitogenicity was abolished by methylation of the cytosines [36]. This effect of methylation was thought to be a consequence of the

Correspondence to: A. M. Krieg (address see [2] above)

disruption of higher ordered structures of these DNA polymers, to which the immune stimulatory effects were attributed.

Around the same time, several groups of investigators working with antisense ODN noted striking sequence-specific immune stimulatory effects of certain ODN [5, 23, 26, 34, 38, 49]. In some cases, these immune stimulatory effects were attributed to an antisense mechanism of action, while other investigators realized that the effects represented a new type of sequence-specific non-antisense mechanism. No common sequence motif was evident from visual comparison of the ODN sequences, and none of these immune stimulatory ODN contained palindromes. However, after testing several hundred ODN, we realized that all of the immune stimulatory ODN contained CpG dinucleotides in particular base contexts, which did not require palindromes. Based on the known differences in CpG frequency and methylation between vertebrate and microbial genomes, we hypothesized that immune stimulation by CpG dinucleotides could represent an immune defense mechanism, in which case it would presumably be abolished by methylation of the CpG, which would make the ODN structurally similar to vertebrate DNA. Indeed, synthesis of ODN containing methylated CpG motifs eliminated their immune stimulatory effects [27]. Finally, we showed that the immune stimulatory effects of bacterial DNA were abolished by methylation, confirming that its immune stimulatory effects were due to the presence of unmethylated CpG motifs rather than to some other type of structure [27].

These data suggested the hypothesis that immune recognition of unmethylated CpG motifs represented a type of pattern recognition receptor (PRR) to detect early evidence of microbial invasion and activate protective defense mechanisms. This hypothesis suggested that treatment with CpG motifs could activate protective immune mechanisms, leading to resistance against invasion. Indeed, we and others have shown a striking ability of CpG DNA treatment to protect against a broad spectrum of intracellular (but not extracellular) bacteria, viruses, and parasites [12, 25, 65]. The effectiveness of the CpG-based immune defenses may be inferred from the fact that intracellular pathogens such as small DNA viruses have extraordinarily low CpG content [20, 42], indicating that this is an evolutionary adaptation to replication in eukaryotic hosts [22].

Mechanisms of cellular binding and uptake of CpG DNA

The PRR which trigger immune system activation are typically located on the surface of the cells, as exemplified by the lipopolysaccharide (LPS) receptors and manose binding protein. This seems intuitively logical since these receptors are optimized for detecting extracellular pathogens. To determine whether the PRR which recognizes CpG DNA is also located on the cell surface, we tested the ability of immobilized ODN to trigger B cell proliferation. These studies demonstrated that B cells on Teflon fibers or avidin-coated plates did not activate B cells in a short-term 4-h stimulation assay [27]. Therefore, we concluded that internalization of ODN was required for CpG-mediated activation, and that cell surface binding was not a sufficient signal. However, Liang et al. [31] reached the opposite conclusion in studies of the response of human B cells to ODN coupled to Sepharose 4B beads which were cultured with the B cells for 4 days, followed by a [^{3}H]thymidine incorporation assay. These "immobilized" ODN nevertheless activated human B cells with equivalent efficiency to unimmobilized ODN, leading to the conclusion that B cell activation was occurring through a cell surface receptor.

Several potential complications prevent the uncritical acceptance of this conclusion. First of all, the ODN may have become dissociated from the beads during the 4-day culture. More importantly, Manzel and Macfarlane (Immune stimulation by CpG-oligodeoxynucleotide requires internalization; submitted) have recently reported that ODN coupled to Sepharose 4B beads by the protocol of Liang et al. [31] are in fact internalized by cells in tissue culture, which of course could cause B cell proliferation even without any surface receptor interaction. On the other hand, Manzel and Macfarlane demonstrated that CpG ODN coupled to Latex, magnetic, or gold beads could not be internalized and did not cause stimulation, supporting the conclusion that cell uptake is required for the action of CpG DNA. The conclusion that CpG DNA stimulation does not require cell surface signaling is further supported by the demonstration that the immune stimulatory effects of CpG DNA are enhanced by lipofection into cells [54]. Taken together, these data support the conclusion that cell surface binding of CpG DNA is not sufficient to mediate its stimulatory activities, and that internalization is required.

This is not to say that CpG DNA does not bind to cell membranes. Indeed, several different groups have independently demonstrated the existence of DNA binding proteins on cell surfaces [1, 30, 32, 52]. However, these proteins appear to bind DNA in a sequence-independent fashion. Studies comparing the cell surface binding of radiolabeled ODN with or without CpG motifs have demonstrated no difference, supporting the conclusion that the cell membrane binding of DNA is a sequence-independent step [27, 54]. ODN uptake by cells demonstrates qualities that are consistent with receptor-mediated endocytosis, especially at low concentrations [3]. As yet, only a single DNA transport protein has been reported [14], leaving open the possibility that ODN uptake could occur through adsorptive endocytosis.

Regardless of the precise mechanism of ODN uptake, their initial intracellular location within the first few minutes after uptake appears to be endosomal [4, 51, 61]. As would be expected, these endosomes become acidified and much of the DNA within them is degraded, unless it contains a nuclease-resistant phosphorothioate backbone. Studies using fluorescently labeled ODN have demonstrated that some fraction of the DNA leaves the endosomes and enters the nucleus [26, 62, 63]. This intracellular trafficking of ODN also appears to be sequence independent.

Essentially all cell types appear to be capable of taking up DNA spontaneously in culture, but the rate of uptake by T cells is much lower than that by B cells or monocyte/macrophage-like cells [16, 24, 63]. ODN uptake by cells is essentially sequence independent, with the exception that poly-G sequences in an ODN lead to higher binding to cell membranes and higher rates of cell uptake [18, 21].

Requirement for endosomal acidification and/or maturation for CpG-induced immune activation

The endosomal localization of internalized CpG ODN could either be a final destination for the ODN, or an essential step in a CpG-mediated signaling pathway. To investigate this question, we treated leukocytes with agents that interfere with endosomal acidification and maturation, including monensin, bafilomycin A, and chloroquine. These agents completely block all of the stimulatory effects of CpG DNA on B cells and monocyte/macrophage/dendritic cells, but do not block the stimulatory effects of other agents, including phorbol myristate acetate, endotoxin, anti-IgM, or anti-CD40 [61]. Quinacrine and other anti-malarial compounds related to chloroquine have recently been demonstrated to be even more potent and selective inhibitors of the stimulatory effects of CpG DNA [33]. We hypothesize that these compounds may somehow interfere with the ability of CpG ODN to exit the endosomes and interact with a CpG binding protein, but the exact mechanism of action of these compounds remains speculative. Several groups are currently seeking to identify the intracellular CpG receptor, and it is hoped that this will lead to a clearer understanding of the mechanism of action of these anti-malarial compounds.

Rapid generation of intracellular reactive oxygen species in response to CpG DNA

The earliest reported alteration in cellular physiology following exposure to CpG DNA is the generation of intracellular reactive oxygen species (ROS), which is already detectable within 5 min [58]. Antioxidants, which block this ROS production, block the stimulatory effects of CpG DNA, suggesting that ROS production may be important in the CpG signaling pathways, rather than a byproduct of activation. ROS generation has also been implicated in signal transduction through the B cell antigen receptor and CD40, leading to either stimulation or apoptosis [10, 11, 29]. Depending on the type and level of ROS generated, either cell activation or apoptosis may result. We hypothesize that the generation of ROS in response to CpG may so alter the redox balance of the cell as to activate redox-sensitive transcription factors such as AP1, NF-κB, p53, and SP-1 [7].

Another signaling intermediate which can be produced in response to CpG DNA is nitric oxide (NO). Bone marrow-derived macrophages that have been primed with IFN-γ show increased expression of the inducible NO synthase (iNOS) gene upon addition of CpG DANN, followed by increased production of NO. However, since this requires priming of the macrophages with IFN-γ, NO production is not a simple and direct consequence of CpG DNA treatment. This is in contrast to the effects of LPS, which induces iNOS expression in the absence of IFN-γ pretreatment [47]. Thus, there are differences in the signaling pathways of LPS and CpG DNA.

Induction of mitogen-activated protein kinase signaling pathways and transcription factors by CpG DNA

Several mitogen-activated protein kinases (MAPK) are rapidly activated in B cells, macrophages, and dendritic cells upon exposure to CpG DNA. The p38 and c-Jun NH_2-terminal kinase (JNK) pathways are activated in B cells and macrophage/dendritic cells within 7 min after CpG DNA exposure [13, 60]. The extracellular receptor kinase (ERK) pathway is also activated in macrophages, although not B cells ([60] and K.J. Stacey and D.A. Hume, personal communication). Activation of the p38 kinase pathway by CpG DNA has been shown to be required for induction of cytokine secretion, which is blocked by the addition of a p38-specific inhibitor [13, 60].

The MAPK pathways lead to the phosphorylation and activation of several transcription factors, including ATF-2 and AP-1. As expected, these transcription factors are indeed phosphorylated and show increased transcriptional activity within approximately 30 min in B cells and macrophages exposed to CpG DNA [13, 60]. Another transcription factor shown to be rapidly activated after CpG stimulation is NF-κB [34, 44, 45, 57, 59]. Inhibition of the activation of NF-κB with antioxidants or specific inhibitors prevents immune stimulation, suggesting a requirement for NF-κB in mediating the effects of CpG DNA [59].

Induction of gene expression by CpG DNA

As expected, given the marked activation of transcription factor activity in CpG-treated cells, gene transcription is induced within 30 min [57, 60]. mRNA levels are increased for several genes which regulate the cell cycle or apoptosis, including myc, myn, Bcl-2, and Bcl-X_L [56–59]. mRNA levels for several transcription factors are also increased, including egr-1, ets-2, C/EBP-β and -δ, and c/Jun [48]. Presumably, these transcription factors are translated and contribute to the induction of other genes, although this has not yet been investigated in detail. This would be consistent with the induction of increased promoter activity for IL-6 and HIV in in vitro assays of macrophages and B cells activated by CpG DNA [48, 58].

The mRNA levels for multiple cytokines are also increased in CpG-treated leukocytes within 15–30 min. These cytokines include IL-1β, IL-1 RA, IL-6, IL-10, IL-12, IL-18, TNF-α, IFN-α/β, IFN-γ, MIP-1β, and MCP-1 [2, 6, 19, 39–41, 44–46, 58, 64]. These cytokine mRNA are translated into protein, with a net effect of marked increases in expression of Th1-like cytokines. In vivo or in vitro, CpG DNA induces a predominantly Th1-like cytokine profile dominated by IL-12, IL-18, and IFN-γ. Although IL-10 is also increased, it may function in a counter-regulatory fashion to control the level of IL-12 secretion in response to CpG DNA [39], which may help to limit CpG-induced toxicity. The effects of CpG DNA on leukocyte gene expression include induction of expression of costimulatory and antigen-presenting molecules such as MHC class II, CD40, CD80, and CD86 and adhesion molecules such as CD54 [9, 17, 19].

Interactions of the CpG signaling pathways with other leukocyte signaling pathways

CpG DNA can drive more than 95% of B cells into the cell cycle at optimal concentrations [27]. However, polyclonal B cell activation of this magnitude would not be expected to be as useful to the immune system as the selective activation of B cells specific for microbial antigens. It is, therefore, of interest that low concentrations of CpG DNA synergize strongly for B cell activation through the antigen receptor, resulting in at least a tenfold increase in B cell proliferation and secretion of IL-6 and Ig [27, 58]. Thus, synergistic costimulation of B cells by CpG DNA and the B cell antigen receptor (BCR) provides a mechanism for the preferential enhancement of antigen-specific antibody responses.

In contrast to this synergy with BCR activation of mature B cells, CpG antagonizes BCR signaling of immature-like B cells, which normally undergo apoptosis instead of activation [37]. A murine B cell line with an immature phenotype, WEHI-231, normally undergoes apoptosis in response to BCR cross-linking, but is rescued from this apoptosis by exposure to CpG DNA [57, 59]. Remarkably, the addition of CpG DNA to WEHI-231 cells can be delayed as long as 8 h after BCR ligation and still show protective effects [57].

CpG shows costimulatory effects with LPS for activation of both B cells and monocytes [15]. In fact, CpG DNA exposure can prime mice for the Schwartzman reaction if the CpG treatment is followed by an otherwise sublethal dose of LPS given 4 h later [8]. This toxicity is likely associated with the synergistic induction of TNF-α expression in mice exposed to both LPS and CpG [8, 43].

The effects of CpG DNA on B cells differ from those of LPS in certain ways. One example is the synergy of CpG DNA with IFN-γ in the activation of B cell proliferation and Ig secretion. IFN-γ normally attenuates LPS-induced B cell activation, but IFN-γ promotes B cell activation by CpG DNA [55].

Conclusions

B cells, monocytes, macrophages and dendritic cells exposed to CpG DNA show the rapid activation of multiple intracellular signaling pathways including the generation of ROS, activation of MAPK, activation of transcription factors such as AP-1 and NF-κB, and increased expression of mRNA and protein for cell cycle regulatory protooncogenes and Th1-like cytokines. The study of the earliest signaling events in these pathways is in its infancy, and it is not yet clear how binding of CpG DNA to the putative intracellular CpG receptor is coupled to the activation of these other pathways. It is expected that these events should become better understood once the CpG receptor has been identified and characterized.

References

1. Aggrarwal SK, Wagner RW, McAllister PK, Rosenberg B (1975) Cell-surface-associated nucleic acid in tumorigenic cells made visible with platinum-pyrimidine complexes by electron microscopy. Proc Natl Acad Sci USA 72:928
2. Anitescu M, Chace JH, Tuetken R, Yi A-K, Berg DJ, Krieg AM, Cowdery JS (1997) Interleukin-10 functions in vitro and in vivo to inhibit bacterial DNA-induced secretion of interleukin-12. J Interferon Cytokine Res 17:781
3. Beltinger C, Saragovi HU, Smith RM, LeSauteur L, Shah N, DeDionisio L, Christensen L, Raible A, Jarett L, Gewirtz AM (1995) Binding, uptake, and intracellular trafficking of phosphorothioate-modified oligodeoxynucleotides. J Clin Invest 95:1814
4. Bennett RM, Gabor GT, Merritt MM (1985) DNA binding to human leukocytes. Evidence for a receptor-mediated association, internalization, and degradation of DNA. J Clin Invest 76:2182
5. Branda RF, Moore AL, Mathews L, McCormack JJ, Zon G (1993) Immune stimulation by an antisense oligomer complementary to the rev gene of HIV-1. Biochem Pharmacol 45:2037
6. Chace JH, Hooker NA, Mildenstein KL, Krieg AM, Cowdery JS (1997) Bacterial DNA-induced NK cell IFN-γ production is dependent on macrophage secretion of IL-12. Clin Immunol Immunopathol 84:185
7. Cotgreave IA, Gerges RG (1998) Recent trends in glutathione biochemistry – glutathione-protein interactions: a molecular link between oxidative stress and cell proliferation? Biochem Biophys Res Commun 242:1
8. Cowdery JS, Chace JH, Yi A-K, Krieg AM (1996) Bacterial DNA induces NK cells to produce interferon-γ in vivo and increases the toxicity of lipopolysaccharides. J Immunol 156:4570
9. Davis HL, Weeranta R, Waldschmidt TJ, Tygrett L, Schorr J, Krieg AM (1998) CpG DNA is a potent adjuvant in mice immunized with recombinant hepatitis B surface antigen. J Immunol 160:870
10. Fang W, Nath KA, Mackey MF, Noelle RJ, Mueller DL, Behrens TW (1997) CD40 inhibits B cell apoptosis by upregulating bcl-x_L expression and blocking oxidant accumulation. Am J Physiol 272:C950
11. Fang W, Rivard JJ, Ganser JA, LeBien TW, Nath KA, Mueller DL, Behrens TW (1995) Bcl-XL rescues WEHI-231 B lymphocytes from oxidant-mediated death following diverse apoptotic stimuli. J Immunol 155:66

12. Gramzinski RA, Sedegah M, Doolan D, Krieg AM, Davis HL, Hoffman SL (2000) IL-12- and IFN-γ-dependent protection of mice against malaria conferred by CpG DNA. Mol Med (in press)
13. Hacker H, Mischak H, Miethke T, Liptay S, Schmid R, Sparwasser T, Heeg K, Lipford GB, Wagner H (1998) CpG-DNA-specific activation of antigen-presenting cells requires stress kinase activity and is preceded by non-specific endocytosis and endosomal maturation. EMBO J 17:6230
14. Hanss B, Leal-Pinto E, Bruggeman LA, Copeland TD, Klotman PE (1998) Identification and characterization of a cell membrane nucleic acid channel. Proc Natl Acad Sci USA 95:1921
15. Hartmann G, Krieg AM (1999) CpG DNA and LPS induce distinct patterns of activation in human monocytes. Gene Therapy 6:893
16. Hartmann G, Krug A, Bidlingmaier M, Hacker U, Eigler A, Albrecht R, Strasburger CJ, Endres S (1998) Spontaneous and cationic lipid-mediated uptake of antisense oligonucleotides in human monocytes and lymphocytes. J Pharmacol Exp Ther 285:920
17. Hartmann G, Weiner G, Krieg AM (1999) CpG DNA as a signal for growth, activation and maturation of human dendritic cells. Proc Natl Acad Sci USA 96:9305
18. Hughes JA, Avrutskaya AV, Juliano RL (1994) Influence of base composition on membrane binding and cellular uptake of 10-mer phosphorothioate oligonucleotides in Chinese hamster ovary (CHRC5) cells. Antisense Res Dev 4:211
19. Jakob T, Walker PS, Krieg AM, Udey MC, Vogel JC (1998) Activation of cutaneous dendritic cells by CpG-containing oligodeoxynucleotides: a role for dendritic cells in the augmentation of Th1 responses by immunostimulatory DNA. J Immunol 161:3042
20. Karlin S, Doerfler W, Cardon LR (1994) Why is CpG suppressed in the genomes of virtually all small eukaryotic viruses but not in those of large eukaryotic viruses? J Virol 68:2889
21. Kimura Y, Sonehara K, Kuramoto E, Makino T, Yamamoto S, Yamamoto T, Kataoka T, Tokunaga T (1994) Binding of oligoguanylate to scavenger receptors is required for oligonucleotides to augment NK cell activity and induce IFN. J Biochem 116:991
22. Krieg AM (1996) Lymphocyte activation by CpG dinucleotide motifs in prokaryotic DNA. Trends Microbiol 4:73
23. Krieg AM, Gause WC, Gourley MF, Steinberg AD (1989) A role for endogenous retroviral sequences in the regulation of lymphocyte activation. J Immunol 143:2448
24. Krieg AM, Gmelig-Meyling F, Gourley MF, Kisch WJ, Chrisey LA, Steinberg AD (1991) Uptake of oligodeoxyribonucleotides by lymphoid cells is heterogeneous and inducible. Antisense Res Dev 1:161
25. Krieg AM, Love-Homan L, Yi A-K, Harty JT (1998) CpG DNA induces sustained IL-12 expression in vivo and resistance to *Listeria monocytogenes* challenge. J Immunol 161:2428
26. Krieg A, Tonkinson J, Matson S, Zhao Q, Saxon M, Zhang L-M, Bhanja U, Yakubov L, Stein CA (1993) Modification of antisense phosphodiester oligodeoxynucleotides by a 5' cholesteryl moiety increases cellular association and improves efficacy. Proc Natl Acad Sci USA 90:1048
27. Krieg AK, Yi A-K, Matson S, Waldschmidt TJ, Bishop GA, Teasdale R, Koretzky G, Klinman D (1995) CpG motifs in bacterial DNA trigger direct B-cell activation. Nature 374:546
28. Kuramoto E, Yano O, Kimura Y, Baba M, Makino T, Yamamoto S, Yamamoto T, Kataoka T, Tokunaga T (1992) Oligonucleotide sequences required for natural killer cell activation. Jpn J Cancer Res 83:1128
29. Lee JR, Koretzky GA (1997) Production of reactive oxygen intermediates following CD40 ligation correlates with c-Jun N-terminal kinase activation and IL-6 secretion in murine B lymphocytes. Eur J Immunol 28:4188
30. Lerner RA, Meinke W, Goldstein DA (1971) Membrane-associated DNA in the cytoplasm of diploid human lymphocytes. Proc Natl Acad Sci USA 68:1212
31. Liang H, Nishioka Y, Reich CF, Pisetsky DS, Lipsky PE (1996) Activation of human B cells by phosphorothioate oligodeoxynucleotides. J Clin Invest 98:1119
32. Loke SL, Stein CA, Zhang XH, Mori K, Nakanishi M, Subasinghe C, Cohen JS, Neckers LM (1989) Characterization of oligonucleotide transport into living cells. Proc Natl Acad Sci USA 86:3474
33. MacFarlane DE, Manzel L (1998) Antagonism of immunostimulatory CpG-oligodeoxynucleotides by quinacrine, chloroquine, and structurally related compounds. J Immunol 160:1122
34. McIntyre KW, Lombard-Gillooly K, Perez JR, Kunsch C, Sarmiento UM, Larigan JD, Landreth KT, Narayanan R (1993) A sense phosphorothioate oligonucleotide directed to the initiation codon of transcription factor NF-κB p65 causes sequence-specific immune stimulation. Antisense Res Dev 3:309
35. Messina JP, Gilkeson GS, Pisetsky DS (1991) Stimulation of in vitro murine lymphocyte proliferation by bacterial DNA. J Immunol 147:1759

36. Messina JP, Gilkeson GS, Pisetsky DS (1993) The influence of DNA structure on the in vitro stimulation of murine lymphocytes by natural and synthetic polynucleotide antigens. Cell Immunol 147:148
37. Norvell A, Mandik L, Monroe JG (1995) Engagement of the antigen-receptor on immature murine B lymphocytes results in death by apoptosis. J Immunol 154:4404
38. Pisetsky DS, Reich CF (1993) Stimulation of murine lymphocyte proliferation by a phosphorothioate oligonucleotide with antisense activity for herpes simplex virus. Life Sci 54:101
39. Redford TW, Yi A-K, Ward CT, Krieg AM (1998) Cyclosporine A enhances IL-12 production by CpG motifs in bacterial DNA and synthetic oligodeoxynucleotides. J Immunol 161:3930
40. Roman M, Martin-Orozco E, Goodman JS, Nguyen M-D, Sato Y, Ronaghy A, Kornbluth RS, Richman DD, Carson DA, Raz E (1997) Immunostimulatory DNA sequences function as T helper-1-promoting adjuvants. Nat Med 3:849
41. Schwartz D, Quinn TJ, Thorne PS, Sayeed S, Yi A-K, Krieg AM (1997) CpG motifs in bacterial DNA cause inflammation in the lower respiratory tract. J Clin Invest 100:68
42. Shpaer EG, Mullins JI (1990) Selection against CpG dinucleotides in lentiviral genes: a possible role of methylation in regulation of viral expression. Nucleic Acids Res 18:5793
43. Sparwasser T, Miethke T, Lipford G, Borschert K, Hacker H, Heet K, Wagner H (1997) Bacterial DNA causes septic shock. Nature 386:336
44. Sparwasser T, Miethe T, Lipford G, Erdmann A, Hacker H, Heeg K, Wagner H (1997) Macrophages sense pathogens via DNA motifs: induction of tumor necrosis factor-α-mediated shock. Eur J Immunol 27:1671
45. Stacey KJ, Sweet MJ, Hume DA (1996) Macrophages ingest and are activated by bacterial DNA. J Immunol 157:2116
46. Sun S, Zhang X, Tough DF, Sprent J (1998) Type I interferon-mediated stimulation of T cells by CpG DNA. J Exp Med 188:2335
47. Sweet MJ, Stacey KJ, Kakuda DK, Markovich D, Hume DA (1998) IFN-γ primes macrophage responses to bacterial DNA. J Interferon Cytokine Res 18:263
48. Sweet MJ, Stacey KJ, Ross IL (1998) Involvement of Ets, rel and Sp1-like proteins in lipopolysaccharide-mediated activation of the HIV-1 LTR in macrophages. J Inflamm 48:67
49. Tanaka T, Chu CC, Paul WE (1992) An antisense oligonucleotide complementary to a sequence in Ic2b increases c2b germline transcripts, stimulates B cell DNA synthesis, and inhibits immunoglobulin secretion. J Exp Med 175:597
50. Tokunaga T, Yamamoto H, Shimada S, Abe H, Fukuda T, Fujisawa Y, Furutani Y, Yano O, Kataoka T, Sudo T, Makiguchi N, Suganuma T (1984) Antitumor activity of deoxyribonucleic acid fraction from *Mycobacterium bovis* BCG. I. Isolation, physicochemical characterization, and antitumor activity. JNCI 72:955
51. Tonkinson JL, Stein CA (1994) Patterns of intracellular compartmentalization, trafficking and acidification of 5'-fluorescein labeled phosphodiester and phosphorothioate oligodeoxynucleotides in HL60 cells. Nucleic Acids Res 22:4268
52. Yakubov LA, Deeva EA, Zarytova VF, Ivanova EM, Ryte AS, Yurchenko LV, Vlassov VV (1989) Mechanism of oligonucleotide uptake by cells: involvement of specific receptors? Proc Natl Acad Sci USA 86:6454
53. Yamamoto S, Yamamoto T, Shimada S, Kuramoto E, Yano O, Kataoka T, Tokunaga T (1992) DNA from bacteria, but not from vertebrates, induces interferons, activates natural killer cells and inhibits tumor growth. Microbiol Immunol 36:983
54. Yamamoto T, Yamamoto S, Kataoka T, Tokunaga T (1994) Lipofection of synthetic oligodeoxyribonucleotide having a palindromic sequence of AACGTT to murine splenocytes enhances interferon production and natural killer activity. Microbiol Immunol 38:831
55. Yi A-K, Chace JH, Cowdery JS, Krieg AM (1996) IFN-γ promotes IL-6 and IgM secretion in response to CpG motifs in bacterial DNA and oligodeoxynucleotides. J Immunol 156:558
56. Yi A-K, Chang M, Peckham DW, Krieg AM, Ashman RF (1998) CpG oligodeoxyribonucleotides rescue mature spleen B cells from spontaneous apoptosis and promote cell cycle entry. J Immunol 160:5898
57. Yi A-K, Hornbeck P, Lafrenz DE, Krieg AM (1996) CpG DNA rescue of murine B lymphoma cells from anti-IgM induced growth arrest and programmed cell death is associated with increased expression of c-myc and bcl-xL. J Immunol 157:4918
58. Yi A-K, Klinman DM, Martin TL, Matson S, Krieg AM (1996) Rapid immune activation by CpG motifs in bacterial DNA: systemic induction of IL-6 transcription through an antioxidant-sensitive pathway. J Immunol 157:5394

59. Yi A-K, Krieg AM (1998) CpG DNA rescue from anti-IgM induced WEHI-231 B lymphoma apoptosis via modulation of IκBα and IκBβ and sustained activation of nuclear factor-κB/c-Rel. J Immunol 160:1240
60. Yi A-K, Krieg AM (1998) Rapid induction of mitogen activated protein kinases by immune stimulatory CpG DNA. J Immunol 161:4493
61. Yi A-K, Tuetken R, Redford T, Kirsch J, Krieg AM (1998) CpG motifs in bacterial DNA activate leukocytes through the pH-dependent generation of reactive oxygen species. J Immunol 160:4755
62. Zhao Q, Matson S, Herrara CJ, Fisher E, Yu H, Waggoner A, Krieg AM (1993) Comparison of cellular binding and uptake of antisense phosphodiester, phosphorothioate, and mixed phosphorothioate and methylphosphonate oligonucleotides. Antisense Res Dev 3:53
63. Zhao Q, Song X, Waldschmidt T, Fisher E, Krieg AM (1996) Oligonucleotide uptake in human hematopoietic cells is increased in leukemia and is related to cellular activation. Blood 88:1788
64. Zhao Q, Temsamani J, Zhou R-Z, Agrawal S (1997) Pattern and kinetics of cytokine production following administration of phosphorothioate oligonucleotides in mice. Antisense Nucleic Acid Drug Dev 7:495
65. Zimmerman S, Egeter O, Hausmann S, Lipford GB, Rocken M, Wagner H, Geeg K (1998) Cutting edge: CpG oligodeoxynucleotides trigger protective and curative Th1 responses in lethal murine *leishmaniasis*. J Immunol 160:3627

Immunostimulatory DNA sequences and cancer therapy

George J. Weiner

University of Iowa Cancer Center, Department of Internal Medicine,
Interdisciplinary Graduate Program in Immunology, 200 Hawkins Drive,
5970 JPP, Iowa City, IA 52242, USA

Introduction

The ability to induce regression of malignant tumors through the stimulation of the immune system has been a goal for decades. Indeed, the first attempts to treat cancer using nonspecific immune stimulants as well as immunization with tumor cells and tumor extracts took place soon after immunization was found to be effective for infectious diseases. Although therapeutic responses to cancer were occasionally reported, such positive results were rare, usually transient and almost always unreproducible. We now understand that most tumors fail to regress following nonspecific immunostimulation. It is also difficult to break tolerance and induce an antigen-specific immune response against self-antigens such as those expressed by tumors. Nevertheless, it is clear in animal models that enhanced innate immunity or induction of antigen-specific immunity can have significant antitumor effects. Clinical trials suggest effective cancer immunotherapy should be possible in patients as well, although we still have much to learn about inducing antitumor immunity without causing unacceptable toxicity. Immunostimulatory DNA Sequences also known as CpG DNA, are one class of compounds that have shown promise in recent years as potent immunostimulatory agents. Preclinical studies suggest they may be useful cancer immunotherapeutic agents. In this chapter the potential of this new class of immunostimulatory agents as cancer therapies with be reviewed.

We continue to learn more about the complex immunologic effects of Immunostimulatory DNA at both the molecular and cellular level. These findings are outlined elsewhere in this volume and will not be discussed here. Instead, we will focus on a number of promising approaches to cancer immunotherapy and how Immunostimulatory DNA might play a role in these approaches. Although the data reviewed below are promising, it is important to point out that evaluation of Immunostimulatory DNA as a cancer therapy is only beginning and no clinical trials have been performed to date. In some cases, there is little or no direct experimental data to support the proposed hypotheses. Thus, much of the discussion that follows is based on indirect evidence and conjecture. Nevertheless, we believe our current understanding of the immune response to tumors, combined with a growing knowledge of the immunologic effects of Immunostimulatory DNA, is enough to warrant discussion of Immunostimulatory DNA as a potential component of cancer therapy.

Immunostimulatory DNA can impact on both innate immunity and induction of an antigen-specific immune response. Approaches discussed below are divided into those that involve innate immunity and nonspecific antitumor activity, and those that involve the development of an active, antigen-specific anti-tumor response. Specifically, potential uses of Immunostimulatory DNA in the treatment of cancer include the following:

1.) Use of Immunostimulatory DNA to enhance innate immunity and increase:
    a) NK-mediated lysis
    b) Antibody dependent cellular cytotoxicity (ADCC)
    c) Adoptive cellular immunotherapy
2.) Use of Immunostimulatory DNA to enhance development of an antigen-specific immune response through
    a) Immunization with tumor-associated antigens
    b) DNA immunization
    c) In vitro activation of antigen-presenting cells.

Innate immunity

The first reported systematic attempt to utilize nonspecific immune stimulation as a therapy for cancer took place in the 1890s when Dr. William Coley, a New York surgeon, performed a series of studies evaluating the antitumor activity of bacteria and bacterial products. Dr. Coley initially injected live streptococci directly into the tumor masses of his patients [10]. This resulted in tumor regression in some cases but proved to be toxic. Indeed, the first patient treated in this manner almost died of erysipelas. In subsequent studies, Coley used a mixture of heat-killed gram-positive and gram-negative organisms [11]. This preparation, known as "Coley's toxin", was non-infectious but still was associated with severe toxicity. Some patients experienced tumor regression, although the response rate was less than that seen with live organisms. We now believe that much of the antitumor activity of Coley's toxin was due to endotoxin [58]. However, Coley's original success was with streptococcus that does not produce endotoxin. Additional bacterial components, such as bacterial DNA, may well have played a role in the observed responses.

The therapeutic effect of Coley's toxin was likely due to production of a number of cytokines. Many of these cytokines are now available in recombinant form, and are known to have anti-tumor effects in vitro and in animal models. A number of such cytokines have undergone clinical evaluation as antitumor agents [22] where they have clear, although limited, antitumor activity [29, 47]. Such studies demonstrate that nonspecific cancer immunotherapy can be effective. Unfortunately, the limited extent of clinical responses and significant toxicity has limited the role recombinant cytokines play in the treatment of cancer.

Immunostimulatory DNA are capable of inducing production of a number of the cytokines that, individually, have anti-tumor activity, including tumor necrosis factor-α (TNF-α), interleukin-12 (IL-12) and IFN-γ [2, 12, 33]. As detailed elsewhere in this volume, Immunostimulatory DNA also have direct effects on immune cell subpopulations that play an important role in antitumor immunity including natural killer (NK) cells [2], B cells [30], monocytes and macrophages [6, 52], dendritic cells [21, 27, 34], and possibly T cells [32]. The immune response normally involves the integrated production of a variety of cytokines that work in concert both locally and systemically. It is rational to hypothesize that agents, such as Immunostimulatory DNA, that are able to orchestrate the production of cytokines by the host both temporally and spatially will be more effective at inducing an antitumor response than individual recombinant cytokines.

NK-mediated lysis

Systemic administration of Immunostimulatory DNA alone can have antitumor effects that appear to be related to enhanced NK activity. Smith and Wickstrom [51] used a murine model of lymphoma to evaluate the antitumor effects of an antisense phosphorothioate DNA designed to block the c-*myc* oncogene. Both antisense DNA and control sequences inhibited tumor growth. Further investigation demonstrated that the immunostimulatory effect of the DNA, and not antisense activity, was responsible for the observed antitumor effects. Ballas et al. (manuscript in preparation) have found Immunostimulatory DNA inhibits the growth of B16 melanoma cells in both immunocompetent and severe combined immunodeficiency mice that lack T or B cells but retain NK function. Removing NK cells eliminated the antitumor response. We have found similar results with the EL4 T-cell lymphoma. Taken together, these results suggest that innate immunity stimulated by Immunostimulatory DNA can have significant antitumor effects in select animal models, and that NK activity plays a key role in this response. While toxicity from Immunostimulatory DNA in these and other animal models has been limited, toxicity from nonspecific anti-cancer therapy often limits clinical efficacy. Clinical trials currently being planned are needed to determine whether Immunostimulatory DNA used to stimulate the innate immune system have promise in the treatment of cancer.

Antibody-dependent cellular cytotoxicity

Enhancement of the innate immune system can be used to increase antitumor activity in a more specific manner if used in combination with agents that allow for tumor targeting. The most logical approach to such combination therapy is to combine Immunostimulatory DNA, which activate NK cells and monocytes/macrophages, with antitumor monoclonal antibodies. Recent advances, such as humanization of monoclonal antibodies, have led to the demonstration that this class of agents has significant clinical antitumor activity in a number of tumor types including lymphoma and breast carcinoma [39, 44]. Despite this success, there continues to be significant room for improvement. Although the mechanisms responsible for the clinical response to antitumor antibody therapy are not yet clear, ADCC mediated by NK cells and monocytes/macrophages likely plays a large role.

A variety of cytokines known to activate cells responsible for ADCC have been evaluated for their ability to enhance the antitumor effects of unlabeled antibody. For example, IL-2 was shown to be modestly effective at enhancing the antitumor activity of antitumor antibody in a mouse lymphoma model [4]. This approach is now being evaluated in clinical trials. Immunostimulatory DNA activate both NK cells and macrophages. They, therefore, would be expected to enhance the efficacy of antibody by increasing effector cell killing of antibody-coated tumor cells. Indeed, we found that Immunostimulatory DNA-activated murine splenocytes or human peripheral blood lymphocytes mediate ADCC more effectively than do unactivated lymphocytes. In vivo, Immunostimulatory DNA alone had no effect on survival of mice inoculated with the 38C13 murine B cell lymphoma. However, a single injection of Immunostimulatory DNA enhanced the antitumor response to antitumor antibody therapy. These antitumor effects were less pronounced when treatment consisted of an identical DNA containing methylated cytosines. The combination of antibody plus a single dose of Immunostimulatory DNA was more effective than antibody with multiple doses of IL-2 at inhibiting tumor growth [59]. More recently, we have found that repeated doses of antibody plus Immunostimulatory DNA can eliminate tumor load estimated to be 30-fold greater than can antibody alone (manuscript in preparation). Thus, use of Immunostimulatory DNA to enhance the efficacy of antibody therapy remains promising. A clinical trial designed to assess this possibility is currently being planned.

Adoptive cellular immunotherapy

Another approach to using the immune system to treat cancer involves infusion of ex vivo activated cells, sometimes referred to as "adoptive immunotherapy". In the 1980s, development of recombinant cytokines, such as IL-2, allowed for the ex vivo expansion and evaluation both in vitro and in vivo of various populations of lymphocytes. Cells from the peripheral blood expanded in this manner were called "lymphokine-activated killer" or LAK cells and had significant in vitro tumoricidal activity. Although initial clinical trials using LAK cells were promising [22], large doses of cytokines were needed to achieve activity, and these resulted in significant toxicity. In addition, LAK cells expanded from the peripheral blood were not tumor specific and did not migrate well to tumor [3]. Nevertheless, some clinical responses were observed, and ongoing studies are exploring approaches to overcome these problems. Much of the antitumor activity observed with LAK cells appears to be due to NK activity. Thus, Immunostimulatory DNA that activate NK cells could play a role in adoptive immunotherapy approaches.

A related approach designed to select tumor-specific T cells is to use "tumor-infiltrating lymphocytes", or TILs, obtained from the tumor mass itself and expanded in vitro using cytokines. Despite enhanced specificity in vitro, clinical trials of TILs have demonstrated little anti-tumor activity [50]. Although TILs are harvested from the tumor mass, many appear to be bystander cells that are not truly specific for the tumor. There is also evidence that the signaling pathways in TILs are abnormal, likely due to the cytokine environment within the tumor mass, which limits the cytotoxic capabilities of TILs [15].

The direct effect of Immunostimulatory DNA on T cells remains controversial. In studies using highly purified T cells, Lipford et al. [32] found that Immunostimulatory DNA enhances proliferation of T cells when the T cell receptor is engaged, suggesting that Immunostimulatory DNA are capable of supplying a co-stimulatory signal directly to the T cell. Ongoing studies are exploring the effect of Immunostimulatory DNA on T cell activation and whether such an effect can be used to enhance T cell-mediated lysis of tumors using TILs or other T cell populations.

Tumor-specific response

While vaccination for infectious diseases has had a major impact on worldwide public health, development of cancer vaccines has been more difficult. Recent advances in the field of immunology are allowing us to understand the challenges associated with development of safe and effective cancer vaccines. Perhaps most challenging is the need to break immune tolerance against an antigen that will allow an immune response strong enough to induce tumor cell destruction [17, 23, 53]. There is now solid evidence that Immunostimulatory DNA can function as immune adjuvants and enhance development of an active immune response when administered with antigen. A number of strategies utilizing Immunostimulatory DNA in cancer vaccination are now being explored.

Immunization with tumor-associated antigens

Tumor-associated antigens have been identified that can serve as acceptable, although not ideal, targets for cancer immunization. The idiotype (Id) expressed by B cell malignancies is one such antigen [26]. A number of proteins associated with melanoma that are relatively tumor specific have also been identified [38]. Other antigens that also serve as tumor markers, such as carcinoembryonic antigen [45] and prostate-specific antigen [24], are also showing early promise as targets for immunization.

Debate continues as to whether a humoral or a cellular antitumor response is most desirable when designing cancer immunization strategies targeted against these and other antigens. Induction of an antibody response is used as an indication of successful immunization in many of the cancer-vaccine studies completed to date. This is based in large part on the relative ease of quantitating the antibody response compared to the cellular response. There is also evidence that the ability to induce a humoral response following immunization can correlate with clinical outcome [35]. However, numerous solid-tumor animal models demonstrate that a cellular immune response is required to induce a significant antitumor response. Overall, there is now general agreement that, for most solid tumors, induction of a potent antitumor cellular response will be required.

Unfortunately, immune adjuvants used most extensively enhance the T helper 2 (Th2) response, and so do not markedly enhance cellular immunity. Aluminum hydroxide is used in many commercial vaccine preparations and has been shown to actually block activation of $CD8^+$ cytotoxic T lymphocytes (CTLs) in mice immunized against hepatitis B surface antigen (HBsAg) [35]. Other adjuvants that induce more of a Th1 response are currently being evaluated in both pre-clinical and clinical studies [1]. These include threonyl-muryl dipeptide [26], a variety of attenuated or killed bacteria [1, 7] and bacterial derivatives [28], BCG [40] and *Quillaja saponaria* 21 (QS21) [35]. Each of these, particularly QS21, has shown some efficacy and promise. However, none is ideal due to toxicity (including both systemic toxicity and local inflammation after repeated immunization), minimal efficacy at stimulating a cellular response or difficulties associated with production. Thus, new adjuvants are needed for vaccine approaches designed to enhance the Th1 response.

Synthetic oligodeoxynucleotides containing Immunostimulatory DNA are particularly attractive as adjuvants for tumor-antigen immunization because of their ease of production and ability to induce a Th1 response. Preliminary studies also suggest minimal toxicity. In a number of murine systems, Immunostimulatory DNA have been evaluated as immune adjuvants and shown to be effective. Although the studies outlined below were not all performed in tumor models, they do point to the promise of Immunostimulatory DNA as adjuvants in immunization with protein and peptide tumor antigens. Using hen-egg lysozyme (HEL) as a model antigen, Chu et al. [8] found that immunization in incomplete Freund's adjuvant (IFA) resulted in Th2-dominated immune response characterized by HEL-specific secretion of Th2 cytokines (i.e. IL-5 but not IFN-γ). In contrast, immunization with HEL and Immunostimulatory DNA switched the immune response to a Th1-dominated cytokine pattern (high levels of IFN-γ and decreased IL-5). Immunostimulatory DNA also enhanced production of anti-HEL IgG2a (a Th1-associated isotype) when compared with IFA-HEL. This Th1 response was more marked than that seen with complete Freund's adjuvant (CFA) despite a lack of local inflammation. Davis et al. [13] also found a marked increase in antigen-specific IgG and IgG2a using HBsAg as the immunogen. Importantly, they also found Immunostimulatory DNA enhanced development of an HBsAg-specific cytotoxic T cell response. Lipford et al. [32] found a similar humoral and cellular response using ovalbumin as the target antigen.

Our studies utilized the Id from the 38C13 murine lymphoma model as the target antigen. Immunostimulatory DNA were as effective as CFA at inducing an antigen-specific antibody response, and were associated with less toxicity. As in the studies outlined above, Immunostimulatory DNA induced a higher titer of antigen-specific IgG2a than CFA. Therapeutically, mice immunized with Immunostimulatory DNA as an adjuvant and Id-keyhole limpet hemocyanin (KLH) as the immunogen were protected from tumor challenge to a degree similar to that seen in mice immunized with CFA and Id-KLH, but with less toxicity [57]. We also found synergy between Immunostimulatory DNA and granulocyte-monocyte colony-stimulating factor (GM-CSF). Immunization using antigen (Id)/GM-CSF fusion protein and Immunostimulatory DNA resulted in remarkable levels of anti-Id, and shifted production towards the IgG2a isotype. This effect was most pronounced after repeat immunizations with Immunostimulatory DNA and Id/GM-CSF fusion protein. A single immunization with Immunostimulatory DNA and Id/GM-CSF fusion protein 3 days prior to tumor inoculation prevented tumor growth, whereas other approaches to vaccination in this model are ineffective under those conditions [34].

Studies in these varied systems indicate that Immunostimulatory DNA enhances an antigen-specific Th1 response after immunization with soluble protein antigen and can lead to development of antigen-specific cellular immunity. Immunostimulatory DNA function at least as well as standard adjuvants such as CFA and have a limited toxicity. Perhaps most importantly, Immunostimulatory DNA are superior at inducing a therapeutic effect. Studies that compare Immunostimulatory DNA to the other adjuvants outlined above are ongoing in animal models to determine whether synergy exists between these adjuvants, as are studies to determine the efficacy of Immunostimulatory DNA as an adjuvant in humans.

DNA immunization

According to classic immunologic teaching, intracellular proteins are processed and presented by MHC class I molecules, and this leads to a cellular immune response. In contrast, extracellular antigens are taken into the cell and presented by MHC class II molecules, which leads to a humoral response. It is now accepted that there is cross-talk between the class I and class II pathways, with some extracellular antigens taken up by antigen-presenting cells (APCs) and processed in a manner that leads to presentation in class I molecules and development of a CTL response [46]. The results outlined above support the concept that such "cross-priming" takes place. In these systems, an effective cellular response can be induced by immunization with an intact tumor antigen plus Immunostimulatory DNA, that activate cells that can process exogenous antigen and present peptides derived from these proteins by MHC class I molecules [13].

Although individual Immunostimulatory DNA differ somewhat in their ability to activate various immune cell populations and induce cytokine production in human and murine systems, it is now clear that both human and murine leukocytes respond to this novel pathway of immune activation [31]. It is important to note that Immunostimulatory DNA are only now being evaluated as immune adjuvants in humans.

In vitro activation of APCs

While it is unclear whether Immunostimulatory DNA can impact directly on T cell activation, there is no doubt that these agents can enhance T cell activity indirectly by APCs and improving antigen presentation. This concept fits well with the recent focus of adoptive immunotherapy studies on the use of APCs to induce an active immune response in the host. Among the most promising recent cancer-immunotherapy studies are those involving dendritic cells (DCs), which are extremely potent APCs [18, 37, 42]. Of particular interest is the ability of DCs to induce a cellular immune response [19, 20, 41, 54]. Levy and colleagues [25] have demonstrated induction of an antigen-specific cellular response following treatment with antigen-pulsed DCs in a small clinical trial. This was in stark contrast to the studies, reported by the same group, which demonstrated that immunization of patients with Id-KLH leads to an intense humoral response [43]. Of particular interest is the suggestion of prolonged survival in the small number of patients treated with Id-pulsed DCs [26].

Immunostimulatory DNA have profound effects and enhance the ability of some subpopulations of DCs to present antigen and induce an antigen-specific cellular response. Sparwasser et al. [52] have shown that Immunostimulatory DNA induces maturation of immature DC obtained from murine bone marrow and activates mature DC to produce cytokines, including IL-12, IL-6 and TNF-α. Jakob et al. [27] found that treatment of DCs derived from murine fetal skin decreased E-cadherin-mediated adhesion, up-regulated MHC class II and co-stimulatory molecules and enhanced accessory cell activity. Injection of Immunostimulatory DNA into murine dermis led to enhanced expression of MHC class II and CD86 by Langerhans' cells [27]. We also found that Immunostimulatory DNA markedly enhances the production of cytokines, including IL-12, from DCs derived from murine bone-marrow using GM-CSF and IL-4 [34]. In addition, Immunostimulatory DNA can enhance the survival, maturation and differentiation of primary human DCs isolated from the peripheral blood, but had little impact on monocyte-derived DCs [21].

Clearly, DCs do not represent a single population of cells. The ideal source of DCs or approach to in vitro expansion, activation, exposure to antigen or re-infusion has yet to be determined. In addition, further studies are needed to determine the potentially important role of Immunostimulatory DNA in activating this cell population.

Another area of intense interest in the field of cancer immunotherapy is the use of DNA immunization using DNA constructs containing sequences that encode for the antigen of interest [9, 53, 56]. The intent of such therapy is to have host cells take up the DNA, produce protein based on the infused DNA, and express peptides derived from that protein in host class I, thereby inducing a cellular immune response directed towards that antigen. Although initial thoughts were that any cells (such as myocytes) could perform these functions, there is now evidence that professional APCs are involved [14, 16]. Irrespective of which cells are responsible, this approach has been evaluated with some success in tumor models [55]. Sato et al. [48] found that human monocytes transfected with plasmid DNA or double-stranded oligonucleotides containing Immunostimulatory DNA transcribed larger amounts of IFN-α, IFN-β, and IL-12 when compared with cells transfected with DNA that did not contain such sequences. Modifying the Immunostimulatory DNA content of vectors intended for DNA immunization can have a significant impact on their ability to induce development of a cellular response [5]. The ability to construct vectors that encode for a specific protein and enhance a Th1 response to peptides derived from that protein would have clear implications in the area of tumor vaccination. This exciting approach to immunization is reviewed in more detail elsewhere in this volume.

Conclusions

The relationship between the immune system and malignancy is extremely complex. Recent advances in our understanding of this interaction, and the success of select monoclonal antibody treatments of cancer, have reawakened interest in the field of cancer immunotherapy. Recent recognition of the potent immunostimulatory effects of select sequences of DNA suggest that such agents may well be important if cancer immunotherapy is to play a major role in our treatment and prevention of malignancy. Preliminary studies suggest these sequences can be effective, alone or in combination with antibodies, at inducing tumor regression. Perhaps even more promising is their ability to enhance development of an antigen-specific antitumor response when used as a vaccine adjuvant, as an agent capable of stimulating APCs or as part of DNA immunization strategy. Further work with Immunostimulatory DNA in both the laboratory and the clinic is needed before we can know their true promise in cancer therapy.

References

1. Baldridge JR, Ward JR (1997) Effective adjuvants for the induction of antigen-specific delayed type hypersensitivity. Vaccine 15:395
2. Ballas ZK, Rasmussen WL, Krieg AM (1996) Induction of NK activity in murine and human cells by CpG motifs in oligodeoxynucleotides and bacterial DNA. J Immunol 157:1840
3. Basse PH (1995) Tissue distribution and tumor localization of effector cells in adoptive immunotherapy of cancer. APMIS Suppl 55:1
4. Berinstein N, Levy R (1987) Treatment of a murine B-cell lymphoma with monoclonal antibodies and IL-2. J Immunol 139:971
5. Brazolot Millan CL, Weeratna R, Krieg AM, Siegrist C A, Davis HL (1998) CpG DNA can induce strong Th1 humoral and cell-mediated immune responses against hepatitis B surface antigen in young mice. Proc Natl Acad Sci USA 15553
6. Chace JH, Hooker NA, Mildenstein KL, Krieg AM, Cowdery JS (1997) Bacterial DNA-induced NK cell IFN-gamma production is dependent on macrophage secretion of IL-12. Clin Immunol Immunopathol 84:185
7. Chen HY, Wu SL, Yeh MY, Chen CF, Mikami Y, Wu JS (1993) Antimetastatic activity induced by *Clostridium butyricum* and characterization of effector cells. Anticancer Res 13:107
8. Chu RS, Targoni OS, Krieg AM, Lehmann PV, Harding CV (1997) CpG oligodeoxynucleotides act as adjuvants that switch on T helper 1 (Th1) immunity. J Exp Med 186:1623
9. Cohen AD, Boyer JD, Weiner DB (1998) Modulating the immune response to genetic immunization. FASEB J 12:1611
10. Coley WB (1893) The treatment of malignant tumors by repeated inoculations of *Erysipelas* with a report of ten original cases. Am J Med Sci 105:487
11. Coley WB (1894) Treatment of inoperable malignant tumors with the toxins of *Erysipelas* and the bacillus *Prodigiosus*. Am J Med Sci 108:183
12. Cowdery JS, Chace JH, Yi AK, Krieg AM (1996) Bacterial DNA induces NK cells to produce IFN-γ in vivo and increases the toxicity of lipopolysaccharides. J Immunol 156:4570

13. Davis HL, Weeratna R, Waldschmidt TJ, Tygrett L, Schorr J, Krieg AM (1998) CpG DNA is a potent adjuvant in mice immunized with recombinant hepatitis B surface antigen. J Immunol 160:870
14. Doe B, Selby M, Barnett S, Baenziger J, Walker CM (1996) Induction of cytotoxic T lymphocytes by intramuscular immunization with plasmid DNA is facilitated by bone marrow-derived cells. Proc Natl Acad Sci USA 93:8578
15. Finke JH, Zea AH, Stanley J, Longo DL, Mizoguchi H, Tubbs RR, Wiltrout RH, Oshea JJ, Kudoh S, Klein E, Bukowski RM, Ochoa AC (1993) Loss of T-cell receptor ζ-chain and p56(lck) in T-cells infiltrating human renal cell carcinoma. Cancer Res 53:5613
16. Fu TM, Ulmer JB, Caulfield MJ, Deck RR, Friedman A, Wang S, Liu X, Donnelly JJ, Liu MA (1997) Priming of cytotoxic T lymphocytes by DNA vaccines: requirement for professional antigen presenting cells and evidence for antigen transfer from myocytes. Mol Med 3:362
17. Gilboa E (1996) Immunotherapy of cancer with genetically modified tumor vaccines. Semin Oncol 23:101
18. Gilboa E, Nair SK, Lyerly HK (1998) Immunotherapy of cancer with dendritic-cell-based vaccines. Cancer Immunol Immunother 46:82
19. Girolomoni G, Ricciardi-Castagnoli P (1997) Dendritic cells hold promise for immunotherapy. Immunol Today 18:102
20. Hamblin TJ (1996) From dendritic cells to tumour vaccines. Lancet 34:7705
21. Hartmann G, Weiner GJ, Krieg AM (1999) CpG DNA: A potent signal for growth, activation, and maturation of human dendritic cells. Proc Natl Acad Sci USA 96:9305
22. Heaton KM, Grimm EA (1993) Cytokine combinations in immunotherapy for solid tumors – a review. Cancer Immunol Immunother 37:213
23. Hellstrom KE, Gladstone P, Hellstrom I (1997) Cancer vaccines – challenges and potential solutions. Mol Med Today 3:286
24. Hodge JW, Schlom J, Donohue SJ, Tomaszewski JE, Wheeler CW, Levine BS, Gritz L, Panicali D, Kantor JA (1995) A recombinant vaccinia virus expressing human prostate-specific antigen (PSA): safety and immunogenicity in a non-human primate. Int J Cancer 63:231
25. Hsu FJ, Benike C, Fagnoni F, Liles TM, Czerwinski D, Taidi B, Engleman EG, Levy R (1996) Vaccination of patients with B-cell lymphoma using autologous antigen-pulsed dendritic cells. Nat Med 2:52
26. Hsu FJ, Caspar CB, Czerwinski D, Kwak LW, Liles T, Syrengelas A, Taidi-Laskowski A, Levy R (1997) Tumor-specific idiotype vaccines in the treatment of patients with B-cell lymphoma – long term results of a clinical trial. Blood 89:3129
27. Jakob T, Walker PS, Krieg AM, Udey MC, Vogel JC (1998) Activation of cutaneous dendritic cells by CpG-containing oligodeoxynucleotides: a role for dendritic cells in the augmentation of Th1 responses by immunostimulatory DNA. J Immunol 161:3042
28. Johnston D, Bystryn JC (1991) Effect of cell wall skeleton and monophosphoryl lipid A adjuvant on the immunogenicity of a murine B16 melanoma vaccine. J Nat Cancer Inst 83:1240
29. Kantarjian HM, Giles FJ, O'Brien SM, Talpaz M (1998) Clinical course and therapy of chronic myelogenous leukemia with interferon-alpha and chemotherapy. Hematol Oncol Clin North Am 12:31
30. Krieg AM, Yi AK, Matson S, Waldschmidt TJ, Bishop GA, Teasdale R, Koretzky GA, Klinman DM (1995) CpG motifs in bacterial DNA trigger direct B-cell activation. Nature 374:546
31. Krieg AM, Matson S, Fisher E (1996) Oligodeoxynucleotide modifications determine the magnitude of B cell stimulation by CpG motifs. Antisense Nucleic Acid Drug Dev 6:133
32. Lipford GB, Bauer M, Blank C, Reiter R, Wagner H, Heeg K (1997) CpG-containing synthetic oligonucleotides promote B and cytotoxic T cell responses to protein antigen: a new class of vaccine adjuvants. Eur J Immunol 27:2340
33. Lipford GB, Sparwasser T, Bauer M, Zimmermann S, Koch ES, Heeg K, Wagner H (1997) Immunostimulatory DNA: sequence-dependent production of potentially harmful or useful cytokines. Eur J Immunol 27:3420
34. Liu HM, Newbrough SE, Bhatia SK, Dahle CE, Krieg AM, Weiner GJ (1998) Immunostimulatory CpG oligodeoxynucleotides enhance the immune response to vaccine strategies involving granulocyte-macrophage colony-stimulating factor. Blood 92:3730
35. Livingston P (1998) Ganglioside vaccines with emphasis on GM2. Semin Oncol 25:636
36. Lotze MT, Rosenberg SA (1986) Results of clinical trials with the administration of interleukin 2 and adoptive immunotherapy with activated cells in patients with cancer. Immunobiology 172:420
37. Lotze MT, Shurin M, Davis I, Amoscato A, Storkus WJ (1997) Dendritic cell based therapy of cancer. Adv Exp Med Biol 417:551

38. Maeurer MJ, Storkus WJ, Kirkwood JM, Lotze MT (1996) New treatment options for patients with melanoma: review of melanoma-derived T-cell epitope-based peptide vaccines. Melanoma Res 6:11
39. Maloney DG, Grillo-lopez AJ, White CA, Bodkin D, Schilder RJ, Neidhart JA, Janakiraman N, Foon KA, Liles TM, Dallaire BK, Wey K, Royston I, Davis T, Levy R (1997) Idec-C2b8 (Rituximab) anti-Cd20 monoclonal antibody therapy patients with relapsed low-grade non-Hodgkin's lymphoma. Blood 90:2188
40. Mastrangelo MJ, Maguire HC Jr, Sato T, Nathan FE, Berd D (1996) Active specific immunization in the treatment of patients with melanoma. Semin Oncol 23:773
41. McCann J (1997) Immunotherapy using dendritic cells picks up steam. J Nat Cancer Institute 89:541
42. Morse MA, Lyerly HK (1998) Immunotherapy of cancer using dendritic cells. Cytokines Cell Mol Ther 4:35
43. Nelson EL, Li XB, Hsu FJ, Kwak LW, Levy R, Clayberger C, Krensky AM (1996) Tumor-specific, cytotoxic T-lymphocyte response after idiotype vaccination for B-cell, non-Hodgkin's lymphoma. Blood 88:580
44. Pegram MD, Lipton A, Hayes DF, Weber BL, Baselga JM, Tripathy D, Baly D, Baughman SA, Twaddell T, Glaspy JA, Slamon DJ (1998) Phase II study of receptor-enhanced chemosensitivity using recombinant humanized anti-p185HER2/neu monoclonal antibody plus cisplatin in patients with HER2/neu-overexpressing metastatic breast cancer refractory to chemotherapy treatment. J Clin Oncol 16:2659
45. Pervin S, Chakraborty M, Bhattacharya-Chatterjee M, Zeytin H, Foon KA, Chatterjee SK (1997) Induction of antitumor immunity by an anti-idiotype antibody mimicking carcinoembryonic antigen. Cancer Res 57:728
46. Rock KL (1996) A new foreign policy: MHC class I molecules monitor the outside world. Immunol Today 17:131
47. Rosenberg SA, Mule JJ, Spiess PJ, Reichert CM, Schwarz SL (1985) Regression of established pulmonary metastases and subcutaneous tumor mediated by the systemic administration of high-dose recombinant interleukin 2. J Exp Med 161:1169
48. Sato Y, Roman M, Tighe H, Lee D, Corr M, Nguyen MD, Silverman GJ, Lotz M, Carson DA, Raz E (1996) Immunostimulatory DNA sequences necessary for effective intradermal gene immunization. Science 273:352
49. Schirmbeck R, Melber K, Kuhrober A, Janowicz ZA, Reimann J (1994) Immunization with soluble hepatitis B virus surface protein elicits murine H-2 class I-restricted $CD8^+$ cytotoxic T-lymphocyte responses in vivo. J Immunol 152:1110
50. Schwartzentruber DJ, Hom SS, Dadmarz R, White DE, Yannelli JR, Steinberg SM, Rosenberg SA, Topalian SL (1994) In vitro predictors of therapeutic response in melanoma patients receiving tumor-infiltrating lymphocytes and interleukin-2. J Clin Oncol 12:1475
51. Smith JB, Wickstrom E (1998) Antisense c-myc and immunostimulatory oligonucleotide inhibition of tumorigenesis in a murine B-cell lymphoma transplant model. J Natl Cancer Inst 90:1146
52. Sparwasser T, Koch ES, Vabulas RM, Heeg K, Lipford GB, Ellwart JW, Wagner H (1998) Bacterial DNA and immunostimulatory CpG oligonucleotides trigger maturation and activation of murine dendritic cells. Eur J Immunol 28:2045
53. Spooner RA, Deonarain MP, Epenetos AA (1995) DNA vaccination for cancer treatment. Gene Ther 2:173
54. Steinman RM (1996) Dendritic cells and immune-based therapies. Exp Hematol 24:859
55. Syrengelas AD, Chen TT, Levy R (1996) DNA immunization induces protective immunity against B-cell lymphoma. Nat Med 2:1038
56. Ulmer JB, Donnelly JJ, Liu MA (1996) Toward the development of DNA vaccines. Curr Opin Biotechnol 7:653
57. Weiner GJ, Liu HM, Wooldridge JE, Dahle CE, Krieg AM (1997) Immunostimulatory oligodeoxynucleotides containing the CpG motif are effective as immune adjuvants in tumor antigen immunization. Proc Natl Acad Sci USA 94:10833
58. Wiemann B, Starnes CO (1994) Coley's toxins, tumor necrosis factor and cancer research: a historical perspective. Pharmacol Ther 64:529
59. Wooldridge JE, Ballas Z, Krieg AM, Weiner GJ (1997) Immunostimulatory oligodeoxynucleotides containing CpG motifs enhance the efficacy of monoclonal antibody therapy of lymphoma. Blood 89:2994

Modulation of asthmatic response by immunostimulatory DNA sequences

David Broide, Jae Youn Cho, Marina Miller, Jyothi Nayar, Greg Stachnick, Diego Castaneda, Mark Roman, Eyal Raz

Department of Medicine, University of California San Diego, Basic Science Building, Room 5090, 9500 Gilman Drive, La Jolla, CA 92093-0635, USA

Current understanding of the pathogenesis of allergic asthma

Asthma is a common disease in the USA affecting approximately 5% of the population. The expression of the allergic asthma phenotype is dependent upon both host genetic factors as well as environmental allergen exposure to inhalant allergens such as house dust mite, cat, grass pollen, and cockroach. Progress in identifying the genes involved in asthma has been assisted by both population-based genetic studies as well as candidate gene approaches. Population-based whole genome wide screen studies in asthmatics have identified linkage to multiple chromosome regions including chromosomes 5q, 6p, 11q, 12q, 13q, and 16q [6, 21], suggesting that multiple genes are associated with the asthma phenotype. Several candidate genes on chromosome 5q (IL-4, IL-5, IL-9, IL-13, β2 adrenergic receptor, corticosteroid receptor), chromosome 11 (beta chain of the high-affinity IgE receptor), chromosome 12 (stem cell factor, IFN-γ, insulin growth factor, and Stat 6), and chromosome 16 (IL-4 receptor) may contribute to asthma and allergy development [6, 21]. In addition, involvement of genes associated with antigen presentation (MHC class II genes) and T cell responses (T cell receptor α chain) have been linked to asthma. These initial genetic studies suggest a complex relationship between genetic susceptibility to asthma, bronchial hyperresponsiveness, and allergic inflammation.

The characteristic features of asthma include airway inflammation, bronchial hyperresponsiveness, and the development of reversible airway obstruction. The inflammatory and immune response associated with allergic asthma has several characteristic features including prominent infiltration of the airways with eosinophils [2, 3] and Th2-type lymphocytes [24]. Th2 lymphocytes express cytokines such as IL-5 (a lineage-specific eosinophil growth factor) and IL-4 (a switch factor for IgE synthesis). The eosinophil contributes to the development of bronchial hyperresponsiveness by releasing its content of pro-inflammatory mediators including preformed cytoplasmic granule mediators (i.e., major basic protein), newly synthesized lipid mediators (leukotriene C4, platelet-activating factor), and cytokines (GM-CSF, TNF, TGF-β, IL-5, as well as many others) [2, 3]. These eosinophil-derived mediators

Correspondence to: D. Broide

contribute to airway smooth muscle contraction, mucus secretion, and denudation of airway epithelium, all hallmarks of asthma [8]. The ongoing inflammatory response in the airway of asthmatics may lead to airway remodeling and a progressive decline in lung function that is exaggerated with respect to the natural decline related to the ageing process [9, 28]. Airway remodeling in asthma is characterized by bronchial wall thickening, smooth muscle hypertrophy, and thickening of the basement membrane due to deposition of collagen types III, V and to a lesser extent collagen type I and fibronectin [25]. There is not much information available on the time of onset of these airway remodelling changes or their rate of progression. Altered airway structure in asthma may result in altered airway function. This altered airway function may be due to the increase in amount of smooth muscle, allowing greater shortening in response to a bronchoconstrictor stimulus, or to the increase in airway adventitial area leading to an uncoupling of the distending forces of parenchymal recoil from the forces tending to narrow the airways [32].

Anti-inflammatory therapy and asthma

The recognition that asthma is an inflammatory disease of the airways which in the long term may result in airway remodeling in some asthmatics has led to early institution of therapy aimed at reducing airway inflammation. Several studies have suggested that a delayed introduction of inhaled anti-inflammatory therapy results in an impaired ability to maximize lung function measures when such therapy is subsequently introduced [9]. Our current most effective anti-inflammatory therapy for asthma is corticosteroids. Despite their effectiveness corticosteroids have been associated with the potential for side effects (cataracts, growth retardation, osteoporosis) resulting in efforts to identify alternate therapies to modulate the airway inflammatory response. Immunotherapy to common airborne allergens (i.e., grass pollen, ragweed, house dust mite) has been shown to be effective in reducing symptoms in patients with allergic rhinitis [1]. However, in patients with allergic asthma the benefits have been more difficult to demonstrate [19] and the potential for side effects (i.e., anaphylaxis to therapy) is greater in patients with moderate to severe asthma, the population most in need of improved therapy.

DNA-based therapy for asthma

While the ability of protein-based immunotherapy to treat grass pollen allergy has been recognized since 1911 [18], the ability of DNA-based therapy to treat asthma has only more recently been investigated. Several approaches to DNA-based therapy for asthma have been identified including antisense therapy, DNA gene therapy (i.e., exon coding immunization), and non-coding DNA immunostimulatory sequence (ISS) therapy (i.e., DNA containing an ISS such as CpG). As the mechanism of action of these DNA-based therapies differ, we will discuss their different mechanisms of action and their potential effectiveness in the therapy of asthma.

Antisense DNA therapy for asthma

Antisense therapy is an attempt to use antisense oligodeoxynucleotide (ODN) sequences complementary to a specific target mRNA to inhibit its expression. In a rabbit model of asthma the ability of antisense targeted to a sequence of the adenosine A1 receptor was used to inhibit the function of the airway adenosine A1 receptor, and assess the subsequent impact on bronchial hyperreactivity in response to inhaled adenosine [20]. Adenosine is a pro-inflammatory mediator released in the lung during episodes of allergic inflammation, and binds to specific adenosine receptors expressed by multiple cell types, including mast cells and airway smooth muscle [22]. Inhalation of adenosine induces bronchoconstriction in asthmatics. Pretreatment of rabbits with inhaled adenosine A1 receptor antisense resulted in at least an order of magnitude increase in the dose of aerosolized adenosine required to reduce dynamic compliance of the lung (a measure of bronchoconstriction) by 50% [20]. Airway smooth muscle derived from the rabbits treated with inhaled adenosine A1 receptor antisense demonstrated an approximately 75% decrease in the A1 receptor density, but not A2 receptor density [20]. These studies suggest that antisense strategies can be used in animal models to target adenosine receptors on airway smooth muscle. The ability to use antisense to treat asthma in humans will require further study.

DNA gene immunization therapy for asthma

In a second approach plasmid DNA coding for a specific antigen or allergen protein, [i.e., β-galactosidase (β-gal), ovalbumin, or dermatophagoides] has been used as DNA gene therapy. The demonstration of the potential to express a protein antigen in vivo by immunizing with DNA encoding the gene instead of the protein was elegantly demonstrated by Wolff et al. [33], who demonstrated the expression of β-gal protein for at least 2 months following injection of the DNA encoding β-gal into mouse muscle cells in vivo. Similar studies utilizing human skin grafted onto nude mice have demonstrated that plasmid DNA can be expressed not only in mice but also in human skin [10]. The immune response to DNA vaccines encoding an allergen have been extensively studied in mice [23, 31]. Intramuscular or intradermal injection of plasmid DNA encoding a specific antigen induces both an antibody and a cellular immune response to the encoded allergen [23, 31]. Studies by Raz et al. [23] demonstrated that mice generated a Th1 immune response to a plasmid DNA construct containing *lacZ*, the gene encoding β-gal. In contrast to the Th1 immune response noted following immunization with β-gal encoded by plasmid DNA, mice immunized with β-gal protein developed a Th2 response. Thus, the immune response to the same antigen differed depending on whether the antigen was delivered as a DNA plasmid or as a protein. In the context of allergic inflammation and asthma, which is characterized by a Th2 response to antigen, the ability to induce a Th1 response by delivering the antigen as a plasmid DNA sequence suggested the potential to use plasmid DNA encoding allergens to down-regulate the Th2 response associated with immune response to allergens. Indeed, primary DNA gene vaccination with plasmid DNA encoding β-gal inhibited the subsequent IgE and IL-5 cytokine response to β-gal protein in alum [4]. Additional studies in a mouse model of asthma induced by ovalbumin (OVA) antigen demonstrated that mice sensitized to develop a Th2 response to OVA protein and pretreated with three intradermal injections of plasmid DNA encoding OVA protein developed significantly less bronchoalveolar lavage fluid eosinophils (84% inhibition), lung eosinophils (70% inhibition), and bone marrow eosinophils (70% inhibition) following inhalation of OVA protein compared to mice pretreated with a control plasmid DNA construct [4]. Moreover, studies in a rat model of asthma have demonstrated that immunization with a plasmid DNA encoding the house dust mite allergen Derp5 inhibits IgE responses, histamine release into bronchoalveolar lavage fluid, and decreases airway hyperreactivity compared to control mice [11].

The mechanism by which plasmid DNA gene immunization induces a Th1 response is probably due both to the intracellular processing of the plasmid DNA gene, as well as to ISS in the plasmid backbone acting as Th1 adjuvants [27]. The fact that DNA plasmid allergen gene immunization converts a normally extracellular expressed protein allergen to an intracellular expressed protein may result in the allergen being presented by MHC class I as opposed to MHC class II antigen pathways. This intracellular processing of allergen via MHC class I antigen presentation causes a much stronger $CD8^+$ T cell response compared to extracellular processing of protein allergen. As $CD8^+$ T cells play an important role in the suppression of IgE formation [16], the potential importance of DNA gene vaccination products interacting with MHC class I antigen presentation and $CD8^+$ T lymphocytes is evident.

The importance of non-coding ISS in the plasmid DNA backbone to the development of Th1 immune responses is suggested from studies by Sato et al. [27]. They demonstrated that the presence or absence of ISS having a CpG motif in the antibiotic resistance gene contained in the plasmid backbone of the DNA vaccine determined whether a Th1 immune response occurred that was independent of the coding sequence of the DNA vaccine. DNA vaccines constructed with a plasmid backbone containing an *amp* R gene (containing the CpG motif) developed Th1 responses, whereas DNA vaccines constructed with a plasmid backbone containing a *kan* R gene (no CpG motifs) did not develop Th1 responses [27]. The demonstration that CpG sequences in the DNA backbone, as opposed to DNA coding sequences, are important attributes in inducing protective Th1, instead of Th2, immune responses to allergens has focused further studies on the potential effect of CpG immunostimulatory DNA sequences alone as a therapy for asthma.

DNA vaccines are currently in phase I studies in human diseases, including infectious diseases (hepatitis, influenza) and cancer [31].

Immunostimulatory CpG sequence DNA therapy for asthma

An alternative DNA-based immunization approach to DNA gene immunization is to utilize non-coding immunostimulatory DNA sequences containing a CpG motif (ISS) to induce a protective Th1 immune response to allergen [5, 13, 26, 29]. Tokunaga et al. [34] identified that CpG motifs in BCG DNA induced interferon-γ and that this CpG effect was mediated by bacterial but not vertebrate DNA. The differences between bacterial and vertebrate DNA include a greater frequency of CpG base pairs in bacterial as compared to vertebrate DNA, and a lower frequency of cytosine methylation in bacterial as compared to vertebrate DNA [14]. As cytosine methylation abolishes the Th1 adjuvant effect of CpG the high frequency of cytosine methylation in vertebrate DNA, as well as the low frequency of CpG sequences, probably both contribute to the reduced ability of vertebrate DNA to act as a Th1 adjuvant. Additional studies have determined that the DNA hexamer sequence having the optimal Th1 adjuvant effect contains the motif 5'-purine-purine-CpG-pyrimidine-pyrimidine, e.g., AACGTT, and activates the secretion of the Th1 cytokine IFN-γ secretion [36]. The effect of CpG on the Th1 response is indirect, as CpG activates the innate immune system including macrophages to up-regulate cytokine expression (IL-12, IL-18, IFN-α, IFN-β), up-regulate MHC molecules, and up-regulate costimulatory molecules [15, 35]. In addition, ISS acts on NK cells to release interferon-γ. These ISS effects on the innate immune response create a cytokine milieu (IFN-γ^+, IL-12^+) which biases the T lymphocyte immune response to a Th1 response to newly encountered antigens.

In a mouse model of allergen-induced airway hyperresponsiveness ISS containing a CpG DNA motif significantly inhibit airway eosinophilia and reduced responsiveness to inhaled methacholine [16, 26]. ISS not only inhibited eosinophilia of the airway (by 93%) and lung parenchyma (91%), but also significantly inhibited blood eosinophilia (86%), suggesting that ISS exerts a significant effect on the bone marrow release and/or production of eosinophils. The inhibition of the bone marrow production of eosinophils by 58% was associated with a significant inhibition of T cell-derived cytokine generation (IL-5, GM-CSF and IL-3). As IL-5 is an important lineage-specific eosinophil growth factor as well as an inducer of the bone marrow release of eosinophils, the inhibitory effect of ISS on the generation of IL-5 plays an important role in mediating the effect of ISS on bone marrow production and/or release of eosinophils. The onset of the ISS effect on reducing the number of tissue eosinophils was both immediate (within 1 day of administration) and sustained (lasted 6 days), and was not due to ISS directly inducing eosinophil apoptosis. ISS is effective in inhibiting eosinophilic airway inflammation when administered either systemically (intraperitoneally), or mucosally (i.e., intranasally or intratracheally).

ISS-ODN administration, via activation of innate immunity, could therefore inhibit pulmonary eosinophilia through at least three different, but additive mechanisms. The first mechanism by which ISS can inhibit pulmonary eosinophilia is through an effect on T cell-derived cytokines important to the bone marrow generation of eosinophils. ISS exerts this inhibitory effect indirectly by stimulating monocytes/macrophages and NK cells to generate IL-12 and IFN that subsequently inhibit T cell generation of IL-5, GM-CSF, and IL-3. The greater inhibition by ISS of peripheral blood eosinophilia (86% inhibition) compared with inhibition of bone marrow eosinophilia (58% inhibition) suggests that ISS may have also inhibited release of eosinophils from the bone marrow. In this regard, IL-5 is known to induce release of eosinophils from the bone marrow, and inhibition of IL-5 generation by ISS could, thus, prevent bone marrow release of eosinophils. A second mechanism by which ISS-induced generation of IFN and IL-12 could inhibit pulmonary eosinophilia is through an effect on eosinophil recruitment, as has previously been demonstrated with IL-12 [7, 30], IFN-α [17], and IFN-γ [12] in models of allergic inflammation and parasitic infection. A third eosinophil-inhibitory mechanism induced by ISS is the generation of an allergen-specific Th1 as opposed to a Th2 response. This would be important for long-term protection and immunological memory. This ISS-induced OVA-specific Th1 response would generate IFN-γ, which further inhibits eosinophil accumulation by biasing naive T cells encountering antigen in an IFN-γ milieu to generate Th1 as opposed to Th2 responses to newly encountered allergens. The first two inhibitory mechanisms affecting pulmonary eosinophilia are most likely mediated by the innate immune response, and are, therefore, primarily immediate and antigen nonspecific in nature. In contrast, the third effect is mediated by the adaptive immune response and requires a longer period of time for differentiation and maturation of antigen-specific Th1 cells from naive $CD4^+$ T cells. Furthermore, while the first two mechanisms lead to a dramatic, but probably temporary reduction in eosinophil recruitment, the third mechanism is involved in the generation of immunological memory that may prevent Th2 cell responses and eosinophil recruitment into the target organ (i.e., the lung) from developing following subsequent airway allergen challenge.

The effect of ISS on reducing the number of tissue eosinophils is both immediate (onset within 1 day) and sustained (over 6 days), and is not due to ISS directly inducing eosinophil apoptosis. Administration of ISS-ODN 6 days before the final OVA inhalation challenge is more effective in inhibiting pulmonary eosinophil infiltration than simultaneous delivery of ISS-ODN and OVA 1 day before the end of the experiment. Administration of ISS-ODN 6 days before the final OVA inhalation challenge also generated OVA-specific Th1 responses (induction of IFN-γ) and attenuated preexisting OVA-specific Th2 responses (i.e., reduction of IL-5). The administration of ISS 1 day before, or together with the final OVA inhalation challenge was sufficient to inhibit pulmonary eosinophil recruitment as well as the generation of eosinophil active cytokines 24 h later. However, this method of ISS administration did not result in OVA-specific Th1 responses, probably because antigen-specific IFN-γ production generally requires more than 24–48 h.

ISS exerts this inhibitory effect on T cell cytokine production indirectly by stimulating monocytes/macrophages and NK cells to generate IL-12 and IFN. Interestingly, a single dose of ISS inhibited airway eosinophilia as effectively as daily injections of corticosteroids for 7 days. Moreover, while both ISS and corticosteroids inhibited IL-5 generation, only ISS was able to induce allergen-specific IFN-γ production and redirect the immune system toward a Th1 response. Sur et al. [29] have demonstrated the importance of IFN-γ production to the in vivo effect of CpG by studying the effectiveness of CpG in IFN-γ-deficient mice. Administration of CpG to IFN-$\gamma^{-/-}$ mice failed to inhibit eosinophil recruitment, indicating a critical role of IFN-γ in mediating the in vivo effects of CpG. Thus, systemic or mucosal administration of ISS prior to allergen exposure could provide a novel form of active immunotherapy in allergic disease.

Conclusion

A variety of DNA-based methods of modulating the immune and/or inflammatory response in animal models of asthma have shown significant promise. Antisense strategies seek to inhibit expression of specific host genes, whereas DNA vaccines aim to modulate the immune response to specific encoded allergens. In contrast, ISS DNA therapy seeks to redirect the host immune response from a Th2 to a Th1 response. Current human studies will help to determine which, if any, of these DNA based therapies is a safe and effective therapy for human asthma.

Acknowledgements This work was supported in part by NIH grants AI45513, AI38425, AI33977, AI40682 and by a University of California Biostar grant (S96-43).

References

1. Adkinson NF, Eggleston PA, Eney D, Goldstein EO, Schuberth KC, Bacon JR, Hamilton RG, Weiss ME, Arshad H, Meinert CL, Tanascia J, Wheeler B (1997) A controlled trial of immunotherapy for asthma in allergic children. N Engl J Med 336:324
2. Broide DH, Gleich GJ, Cuomo A, Coburn D, Federman E, Schwartz L, Wasserman SI (1991) Evidence of ongoing mast cell and eosinophil degranulation in symptomatic asthma airway. J Allergy Clin Immunol 88:637
3. Broide DH, Paine MM, Firestein GS (1992) Eosinophils express interleukin 5 and granulocyte macrophage-colony-stimulating factor mRNA at sites of allergic inflammation in asthmatics. J Clin Invest 90:1414
4. Broide D, Orozco EM, Roman M, Carson DA, Raz E (1997) Intradermal gene vaccination down-regulates both arms of the allergic response. J Allergy Clin Immunol 99:S129
5. Broide D, Schwarze J, Tighe H, Gifford T, Nguyen MD, Malek S, Van Uden J, Martin-Orozco E, Gelfand EW, Raz E (1998) Immunostimulatory DNA sequences inhibit IL-5, eosinophilic inflammation, and airway hyperresponsiveness in mice. J Immunol 161:7054
6. Collaborative study of the genetics of asthma (1997) A genome-wide search for asthma susceptibility loci in ethnically diverse populations. Nat Genet 15:389
7. Gavett SH, O'Hearn DJ, Li X, Huang SK, Finkelman FD, Wills-Karp M (1995) Interleukin 12 inhibits antigen-induced airway hyperresponsiveness, inflammation, and Th2 cytokine expression in mice. J Exp Med 182:1527
8. Gleich GJ, Flavahan NA, Fujisawa T, Vanhoutte PM (1988) The eosinophil as a mediator of damage to respiratory epithelium: a model for bronchial hyperreactivity. J Allergy Clin Immunol 81:776
9. Haahtela T, Jarvinen M, Kava T, Kiviranta K, Koskinen S, Lehtonen K, Nikander K, Persson T, Selroos O, Sovijarvi A, Stenius-Aarniala B, Svahn T, Tammivaara R, Laitinen L (1994) Effects of reducing or discontinuing inhaled budesonide in patients with mild asthma. N Engl J Med 331:700
10. Hengge UR, Walker PS, Vogel JC (1996) Expression of naked DNA in human pig, and mouse skin. J Clin Invest 97:2911
11. Hsu CH, Chua KY, Tao MH, Lai YL, Wu HD, Huang SK, Hsieh KH (1996) Immunoprophylaxis of allergen-induced immunoglobulin E synthesis and airway hyperresponsiveness in vivo by genetic immunization. Nat Med 2:540
12. Iwamoto I, Nakajima H, Endo H, Yoshida S (1993) Interferon γ regulates antigen-induced eosinophil recruitment into the mouse airways by inhibiting the infiltration of $CD4^+$ T cells. J Exp Med 177:573
13. Kline JN, Waldschmidt TJ, Businga TR, Lemish JE, Weinstock JV, Thorne PS, Krieg AM (1998) Modulation of airway inflammation by CpG oligodeoxynucleotides in a murine model of asthma. J Immunol 160:2555
14. Klinman DM, Yi AK, Beaucage SL, Conover J, Krieg AM (1996) CpG motifs present in bacterial DNA rapidly induce lymphocytes to secrete interleukin 6, interleukin 12, and interferon γ. Proc Natl Acad Sci USA 93:2879
15. Krieg AM, Yi AK, Matson S, Waldschmidt TJ, Bishop GA, Teasdale R, Koretzky GA, Klinman DM (1995) CpG motifs in bacterial DNA trigger direct B-cell activation. Nature 374:546
16. MacAry PA, Holmes BJ, Kemeny DM (1998) Ovalbumin-specific MHC class I-restricted $\alpha\beta$-positive, TcI and TcO $CD8^+$ T cell clones mediate the in vivo inhibition of rat IgE. J Immunol 160:580
17. Nakajima H, Nakao A, Watanabe Y, Yoshida S, Iwamoto I (1994) IFN-α inhibits antigen-induced eosinophil and $CD4^+$ T cell recruitment into tissue. J Immunol 153:1264
18. Noon L (1911) Prophylactic inoculation against hay fever. Lancet I:1572
19. Norman PS (1998) Immunotherapy past and present. J Allergy Clin Immunol 102:1
20. Nyce JW, Metzger WJ (1997) DNA antisense therapy for asthma in an animal model [published erratum appears in Nature (1997) 27:390]. Nature 385:721
21. Ober C, Cox NJ, Abney M, Di Rienzo A, Lander ES, Changyaleket B, Gidley H, Kurtz B, Lee J, Nance M, Pettersson A, Prescott J, Richardson A, Schlenker E, Summerhill E, Willadsen S, Parry R (1998) Genome-wide search for asthma susceptibility loci in a founder population. The Collaborative Study on the Genetics of Asthma. Hum Mol Gen 7:1393
22. Peachell PT, Columbo M, Kagey-Sobotka A, Lichtenstein LM, Marone G (1988) Adenosine potentiates mediator release from human lung mast cells. Am Rev Respir Dis 138:1143
23. Raz E, Tighe H, Sato Y, Corr MP, Dudler JA, Roman M, Swain SL, Spiegelberg HL, Carson DA (1996) Preferential induction of a TH1 immune response and inhibition of specific IgE antibody formation by plasmid DNA immunization. Proc Natl Acad Sci USA 93:5141

24. Robinson DS, Hamid Q, Ying S, Tsicopoulos A, Barkans J, Bentley AM, Corrigan C, Durham SR, Kay AB (1992) Predominant TH2-like bronchoalveolar T-lymphocyte population in atopic asthma. N Engl J Med 326:298
25. Roche WR, Beasley R, Williams JH, Holgate ST (1989) Subepithelial fibrosis in the bronchi of asthmatics. Lancet I:520
26. Roman M, Orozco EM, Goodman J, Nguyen MD, Sato Y, Ronaghy A, Kornbluth RS, Richman DD, Carson DA, Raz E (1997) Immunostimulatory DNA sequences function as T helper-1 promoting adjuvants. Nat Med 3:849
27. Sato Y, Roman M, Tighe H, Lee D, Corr MP, Nguyen MD, Silverman GJ, Lotz M, Carson DA, Raz E (1996) Immunostimulatory DNA sequences necessary for effective intradermal gene immunization. Science 273:352
28. Schachter EN, Doyle CA, Beck GJ (1984) A prospective study of asthma in a rural community. Chest 85:623
29. Sur S, Wild JS, Choudhury BK, Sur N, Alam R, Klinman DM (1999) Long-term prevention of allergic lung inflammation in a mouse model of asthma by CpG oligodeoxynucleotides. J Immunol 162:6284
30. Trinchieri G (1995) Interleukin-12: a proinflammatory cytokine with immuno-regulatory functions that bridge innate resistance and antigen-specific adaptive immunity. Annu Rev Immunol 13:251
31. Weiner DB, Kennedy RC (1999) Genetic vaccines. Sci Am 281:34
32. Wiggs BR, Moreno R, Hogg JC, Hilliam C, Pare PD (1990) A model of the mechanics of airway narrowing. J Appl Physiol 69:849
33. Wolff JA, Malone RW, Williams P, Chong W, Ascadi G, Jani A, Felgner PL (1990) Direct gene transfer into mouse muscle in vivo. Science 247:1465
34. Yamamoto S, Kuramoto E, Shimada S, Tokunaga T (1988) In vitro augmentation of natural killer cell activity and production of interferon-α/β and γ with deoxyribonucleic acid fraction from *Mycobacterium bovis* BCG. Jpn J Cancer Res 79:866
35. Yamamoto S, Yamamoto T, Kataoka T, Kuramoto E, Yano O, Tokunaga T (1992) Unique palindromic sequences in synthetic oligonucleotides are required to induce IFN and IFN-mediated natural killer activity. J Immunol 148:4072
36. Yamamoto T, Yamamoto S, Kataaoka T, Komuro K, Kohase M, Tokunaga T (1994) Synthetic oligonucleotides with cerain palindromes stimulate interferon production of human peripheral blood lymphocytes in vitro. Jpn J Cancer Res 85:775

The role of CpG in DNA vaccines

Michael J. McCluskie[1], Risini D. Weeratna[1], Heather L. Davis[1–4]

[1] Loeb Health Research Institute at the Ottawa Hospital, 725 Parkdale Avenue, Ottawa, K1Y 4E9, Canada
[2] Department of Biochemistry, Microbiology and Immunology, Faculty of Medicine, University of Ottawa, Ottawa, Canada
[3] School of Rehabilitation Sciences, Faculty of Health Sciences, University of Ottawa, Ottawa, Canada
[4] Coley Pharmaceutical Group, Wellesley, Massachusetts, USA

Abstract. One of the most exciting developments in the field of vaccine research in recent years has been DNA vaccines, with which immune responses are induced subsequent to the in vivo expression of antigen from directly introduced plasmid DNA. Strong immune responses have been demonstrated in a number of animal models against many viral, bacterial and parasitic pathogens, and several human clinical trials have been undertaken. The strong and long-lasting antigen-specific humoral (antibodies) and cell-mediated (T help, other cytokine functions and cytotoxic T cells) immune responses induced by DNA vaccines appear to be due to the sustained in vivo expression of antigen, efficient antigen presentation and the presence of stimulatory CpG motifs. These features are desirable for the development of prophylactic vaccines against numerous infectious agents. Furthermore, the strong cellular responses are also very desirable for the development of therapeutic DNA vaccines to treat chronic viral infections or cancer. Efforts are now focusing on understanding the mechanisms for the induction of these immune responses, which in turn should aid in the optimization of DNA vaccines. This review will focus on the role of CpG motifs in DNA vaccines.

Introduction

A DNA vaccine is one with which antigen is synthesized in vivo upon introduction into the body of an antigen-encoding plasmid, which leads to the induction of antigen-specific immune responses. Early studies by Wolff et al. [57] demonstrated that injection of plasmid DNA in saline ("naked" DNA) encoding a luciferase reporter gene into muscles of mice, resulted in long-term reporter gene expression in transfected muscle fibers. Subsequently it was shown that if the plasmid encoded an antigenic protein, such as human growth hormone in a mouse, immune responses were induced [53]. A large number of different routes and methods of DNA delivery have been reported [9, 38]. Nevertheless, most DNA vaccines are delivered into the muscle by intramuscular (IM) injection or into the skin by epidermal gene-gun delivery

Correspondence to: H.L. Davis (address see [1] above)

or intradermal (ID) injection. Disease-specific DNA-based immunization has now been demonstrated in numerous animal models against many viral, bacterial and parasitic diseases [9], and several human clinical trials have been completed or are underway [4, 35, 52, 54, 55].

The strong immune responses that DNA vaccines can generate appear to be due to a combination of (1) the sustained in vivo synthesis of antigen [8], (2) antigen expression, possibly in antigen-presenting cells (APC), that results in major histocompatibility complex (MHC) class I and II presentation of antigen [6, 7], and (3) the potent adjuvant effect of immunostimulatory CpG motifs (CpG-S) present in the DNA backbone [28, 49]. In addition, DNA vaccines offer several advantages over the traditional antigen-based vaccines: low cost and relative ease of manufacturing; heat stability, thereby negating the need for a "cold-chain"; the possibility to make multivalent vaccines against several pathogens by cloning genes encoding different antigens into a single vector (for co-linear expression), or by mixing different plasmids together; and the ease of cloning which would allow new vaccines to be created quickly, for example in response to new or changing strains of pathogens.

The basic components of DNA vaccine vectors include: (1) a bacterial origin of replication (ori); (2) a prokaryotic selectable marker gene such as an antibiotic resistance gene; (3) antigen-encoding sequences; (4) eukaryotic transcription regulatory elements (e.g., promoter and enhancer sequences); (5) a transcription termination element; and (6) optional elements that may be included in DNA vaccines (e.g., introns, unrelated Th epitopes to provide additional T help, immunostimulatory CpG sequences, or additional genes expressing cytokines or co-stimulatory molecules) [9].

The role of CpG in DNA vaccines

DNA vaccines possess their own adjuvant activity owing to the presence of unmethylated CpG dinucleotides in particular base contexts (CpG-S motifs) [28]. Such CpG-S motifs are found at the expected frequency (1/16) in bacteria, but are underrepresented (1/60) and methylated in vertebrate DNA. It appears that CpG-S motifs are an evolutionary adaptation to augment innate immunity in response to bacterial infection. CpG DNA has many effects on the immune system including stimulation of B cells to proliferate, secrete immunoglobulin (Ig), IL-6 and IL-12, and to be protected from apoptosis [24, 28, 61]. In addition, it enhances expression of MHC class II and B7 co-stimulatory molecules [10, 51]. CpG DNA also directly activates monocytes, macrophages and dendritic cells to secrete various cytokines and chemokines [13, 24].

Overall, CpG DNA induces a Th1-like pattern of cytokine production dominated by IL-12 and IFN- γ with little secretion of Th2 cytokines [24], and are thought to account for the strong CTL responses frequently seen with DNA vaccines [29]. Although such responses are T cell independent and antigen nonspecific, the B cell activation by CpG DNA synergizes strongly with signals delivered through the B cell antigen receptor for both B cell proliferation and Ig secretion [28]. This synergy promotes antigen-specific immune responses and accounts for the strong Th1-like adjuvant effect of CpG-containing oligonucleotides given with a protein vaccine after IM or intranasal (IN) administration [10, 37, 39].

DNA vaccines and role of CpG motifs

Plasmids contain many CpG-S motifs and have been shown to be essential for the immunogenicity of DNA vaccines [24, 49]. Furthermore the DNA backbone itself provides an immunostimulatory effect since injection of a non-coding DNA vector can significantly enhance immune responses to a co-administered DNA or protein vaccine [12, 25, 31, 33, 45]. Not only did the non-coding vector enhance immune responses, but it was also responsible for establishing the Th1 bias of the response to a protein antigen [31]. The immunomodulatory effect of the plasmid is diminished upon methylation [12, 25, 31], indicating the requirement of unmethylated CpG motifs.

However, not all DNA sequences containing CpG motifs have stimulatory effects on the immune system. The CpG dinucleotide in a CpG-S motif is generally preceded on the 5' side by two purines such as ApA, GpA or a purine and a T such as GpT, and followed on the 3' side by two pyrimidines, most commonly TpT. However, DNA sequences containing CpG dinucleotides that can counteract the stimulatory effect of CpG-S have been identified. These neutralizing motifs (CpG-N) contain sequences where the CpG dinucleotide is typically preceded by a C (CCG), followed by a G (CGG), or contain CG repeats (CGCGCG). Interestingly, high numbers of CpG-N motifs are found in certain serotypes of adenovirus (e.g., types 2 and 5) and appear to have evolved as a defense mechanism of the virus to suppress the immunostimulatory properties of their genomic CpG-S motifs [27]. In addition, CpG-N motifs are overrepresented in the human genome (especially CCG), where they are two- to fivefold more frequent than the CpG-S motifs. These may function to down-regulate any immunostimulatory effect of unmethylated CpGs present in CpG islands within vertebrate DNA.

Therefore, to optimize immune responses to DNA vaccines, it is necessary to increase the number of CpG-S motifs and/or reduce the number of CpG-N motifs so that the net balance between stimulatory and neutralizing sequences is enhanced. While it would be highly desirable to improve the function of DNA vaccines by simply adding oligodeoxynucleotides (ODN) containing CpG-S motifs, this, unfortunately, is not possible. Mixing of CpG DNA with antigen-encoding plasmid DNA prior to injection results in a dose-dependent reduction in gene expression [56], which is likely due to competitive interference by the synthetic backbone of the ODN at DNA binding sites on the surface of target cells [63], which in turn would decrease transfection efficiency. Thus, to optimize the CpG content, it is necessary to clone the CpG-S motifs into the vector backbone.

We have demonstrated that removal of 52 of 134 identified CpG-N motifs in a DNA vaccine markedly enhanced its Th1-like function in vivo, and that this could be further enhanced by the addition of CpG-S motifs [27]. Interestingly, the addition of 50 CpG-S motifs was inferior to that with 16 motifs for induction of antigen-specific humoral responses, despite the fact that this vector gave the best CTL responses [27]. Interferon-γ (IFN-γ) is known to down-regulate viral (e.g., cytomegalovirus, CMV) [14, 46, 58] as well as some non-viral promoters [60]. Thus, it is possible that the high levels of IFN-γ induced by CpG DNA may have reduced the amount of antigen expressed in this study by down-regulation of the CMV promoter.

Most DNA vaccines to date have been delivered by parenteral immunization (i.e., IM, ID or SC injection). Nevertheless, in recent years a number of studies have reported the use of DNA vaccines for mucosal delivery particularly to the respiratory tract [38]. A number of groups have demonstrated that DNA delivery to the lungs or nasal epithelium, results in high levels of gene expression for only a limited period (days 2 to 4 after gene transfer), although very low levels of gene expression persist for at least several weeks [1, 5, 22, 36, 41]. It appears that the transient gene expression in mucosal tissues is largely due to a combination of cell turnover, which is possibly enhanced by vaccine delivery and promoter turn-off, and is due, at least in part, to the elevated levels of Th1 cytokines. IFN-γ and TNF-α are found in the bronchoalveolar lavage fluid of mice following IN administration of plasmid DNA [11, 32, 50, 59] and this appears to be caused by the presence of CpG-S motifs within the plasmid [11]. The short-lived expression may not be a problem for DNA immunization; however, it would present more difficulties in gene therapy applications as discussed below. In any event, CpG-S motifs do have potent adjuvant function when delivered to a mucosal surface in the form of an ODN [17, 37, 39, 42]. If the other problems associated with delivery of DNA vaccines to mucosal surfaces can be overcome, their immunostimulatory function should be adequate.

Furthermore, it appears that the CpG content of the DNA vector may influence the Th bias of the immune response and may explain, at least in part, why different plasmids induce predominantly Th1 [19, 30], Th2 [2, 42, 47, 48] or mixed Th1/Th2 [22] responses when naked DNA is delivered to the lungs. Other factors which appear to determine whether a Th1 or Th2 response predominates after immunization include (1) the antigen, (2) the dose of antigen, (3) the route and method of DNA administration, (4) co-expression of cytokines, and (5) whether another adjuvant is used.

Therapeutic uses of plasmid DNA and role of CpG motifs

There are several potential applications for direct gene transfer for therapeutic purposes. Perhaps the most obvious is gene therapy for inborn errors of metabolism, such as delivery of the cystic fibrosis (CF) transmembrane conductance regulator gene (CFTR) to treat CF [1, 5]. However, the successful application of DNA vectors for gene therapy will depend on the safety of repeatedly delivering high doses of DNA. Human gene therapy trials have had disappointing results and this appears to be due, at least in part, to immune responses against the therapeutic gene product or other foreign proteins expressed from viral vectors. CF patients given repeated administrations of a modified adenovirus containing the CFTR gene exhibited partial corrective responses early in therapy, but this was lost after repeated administrations, most likely because of neutralizing antibodies against vector proteins [26]. Similarly, trials of myoblast transplant for Duchenne muscular dystrophy have been unsuccessful due to the immune-mediated destruction of dystrophin-expressing myofibers in transplanted patients [20, 40].

To reduce the immune activation in gene therapy applications, it may be helpful to reduce the number of CpG-S motifs and increase the number of CpG-N motifs. We have produced such vectors and have shown that they induce less IL-6 production from mouse splenocytes in vivo than unmodified vectors (Davis and Krieg, unpublished results). It is also possible that use of tissue-specific promoters that are not active in APC, and thus prevent immune induction, will improve longevity of gene expression (Weeratna, unpublished data).

It is also possible that cytokines produced as a result of immune stimulation may reduce gene expression by down-regulation of promotor activity [14, 46, 58, 60] and thus reduce the levels of therapeutic gene products. It is not possible to simply methylate the stimulatory CpG motifs in gene therapy plasmids, since expression is greatly reduced if the antigen-encoding sequences are methylated [43], and virtually abolished if the promoter region is methylated [18, 62]. Nor can all stimulatory CpG motifs be deleted in gene therapy vectors since many are located in the origin of replication, where even single base changes can greatly reduce plasmid replication.

There is also considerable interest in the use of cytokine-expressing plasmids for therapeutic purposes, particularly in the treatment of pulmonary allergic responses [15, 34]. Asthma is associated with Th2 responses [16, 21], and thus Th1 cytokines may help reduce allergic responses. Indeed, mucosal IL-12 or IFN-γ gene transfer inhibits pulmonary allergic responses [15, 34] and restores local antiviral immunity [15]. Interestingly, inhibition of airway allergic responses is also seen by administration of synthetic immunostimulatory CpG ODN [3, 23], which preferentially induce Th1 responses [24, 29]. It is, therefore, highly likely that through rational optimization of CpG content in DNA vaccines it will be possible to develop better therapies for the treatment of asthmatic conditions.

Conclusions

As illustrated in this review, CpG-S and CpG-N motifs play pivotal roles in plasmid DNA technology, both for DNA vaccines and gene therapy vectors. Knowledge of the effects of CpG motifs in plasmid DNA helps explain the poor responses generated with gene therapy and DNA vaccines in humans but it also provides strategies for improvement. Therefore it is important to pay careful consideration to vector design to fully take advantage of this exciting new technology.

References

1. Alton EWFW, Middleton PG, Caplen NJ, Smith SN, Steel DM, Munkonge FM, Jeffery PK, Geddes DM, Hart SL, Williamson R, Fasold KI, Miller AD, Dickinson P, Stevenson BJ, McLachlan G, Dorin JR, Porteous DJ (1993) Non-invasive liposome-mediated gene delivery can correct the ion transport defect in cystic fibrosis mutant mice. Nat Genet 5: 135
2. Asakura Y, Hinkula J, Leandersson AC, Fukushima J, Okuda K, Wahren B (1997) Induction of HIV-1 specific mucosal immune responses by DNA vaccination. Scand J Immunol 46: 326
3. Broide D, Schwarze J, Tighe H, Gifford T, Nguyen MD, Malek S, Van Uden J, Martin-Orozco E, Gelfand EW, Raz E (1998) Immunostimulatory DNA sequences inhibit IL-5, eosinophilic inflammation, and airway hyperresponsiveness in mice. J Immunol 161: 7054
4. Calarota S, Bratt G, Nordlund S, Hinkula J, Leandersson AC, Sandstrom E, Wahren B (1998) Cellular cytotoxic response induced by DNA vaccination in HIV-1-infected patients. Lancet 351: 1320
5. Caplen NJ, Alton EWFW, Middleton PG, Dorin JR, Stevenson BJ, Gao X, Durham SR, Jeffrey PK, Hodson ME, Coutelle C, Huang L, Porteous DJ, Williamson R, Geddes DM (1995) Liposome mediated CFTR gene transfer to the nasal epithelium of patients with cystic fibrosis. Nat Med 1: 39
6. Casares S, Inaba K, Brumeanu TD, Steinman RM, Bona CA (1997) Antigen presentation by dendritic cells after immunization with DNA encoding a major histocompatibility complex class II-restricted viral epitope. J Exp Med 186: 1481
7. Condon C, Watkins SC, Celluzzi CM, Thompson K, Falo LD Jr (1996) DNA-based immunization by in vivo transfection of dendritic cells. Nat Med 2: 1122
8. Davis HL, Brazolot Millan CL, Watkins SC (1997) Immune-mediated destruction of transfected muscle fibers after direct gene transfer with antigen-expressing plasmid DNA. Gene Ther 4: 181
9. Davis HL, McCluskie MJ (1999) DNA vaccines for viral diseases. Microbes Infect 1: 7

10. Davis HL, Weeranta R, Waldschmidt TJ, Tygrett L, Schorr J, Krieg AM (1998) CpG DNA is a potent enhancer of specific immunity in mice immunized with recombinant hepatitis B surface antigen. J. Immunol 160:870
11. Freimark BD, Blezinger HP, Florack VJ, Nordstrom JL, Long SD, Deshpande DS, Nochumson S, Petrak KL (1998) Cationic lipids enhance cytokine and cell influx levels in the lung following administration of plasmid: cationic lipid complexes. J Immunol 160: 4580
12. Gursel M, Tunca S, Ozkan M, Ozcengiz G, Alaeddinoglu G (1999) Immunoadjuvant action of plasmid DNA in liposomes. Vaccine 17: 1376
13. Halpern MD, Kurlander RJ, Pisetsky DS (1996) Bacterial DNA induces murine interferon-γ production by stimulation of interleukin-12 and tumor necrosis factor-α. Cell Immunol 167: 72
14. Harms JS, Splitter GA (1995) Interferon-gamma inhibits transgene expression driven by SV40 or CMV promoters but augments expression driven by the mammalian MHC I promoter. Hum Gene Ther 6: 1291
15. Hogan SP, Foster PS, Tan X, Ramsay AJ (1998) Mucosal IL-12 gene delivery inhibits allergic airways disease and restores local antiviral immunity. Eur J Immunol 28: 413
16. Hogg J. C. (1997) The pathology of asthma. APMIS 105: 735
17. Horner AA, Ronaghy A, Cheng PM, Nguyen MD, Cho HJ, Broide D, Raz E (1998) Immunostimulatory DNA is a potent mucosal adjuvant. Cell Immunol 190: 77
18. Hug M, Silke J, Georgiev O, Rusconi S, Schaffner W, Matsuo K (1996) Transcriptional repression by methylation: cooperativity between a CpG cluster in the promoter and remote CpG-rich regions. FEBS Lett 379: 251
19. Ishii N, Fukushima J, Kaneko T, Okada E, Tani K, Tanaka SI, Hamajima K, Xin KQ, Kawamoto S, Koff W, Nishioka K, Yasuda T, Okuda K (1997) Cationic liposomes are a strong adjuvant for a DNA vaccine of human immunodeficiency virus type 1. AIDS Res Hum Retroviruses 13: 1421
20. Karpati G, Ajdukovic D, Arnold D, Glendhill RB, Guttmann R, Holland P, Koch PA, Shoubridge E, Spence D, Vanasse M, Watters GV, Abrahamowicz M, Duff C, Worton RG (1993) Myoblast transfer in Duchenne muscular dystrophy. Ann Neurol 34: 8
21. Kay AB (1996) TH2-type cytokines in asthma. Ann N Y Acad Sci 796: 1
22. Klavinskis LS, Barnfield C, Gao L, Parker S (1999) Intranasal immunization with plasmid DNA-lipid complexes elicits mucosal immunity in the female genital and rectal tracts. J Immunol 162: 254
23. Kline JN, Waldschmidt TJ, Businga TR, Lemish JE, Weinstock JV, Thorne PS, Krieg AM (1998) Modulation of airway inflammation by CpG oligodeoxynucleotides in a murine model of asthma. J Immunol 160: 2555
24. Klinman DM, Yamshchikov G, Ishigatsubo Y (1997) Contribution of CpG motifs to the immunogenicity of DNA vaccines. J Immunol 158: 3635
25. Klinman DM, Yi AK, Beaucage SL, Conover J, Krieg AM (1996) CpG motifs present in bacteria DNA rapidly induce lymphocytes to secrete interleukin 6, interleukin 12, and interferon gamma. Proc Natl Acad Sci USA 93:2879
26. Knoell, DL, Yiu IM (1998) Human gene therapy for hereditary diseases: a review of trials. Am J Health Syst Pharm 55: 899
27. Krieg AM, Wu T, Weeratna R, Efler SM, Love-Homan L, Yang L, Yi AK, Short D, Davis HL (1998) Sequence motifs in adenoviral DNA block immune activation by stimulatory CpG motifs. Proc Natl Acad Sci USA 95: 12631
28. Krieg AM, Yi AK, Matson S, Waldschmidt TJ, Bishop GA, Teasdale R, Koretzky GA, Klinman DM (1995) CpG motifs in bacterial DNA trigger direct B-cell activation. Nature 374: 546
29. Krieg AM, Yi AK, Schorr J, Davis HL (1998) The role of CpG dinucleotides in DNA vaccines. Trends Microbiol 6: 23
30. Kuklin N, Daheshia M, Karem K, Manickan E, Rouse BT (1997) Induction of mucosal immunity against herpes simplex virus by plasmid DNA immunization. J Virol 71: 3138
31. Leclerc C, Deriaud E, Rojas M, Whalen RG (1997) The preferential induction of a Th1 immune response by DNA-based immunization is mediated by the immunostimulatory effect of plasmid DNA. Cell Immunol 179: 97
32. Lee ER, Marshall J, Siegel CS, Jiang CW, Yew NS, Nichols MR, Nietupski JB, Ziegler RJ, Lane MB, Wang KX, Wan NC, Scheule RK, Harris DJ, Smith AE, Cheng SH (1996) Detailed analysis of structures and formulations of cationic lipids for efficient gene transfer to the lung. Hum Gene Ther 7: 1701
33. Lee SW, Sung YC (1998) Immuno-stimulatory effects of bacterial-derived plasmids depend on the nature of the antigen in intramuscular DNA inoculations. Immunology 94: 285

34. Li XM, Chopra RK, Chou TY, Schofield BH, Wills-Karp M, Huang SK (1996) Mucosal IFN-gamma gene transfer inhibits pulmonary allergic responses in mice. J Immunol 157: 3216
35. MacGregor RR, Boyer JD, Ugen KE, Lacy KE, Gluckman SJ, Bagarazzi ML, Chattergoon MA, Baine Y, Higgins TJ, Ciccarelli RB, Coney LR, Ginsberg RS, Weiner DB (1998) First human trial of a DNA-based vaccine for treatment of human immunodeficiency virus type 1 infection: safety and host response. J Infect Dis 178: 92
36. McCluskie MJ, Chu Y, Xia JL, Jessee J, Gebyehu G, Davis HL (1998) Direct gene transfer to the respiratory tract of mice with pure plasmid and lipid-formulated DNA. Antisense Nucleic Acid Drug Dev 8: 401
37. McCluskie MJ, Davis HL (1998) CpG DNA is a potent enhancer of systemic and mucosal immune responses against hepatitis B surface antigen with intranasal administration to mice. J Immunol 161: 4463
38. McCluskie MJ, Davis HL (1999) Novel strategies using DNA for the induction of mucosal immunity. Crit Rev Immunol 19:303
39. McCluskie MJ, Wen Y-M, Di Q, Davis HL (1998) Immunization against hepatitis B virus by mucosal administration of antigen-antibody complexes. Viral Immunol 11: 245
40. Mendell JR, Kissel JT, Amato AA, King W, Signore L, Prior TW, Sahenk Z, Benson S, McAndrew PE, Rice R, Nagaraja H, Stephens R, Lantry L, Morris GE, Burghes AHM (1995). Myoblast transfer in the treatment of Duchenne's muscular dystrophy. N Engl J Med 333: 832
41. Meyer KB, Thompson M, Levy M, Barron L, Szoka FJ (1995) Intratracheal gene delivery to the mouse airway: characterization of plasmid DNA expression and pharmacokinetics. Gene Ther 2: 450
42. Moldoveanu Z, Love-Homan L, Huang WQ, Krieg AM (1998) CpG DNA, a novel immune enhancer for systemic and mucosal immunization with influenza virus. Vaccine 16: 1216
43. Okada E, Sasaki S, Ishii N, Aoki I, Yasuda T, Nishioka K, Fukushima J, Miyazaki J, Wahren B, Okuda K (1997) Intranasal immunization of a DNA vaccine with IL-12- and granulocyte-macrophage colony-stimulating factor (GM-CSF)-expressing plasmids in liposomes induces strong mucosal and cell-mediated immune responses against HIV-1 antigens. J Immunol 159: 3638
44. Parker SE, Vahlsing HL, Serfilippi LM, Franklin CL, Doh SG, Gromkowski SH, Lew D, Manthorpe M, Norman J (1995) Cancer gene therapy using plasmid DNA: safety evaluation in rodents and non-human primates. Hum Gene Ther 6: 575
45. Porter KR, Kochel TJ, Wu SJ, Raviprakash K, Phillips I, Hayes CG (1998) Protective efficacy of a dengue 2 DNA vaccine in mice and the effect of CpG immuno-stimulatory motifs on antibody responses. Arch Virol 143: 997
46. Romero R, Lavine JE (1996) Cytokine inhibition of the hepatitis B virus core promoter. Hepatology 23: 17
47. Sasaki S, Hamajima K, Fukushima J, Ihata A, Ishii N, Gorai I, Hirahara F, Mohri H, Okuda K (1998) Comparison of intranasal and intramuscular immunization against human immunodeficiency virus type 1 with a DNA-monophosphoryl lipid A adjuvant vaccine. Infect Immun 66: 823
48. Sasaki S, Sumino K, Hamajima K, Fukushima J, Ishii N, Kawamoto S, Mohri H, Kensil CR, Okuda K (1998) Induction of systemic and mucosal immune responses to human immunodeficiency virus type 1 by a DNA vaccine formulated with QS-21 saponin adjuvant via intramuscular and intranasal routes. J Virol 72: 4931
49. Sato Y, Roman M, Tighe H, Lee D, Corr M, Nguyen MD, Silverman GJ, Lotz M, Carson DA, Raz E (1996). Immunostimulatory DNA sequences necessary for effective intradermal gene immunization. Science 273: 352
50. Scheule RK, St George JA, Bagley RG, Marshall J, Kaplan JM, Akita GY, Wang KX, Lee ER, Harris DJ, Jiang C, Yew NS, Smith AE, Cheng SH (1997) Basis of pulmonary toxicity associated with cationic lipid-mediated gene transfer to the mammalian lung. Hum Gene Ther 8: 689
51. Sparwasser T, Koch ES, Vabulas RM, Heeg K, Lipford GB, Ellwart JW, Wagner H (1998) Bacterial DNA and immunostimulatory CpG oligonucleotides trigger maturation and activation of murine dendritic cells. Eur J Immunol 28: 2045
52. Tacket CO, Roy MJ, Widera G, Swain WF, Broome S, Edelman R (1999) Phase 1 safety and immune response studies of a DNA vaccine encoding hepatitis B surface antigen delivered by a gene delivery device. Vaccine 22: 2826
53. Tang DC, De Vit M, Johnston SA (1992) Genetic immunization is a simple method for eliciting an immune response. Nature 356: 152-154
54. Ugen KE, Nyland SB, Boyer JD, Vidal C, Lera L, Rasheid S, Chattergoon M, Bagarazzi ML, Ciccarelli R, Higgins T, Baine Y, Ginsberg R, Macgregor RR, Weiner DB (1998) DNA vaccination with HIV-1 expressing constructs elicits immune responses in humans. Vaccine. 16: 1818

55. Wang R, Doolan DL, Le TP, Hedstrom RC, Coonan KM, Charoenvit Y, Jones TR, Hobart P, Margalith M, Ng J, Weiss WR, Sedegah M, de Taisne C, Norman JA, Hoffman SL (1998) Induction of antigen-specific cytotoxic T lymphocytes in humans by a malaria DNA vaccine. Science 282: 476
Weeratna R, Brazolot-Millan CL, Krieg AM, Davis HL (1998) Reduction of antigen expression from DNA vaccines by co-administered oligonucleotides. Antisense Nucleic Acid Drug Dev 8: 351
57. Wolff JA, Malone RW, Williams P, Chong W, Acsadi G, Jani A, Felgner PL (1990) Direct gene transfer into mouse muscle *in vivo*. Science 247: 1465
58. Xiang ZQ, He Z, Wang Y, Ertl HCJ (1997) The effect of interferon-γ on genetic immunization. Vaccine 15: 896
59. Yew NS, Wang KX, Przybylska M, Bagley RG, Stedman M, Marshall J, Scheule RK, Cheng SH (1999) Contribution of plasmid DNA to inflammation in the lung after administration of cationic lipid:pDNA complexes. Hum Gene Ther 10: 223
60. Yew NS, Wysokenski DM, Wang KX, Ziegler RJ, Marshall J, Mcneilly D, Cherry M, Osburn W, Cheng SH (1997) Optimization of plasmid vectors for high-level expression in lung epithelial cells. Hum Gene Ther 8: 575
61. Yi AK, Klinman DM, Martin TL, Matson S, Krieg AM (1996) Rapid immune activation by CpG motifs in bacterial DNA. Systemic induction of IL-6 transcription through an antioxidant-sensitive pathway. J Immunol 157: 5394
62. Zabner J, Cheng SH, Meeker D, Launspach J, Balfour R, Perricone MA, Morris JE, Marshall J, Fasbender A, Smith AE, Welsh MJ (1997) Comparison of DNA-lipid complexes and DNA alone for gene transfer to cystic fibrosis airway epithelia in vivo. J Clin Invest 100: 1529
63. Zhao Q, Matson S, Herrera CJ, Fisher E, Yu H, Krieg AM (1993) Comparison of cellular binding and uptake of antisense phosphodiester, phosphorothioate and mixed phosphorothioate and methylphosphonate oligonucleotides. Antisense Res Develop 3: 53

Mucosal adjuvanticity of immunostimulatory DNA sequences

Anthony A. Horner, Nadya Cinman, Arash Ronaghy, Eyal Raz

Department of Medicine and The Sam and Rose Stein Institute for Aging, University of California, San Diego, 9500 Gilman Drive, La Jolla, CA 92093-0663, USA

Introduction

Unlike the skin which is relatively impermeable, mucosal surfaces allow for the intake of oxygen, water, and other nutrients, and the excretion of metabolic byproducts. This relatively permeable nature places unique constraints and requirements on the immunocytes which protect mucosal surfaces, and makes these sites particularly susceptible to penetration by infectious agents. Despite the relative efficiency of the mucosal immune system in preventing infection, the respiratory, gastro-intestinal and vaginal mucosa represent major portals of entry for pathogens [8, 37]. Locally produced and secreted IgA and cytotoxic T lymphocytes (CTL) within the mucosal tissue and draining lymph nodes protect against microbial infection [1, 8, 12, 37]. Because the mucosal immune system serves a front line role in protecting us from infection, there is a great deal of interest in developing strategies for stimulating protective mucosal immune responses. Unfortunately, traditional vaccination methods are not effective, and at present there is no simple, safe, and generally applicable approach for the induction of mucosal immune responses.

Mucosal delivery of replicating immunogens such as live attenuated vaccines elicits robust and long-lasting immune responses, which include the production of mucosal IgA, serum antibody, and a CTL response [8, 37]. However, simple protein antigens are often used for research purposes and clinical applications, and they are much less immunogenic. Systemic (i.e., intradermal; i.d.) vaccination with monomeric proteins elicits serum antibody production, but many arms of the immune response such as mucosal IgA synthesis and CTL activity are not elicited. On the other hand, mucosal vaccination with protein alone generally will not elicit any immune response and may even induce tolerance [8, 13, 37]. In general, to elicit a mucosal IgA response, monomeric protein antigens need to be delivered to mucosal surfaces with an adjuvant [8, 37]. Cholera toxin (CT) is the best-studied and most potent mucosal adjuvant identified to date. Unfortunately, like many adjuvants it has unacceptable toxicity for use in humans [37]. In addition, CT biases systemic immune responses toward a Th_2 phenotype, potentially leading to IgE production and allergic hypersensitivity toward the antigen [20, 35].

Correspondence to: A. A. Horner

Immunostimulatory sequence DNA contained within plasmids and oligodeoxynucleotides (ISS-ODN) has previously been shown to have potent adjuvant activity for systemic immune responses to protein antigens. The immune response seen after systemic vaccination with simple proteins and ISS-ODN shares many features with the immune response seen after viral infections. It characteristically has a Th_1 bias, is robust and long lasting, and generally includes CTL activity [9, 31, 32, 41]. Here we review our recent observations which lead us to conclude that ISS-ODN is a potent mucosal adjuvant that induces secretory IgA, a Th_1-biased serum antibody profile, a heterogeneous antigen-specific cytokine response, and a CTL response following intranasal (i.n.) co-delivery with antigen [15].

ISS-ODN is an adjuvant for Th_1-biased systemic immune responses

ISS-ODN containing the hexamer 5'-pyrimidine-pyrimadine-CpG-purine-purine-3' have been shown to provide effective adjuvant activity for the induction of systemic Th_1-biased immune responses toward protein antigens co-administered via i.d. and intramuscular routes. The immune response includes the induction of a Th_1 cytokine profile (IFN-γ but not IL-4), the production of high IgG2a and low IgG1 titers (IFN-γ- and IL-4-dependent isotypes, respectively), and a CTL response. In contrast, immunization with protein alone leads to a relatively Th_2-biased immune response without CTL activity [9, 15, 31,41].

Insights into how ISS-ODN functions as an adjuvant

The mechanisms underlying the Th_1-biased adjuvant activity of ISS-ODN are not well understood at the molecular level. However, at the cellular level, we do have some mechanistic insights. Research suggests that much of the adjuvant effect of ISS-ODN on adaptive immunity is due to its ability to induce an innate immune response. ISS-ODN can induce the production of type 1 IFNs, IL-12, and IL-18, from macrophages, and IFN-γ from NK cells in an antigen-independent manner [18, 28, 31,40]. These cytokines are known to promote Th_1-biased immune responses [7, 25]. In addition, ISS-ODN stimulates IL-6 production from B cells and IL-10 production from macrophages [2, 18]. IL-6 stimulates polytypic antibody production, while IL-10 promotes IgA synthesis specifically [10, 26]. However, neither IL-6 nor IL-10 has historically been considered to be a typical Th_1 cytokine [7, 25].

Along with the induction of an innate cytokine response, ISS-ODN induces or increases the expression of a variety of cell surface proteins important for productive adaptive immune responses, in an antigen-independent manner. Incubation of naive splenocytes with ISS-ODN leads to expression of B7.1 and B7.2 on B cells and macrophages. This molecule in turn provides important co-stimulatory signals for T cells via CD28 engagement [16, 22, 33, 36]. In addition, ISS-ODN increases CD40 expression on B cells and macrophages. CD40 ligation by CD154 (CD40 ligand) stimulates isotype switching by B cells and activates antigen-presenting cells (APCs) [11, 22, 36]. Furthermore, ISS-ODN increases B cell and macrophage expression of class I and class II molecules, further increasing their capacity to function as APCs [16, 17, 22, 36]. Lastly, cytokine receptor expression (IL-2R and IFN-γR) is increased on B cells and macrophages, increasing their potential to respond to cytokines in their local environment [22].

A central dogma in immunology is that T cells direct the Th bias of antigen-specific immune responses. However, while cytokine production and expression of cell surface molecules by B cells, NK cells, macrophages, and other APCs are promoted by incubation with ISS-ODN, purified T cells do not demonstrate these responses when incubated with ISS-ODN [2, 16, 17, 18, 22, 28, 31, 36, 40]. We believe that the innate immune response of these cells toward ISS-ODN provides important upstream signals, which both promote and bias subsequent antigen-dependent and specific T cell and B cell immune responses. If correct, this model implies that the Th_1-biased immune response which develops toward antigen delivered with ISS-ODN is initiated and shaped by B cells, NK cells, and macrophages, and other APCs, but not directly by T cells.

The mucosal immune system

Mucosal immunity clearly plays an important front line role in protecting man from his/her environment. However, adjuvants and mucosal delivery are needed for the induction of mucosal immune responses to many antigens including most monomeric proteins [8, 37]. Research suggests that lymphocytes involved in mucosal immune responses express a unique set of surface proteins, such as integrin $\alpha_4\beta_7$, which direct these cells to mucosal organs. These homing receptors allow lymphocytes from the site of primary contact with antigen to traffic to multiple mucosal sites, leading to both local and distal mucosal immunity [5, 29]. Therefore, the mucosal immune system can be considered to be made up of a unique population of lymphocytes that can function semi-independently of lymphocytes involved in systemic immune responses.

Mucosal immunization with ISS-ODN induces a strong secretory IgA response

To further characterize the adjuvant potential and clinical utility of ISS-ODN, we assessed its ability to function as a mucosal adjuvant. CT is the best-studied and most potent known mucosal adjuvant for the induction of secretory IgA [37]. Therefore, the IgA response of mice mucosally immunized with protein and ISS-ODN was compared to the IgA response when mice were mucosally immunized with protein and CT. Both ISS-ODN and CT were found to be effective mucosal adjuvants for a variety of antigens and mouse strains. In Fig. 1, the mucosal IgA response of BALB/c mice i.n. immunized with β-galactosidase (β-gal) is presented. While direct comparison of the IgA levels from different mucosal sites can not be made due to differences in sample collection techniques, the data clearly demonstrate that β-gal/ISS-ODN and β-gal/CT immunized mice had equivalent-antigen specific IgA levels in bronchial, intestinal and vaginal, secretions. To establish that a mucosal adjuvant was needed for the induction of mucosal IgA, mice were i.n. immunized with β-gal alone or with a mutated oligodeoxynucleotide (M-ODN). However, i.n. vaccination without mucosal adjuvant resulted in no detectable IgA (data for i.n. β-gal immunization with M-ODN not shown). To evaluate whether contact with the respiratory mucosa was required for ISS-ODN to have mucosal adjuvant activity, mice were immunized with β-gal and ISS-ODN via intragastric (i.g.) and i.d. routes. These routes of immunization did not lead to measurable IgA in mucosal secretions

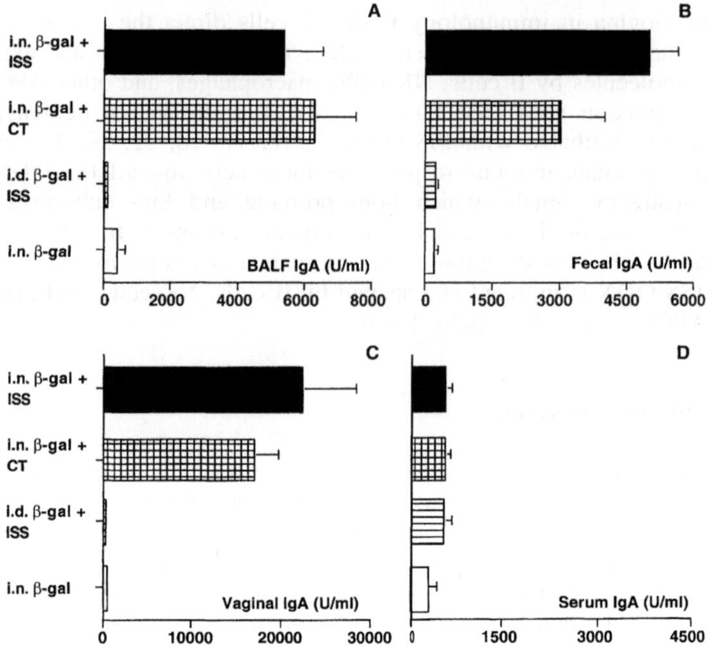

Fig. 1A–D. IgA responses. Mice received three immunizations with β-gal (50 μg) alone, or with ISS-ODN (50 μg), or CT (10 μg) via the i.n. or i.d. route. The immunostimulatory oligodeoxynucleotide used in these experiments has the sequence 5'-TGACTGTG*AACGTTCG*AGATGA-3'. Immunization, sample collection, and ELISA methods are described in [14, 15]. Results were obtained by ELISA and represent mean values for four mice per group, and *error bars* reflect the standard errors of the means. Results are representative of three similar and independent experiments. **A** BALF IgA. BALF (800 μl lavage) was obtained at sacrifice during week 7. There were no significant differences in BALF anti-β-gal IgA levels between i.n. β-gal/ISS-ODN and i.n. β-gal/CT immunized mice. **B** Fecal IgA. Feces were collected at 7 weeks and IgA extracted. There were no significant differences in fecal anti-β-gal IgA levels between i.n. β-gal/ISS-ODN and i.n. β-gal/CT immunized mice. **C** Vaginal IgA. Vaginal washes (50 μl lavage) were obtained at sacrifice during week 7. There were no significant differences in vaginal anti-β-gal IgA levels between i.n. β-gal/ISS-ODN and β-gal/CT immunized mice. **D** Serum IgA. Serum was obtained at week 7. Serum levels of IgA were consistently more than fivefold lower than levels in mucosal samples (β-gal, β-galactosidase; ISS-ODN, immunostimulatory sequence oligodeoxynucleotides; CT, cholera toxin; i.n., intranasal; i.d., intradermal; BALF, bronchoalveolar lavage fluid)

(data for i.g. immunization not shown). To confirm that IgA detected in BALF, fecal material, and vaginal washes of immunized mice was actively secreted by mucosal tissue and did not passively diffuse from serum, anti-β-gal IgA levels in serum, and mucosal sites were compared. It should be noted that initial acquisition of BALF, fecal samples, and vaginal washes requires an unmeasurable dilution of the IgA contained in the material, which does not occur when obtaining serum. Despite this fact, i.n. β-gal/ISS-ODN and i.n. β-gal/CT immunized mice produced higher levels of anti-β-gal IgA in feces, vaginal washes, and BALF than in serum, demonstrating the active secretion of antigen-specific IgA from the mucosal surfaces of these mice.

These results show that ISS-ODN and CT have equivalent mucosal adjuvant activity with a test antigen that has no capacity to induce mucosal IgA production when delivered alone. In addition, mucosal delivery of antigen with ISS-ODN is shown to

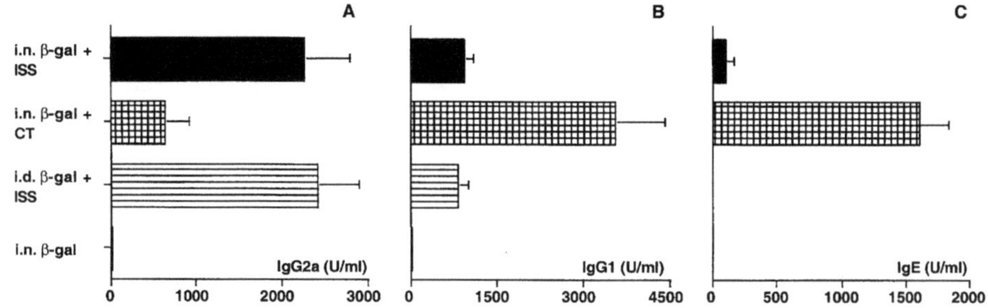

Fig. 2A–C. Serum IgG subclass profiles and IgE. Mice received three immunizations with β-gal (50 μg) alone, or with ISS-ODN (50 μg), via the i.n. or i.d. route. The sequence of the ODN used in these experiments is provided in the legend to Fig. 1. Serum was collected at 7 weeks from immunized mice and assayed by ELISA [15]. Results represent mean values for four mice per group, and *error bars* reflect standard errors of the means. Results are representative of three similar and independent experiments. **A** Serum IgG2a. Serum IgG2a levels were statistically higher in i.n. β-gal/ISS-ODN versus i.n. β-gal/CT immunized mice (P=0.036). **B** Serum IgG1. Serum IgG1 levels were statistically higher in i.n. β-gal/CT versus i.n. β-gal/ISS-ODN immunized mice (P=0.028). **C** Serum IgE. Serum IgE levels were statistically higher in i.n. β-gal/CT versus i.n. β-gal/ISS-ODN immunized mice (P=0.0002)

lead to a secretory IgA response, while i.d. delivery does not. Taken together these findings demonstrate that ISS-ODN is an excellent adjuvant for the induction of both local and distal mucosal immunity when co-delivered with antigen via the nose.

Mucosal immunization with ISS-ODN leads to a Th_1-biased antibody response

The serum antibody response induced by i.n. immunization with ISS-ODN was next evaluated. Again the mucosal adjuvant CT was used for comparison. We found that i.n. delivery of β-gal with ISS-ODN and i.n. delivery of β-gal with CT led to divergent serum antibody profiles. As can be seen in Fig. 2, i.n. vaccination with ISS-ODN and β-gal led to high levels of IgG2a and low levels of IgG1 when compared to i.n. β-gal/CT vaccination. In addition, IgE production in i.n. β-gal/ISS-ODN and i.n. β-gal/CT-immunized mice was evaluated. As seen in Fig. 2, only β-gal/CT-immunized mice produced IgE. The serum antibody profiles induced by i.n. and i.d. delivery of β-gal with ISS were also compared. As demonstrated in Fig. 2, i.n. and i.d. delivery of β-gal with ISS-ODN led to similar serum antibody profiles. Again, the requirement for i.n. immunization with an adjuvant was demonstrated, as i.n. delivery of β-gal alone or with M-ODN did not induce a serum antibody response (data on i.n. β-gal/M-ODN delivery not shown).

A dichotomy in T helper cell function described by a number of investigators has led to the concept of Th_1 cells which produce IFN-γ but not IL-4, and Th_2 cells which produce IL-4 but not IFN-γ [7, 25]. In mice, Th_1-biased immune responses are also associated with the production of IgG2a (IFN-γ dependent), but not IgG1 or IgE (IL-4 dependent) [7]. In contrast, Th_2-biased immune responses are associated with the synthesis of IgG1 and IgE [25, 35]. ISS-ODN is considered to be a Th_1 adjuvant when delivered systemically, while CT is considered to be a Th_2 adjuvant when delivered mucosally [9, 15, 20, 23, 31, 35]. The serum antibody profile after i.n. ISS-ODN/antigen immunization is consistent with these previously published re-

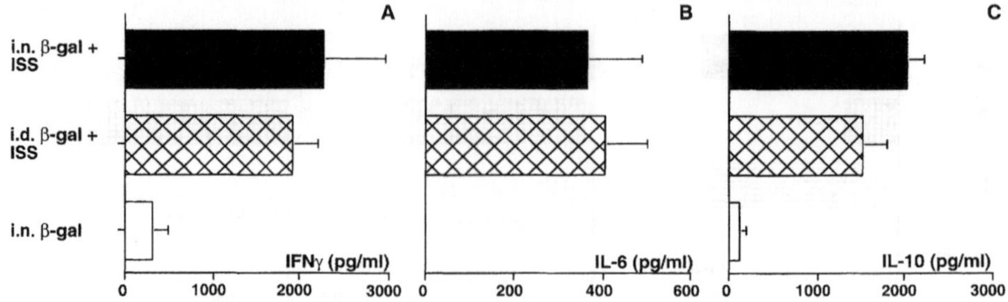

Fig. 3A–C. Antigen-induced splenocyte cytokine profiles. Mice received three immunizations with β-gal (50 μg) alone, or with ISS-ODN (50 μg), via the i.n. or i.d. routes. The sequence of the ODN used in these experiments is provided in the legend to Fig. 1. Splenocytes were harvested from sacrificed mice during week 7, cultured in media with or without β-gal (10 μg/ml), and 72-h supernatants were assayed by ELISA [15]. Splenocytes from immunized mice cultured without β-gal produced negligible amounts of cytokines (data not shown). Results represent the mean for four mice in each group and similar results were obtained in two other independent experiments. *Error bars* reflect standard errors of the means. **A** IFN-γ. **B** IL-6. **C** IL-10

sults, suggesting that ISS-ODN has Th_1-biasing activity which is independent of the route of delivery. More importantly, the present results show that i.n. delivery of antigen with ISS-ODN is just as effective as i.d. delivery of these same reagents for the induction of serum IgG2a synthesis. Considered in conjunction with the IgA data presented previously, the data further demonstrate that mucosal IgA synthesis can occur in the context of both Th_1- and Th_2-biased antibody production.

Mucosal immunization with ISS-ODN induces an antigen-specific IFN-γ, IL-6, and IL-10 response

The adjuvants ISS-ODN and CT have previously been considered to promote antigen-specific Th_1- and Th_2-biased cytokine profiles, respectively [9, 15, 20, 23, 31, 35]. To confirm that i.n. immunization with β-gal and ISS-ODN leads to a similar cytokine profile as systemic delivery, the cytokine profiles of mucosally vaccinated mice were next evaluated. Splenocytes from immunized mice were incubated with β-gal, and culture supernatants were assayed for the production of IFN-γ and IL-4. Splenocytes from mice immunized with β-gal and ISS-ODN by either the i.n. or i.d. route produced equivalent levels of IFN-γ (Fig. 3) but no IL-4 or IL-5 (data not shown). Splenocytes from mice i.n. immunized with β-gal alone or with M-ODN did not demonstrate any detectable antigen-specific cytokine production, further demonstrating the need for an adjuvant in the induction of productive immune responses at mucosal sites.

IFN-γ has not been shown to induce mucosal IgA production. However, IL-6 and IL-10 are known to support IgA synthesis [6, 10, 26, 27]. Because these cytokines are known to be induced during antigen-independent stimulation of mononuclear cells with ISS, we next evaluated the antigen-specific IL-6 and IL-10 responses of immunized mice [2, 18, 28]. Splenocytes from mice i.n. and i.d. immunized with β-gal and ISS-ODN produced significant and equivalent levels of IL-6 and IL-10 (Fig. 3). However, local mucosal T cells are thought to play a greater role than splenic

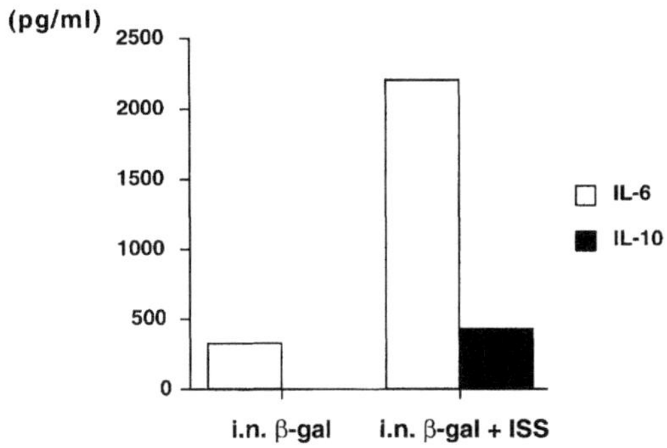

Fig. 4. Antigen-induced pulmonary lymphocyte cytokine profiles. Mice received three immunizations with β-gal (50 μg) alone, or with ISS-ODN (50 μg), via the i.n. route. The sequence of the ODN used in this experiment is provided in the legend to Fig. 1. Lymphocyte-enriched cell populations were harvested from sacrificed mice during week 7 by grinding lung through a fine nylon sieve. These cells were cultured in media with or without β-gal (10 μg/ml), and 72-h supernatants were assayed by ELISA [15]. Cells from immunized mice cultured without β-gal produced negligible amounts of cytokines (data not shown). To obtain enough cells for these cultures, cells from four mice were pooled for each experimental condition

T cells in providing T cell help for secretory IgA production [37]. Therefore, the local cytokine responses that developed after i.n. β-gal delivery with ISS-ODN were next evaluated. Significant amounts of antigen-specific IL-6 and IL-10 were produced by lymphocytes residing in the lung parenchyma of i.n. β-gal/ISS-ODN-immunized mice (Fig. 4). In addition, pulmonary lymphocytes from these mice produced IFN-γ (data not shown). However, pulmonary lymphocytes from mice i.n. immunized with β-gal alone produced only low levels of IL-6 and no detectable IL-10 or IFN-γ.

Analysis of the antigen-specific cytokine profiles of immunized mice demonstrates that i.n. and i.d. β-gal/ISS-ODN immunization are equally effective in the induction of antigen-specific IFN-γ synthesis but neither route of immunization elicits IL-4 or IL-5 responses. Furthermore, β-gal/ISS-ODN immunization induces the development of antigen-specific IL-6 and IL-10 responses. The promotion of IL-6 and IL-10 synthesis both at mucosal and systemic sites may at least partially explain the IgA response seen after i.n. delivery of ISS-ODN with antigen.

Mucosal immunization with ISS-ODN induces a splenic CTL response

Although development of antigen-specific CTL activity is associated with Th_1-biased immunity, not all Th_1-biased immune responses include the development of cytotoxic T cells [1, 37]. Therefore, the ability of i.n. co-delivery of β-gal and ISS-ODN to induce a CTL response was evaluated. As demonstrated in Fig. 5, mice immunized with β-gal and ISS-ODN by either the i.n. or i.d. route displayed vigorous and equivalent splenic CTL activity. Again, i.n. immunization with β-gal alone or with M-ODN led to poor or undetectable CTL responses (data for i.n. β-gal/M-ODN immunization not presented). Considered in conjunction with the splenic cytokine and serum antibody responses previously presented, this data confirms that i.d. and i.n. vaccination with β-gal and ISS-ODN lead to systemic immune responses of equivalent magnitude.

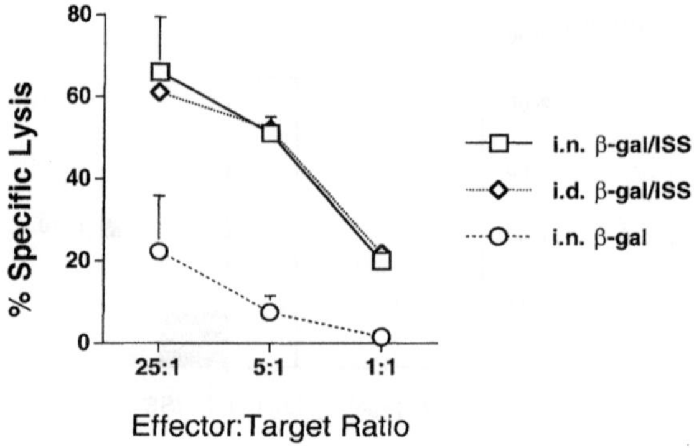

Fig. 5. Splenic CTL responses. Mice received three immunizations with β-gal (50 μg) alone, or with ISS-ODN (50 μg), via the i.n. or i.d. routes. The sequence of the ODN used in this experiment is provided in the legend to Fig. 1. Results were obtained by ELISA using a substrate that is metabolized by lactate dehydrogenase from lysed cells to a colored byproduct [15]. Results represent mean values for four mice per group, and *error bars* reflect the standard errors of the means. Results are representative of three similar and independent experiments. The CTL responses induced by i.n. β-gal/ISS-ODN and i.d. β-gal/ISS-ODN immunizations were not significantly different (CTL, cytotoxic T lymphocyte)

Table 1. Anti-β-gal Ig production induced by mucosal pre-priming

ISS-ODN	β-gal	Serum IgG2a (U/ml)	BALF IgA (U/ml)
	+	<5	<50
Day (0)	+	2390±715	2940±825
Day (–1)	+	3220±1120	463±47
Day (–3)	+	380±34	398±38
Day (–7)	+	178±48	459±183
Day (–14)	+	<5	<50

Mice received i.n. ISS-ODN (50 μg) on a single occasion the specified number of days before or with i.n. β-gal (50 μg). The sequence of the oligodeoxynucleotide used in these experiments is provided in the Fig. 1 legend. Serum and BALF were obtained at week 8 and were analyzed by ELISA as outlined in the legends to Figs. 1 and 2. Ig levels from mice receiving ISS-ODN with or up to 7 days before β-gal were significantly higher than those from mice receiving β-gal alone ($P<0.05$)
ISS-ODN, Immunostimulatory sequence oligodeoxynucleotides; β-gal, β-galactosidase; BALF, bronchoalveolar lavage fluid

Mucosal ISS-ODN pre-priming

We have recently found that ISS-ODN activates the innate immune system for an extended period of time after delivery ([22], see Kobayashi et al. in this issue). Therefore, we considered the possibility that pre-priming with ISS-ODN would lead to an extended period of Th_1 adjuvant activity for antigen-specific immune responses. Work by Kobayashi and colleagues demonstrates that, in fact, i.d. injection of ISS-ODN up to 2 weeks before β-gal delivery leads to an improved immune response compared to immunization with β-gal alone, and that ISS-ODN pre-priming from 3 to 7 days before β-gal delivery is more effective than co-administration. In addition, we have found that there is a 7-day window of adjuvant activity after i.n. ISS-ODN delivery. In Table 1 and Fig. 6, data are presented that detail this observa-

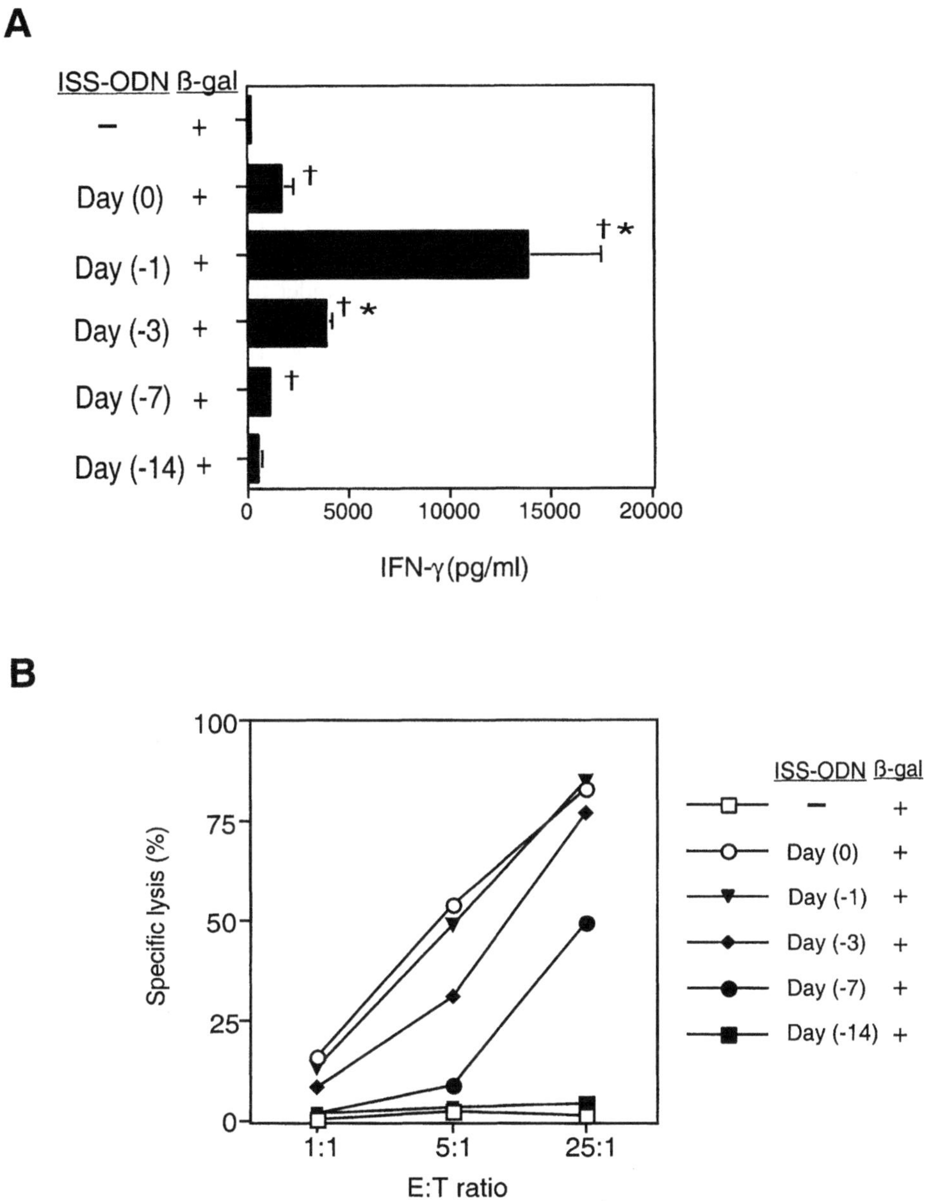

Fig. 6. Splenocyte CTL and IFN-γ response after i.n. ISS pre-priming. Mice received i.n. ISS-ODN (50 μg) on a single occasion the specified number of days before i.n. β-gal (50 μg). The sequence of the ODN used in these experiments is provided in the legend to Fig. 1 and the specifics of the splenocyte cytokine and CTL assays are outlined in Figs. 3 and 5. Results represent the mean±SE for four mice in each group. Similar results were obtained in two other independent experiments. **A** IFN-γ response. Mice pre-primed with ISS up to 7 days prior to β-gal demonstrated an increased IFN-γ response when compared to mice immunized with β-gal alone (†; $P \leq 0.05$). Delivery of ISS from 1–3 days before β-gal led to an elevated IFN-γ response when compared to mice receiving ISS/β-gal co-immunization (★; $P \leq 0.05$) **B** CTL response. Mice pre-primed with ISS up to 7 days prior to β-gal demonstrated statistically improved CTL responses at effector:target ratios of 5:1 and 25:1 when compared to mice immunized with β-gal alone ($P \leq 0.05$)

tion. The mechanisms underlying ISS-ODN pre-priming are discussed in detail in Dr. Kobayashi's review.

Discussion

In summary, the data presented demonstrate that ISS-ODN is a potent mucosal adjuvant. I.n. delivery of antigen with either ISS-ODN or CT leads to equivalent and vigorous mucosal IgA responses, while i.d. co-delivery of antigen with ISS-ODN does not lead to mucosal IgA production. However, under the experimental conditions employed, i.d. and i.n. vaccination with target antigen and ISS-ODN induce equivalent systemic Th_1-biased immune responses characterized by high levels of antigen-specific IFN-γ but no IL-4 production from cultured splenocytes, high IgG2a and low IgG1 and IgE serum concentrations, and vigorous CTL responses. In contrast, i.n. co-delivery of antigen with CT leads to secretory IgA synthesis in conjunction with a Th_2-biased systemic antibody response characterized by high IgG1 and IgE and low IgG2a levels in the serum. In addition, we found that the antigen-specific cytokine response of mice immunized with ISS-ODN includes IL-6 and IL-10 production. These cytokines are known to promote IgA synthesis. Therefore, the production of IL-6 and IL-10 by mucosal T cells may play a role in the mucosal IgA response seen in mice i.n. immunized with β-gal and ISS-ODN. Further studies demonstate that the adjuvant effect of ISS-ODN persists for at least 7 days after i.n. delivery. While initial work utilized BALB/c mice and β-gal as antigen, subsequent studies have demonstrated the generalizability of this phenomenon to other mouse strains and protein antigens ([23, 24] and personal observations).

Consistent with our findings, Moldoveanu et al. [24] have shown that ISS-ODN is an effective mucosal adjuvant for IgA production against a formalin-inactivated influenza vaccine. Interestingly, under the experimental conditions utilized in these studies, the inactivated influenza vaccine stimulated secretory IgA production even without an adjuvant. The multimeric nature of the antigen preparation and the epithelial binding properties of the influenza virus may help explain this observation [34]. These investigators were unable to elicit a CTL response against influenza virus. Formalin inactivation leads to cross-linking of protein. This in turn could limit peptide processing and presentation by MHC molecules leading to relatively weak T cell responses as suggested by the authors [24, 34]. McCluskie et al. [23] have also recently shown that ISS-ODN serves as an effective mucosal adjuvant for the induction of an IgA response, using the hepatitis B surface antigen. Unlike the influenza vaccine, but consistent with antigens used in our studies, hepatitis B surface antigen did not induce an IgA response when mucosally delivered without adjuvant. However, in contrast to our findings, these investigators were also unable to elicit a significant CTL response if ISS-ODN was the only adjuvant used to immunize mice. Our experience suggests that the low doses of antigen and ISS-ODN used in these experiments may have played a role in the poor CTL responses reported.

The fact that equivalent mucosal IgA levels can develop in the context of Th_1-biased and Th_2-biased antibody responses with i.n. β-gal/ISS-ODN and β-gal/CT immunizations, respectively, is consistent with other published results. Marinaro et al. [21] recently demonstrated that oral delivery of tetanus toxoid with CT leads to mucosal IgA production in conjunction with a Th_2-biased antibody profile. However, when tetanus toxoid and CT are co-administered with oral IL-12 the systemic antibody response is skewed toward a Th_1 phenotype, while mucosal IgA production is unaffected (21). Taken together, these findings document that synthesis of mucosal IgA can occur in the context of both Th_1- and Th_2-biased antibody production.

It is intriguing that previous studies have shown that IFN-γ, IL-6, and IL-10 are produced by naive immunocytes incubated with ISS-ODN, while the present experiments demonstrate that these cytokines are also produced as part of the antigen-specific immune response that develops after antigen co-immunization with this adjuvant. Further work will be needed to better understand the basis for this immunologic symmetry. In addition, while earlier studies suggested that IL-6 and IL-10 are produced exclusively by Th_2 cells [7, 25], the present results show that IL-6 and IL-10 synthesis can occur in conjunction with highly Th_1-biased serum antibody responses. This finding adds to a growing body of evidence that IL-6 and IL-10 production are not isolated to either Th_1-biased or Th_2-biased immune responses [3, 6, 7, 25].

Mucosal IgA and CTL responses are known to provide protection against a number of infectious agents. HIV is but one important example [1, 8, 12, 19, 37, 38]. There are a number of strategies available for the development of vaccines which induce these immune parameters. However, none appears to be globally applicable. Live attenuated vaccines induce robust immune responses, including mucosal IgA synthesis and CTL activity. Unfortunately, difficulty in attenuating many pathogens and the risk of iatrogenic disease limits the use and development of live attenuated vaccines [8, 13, 19, 37]. On the other hand, recombinant proteins from infectious agents are generally safe, but induce relatively poor immune responses, and generally none when delivered to mucosal surfaces. However, mucosal adjuvants can improve immune responses towards co-administered protein antigens substantially [8, 13, 37].

CT is an extremely potent mucosal adjuvant, but is inherently toxic and induces a Th_2-biased antibody response which can include the development of IgE and consequent allergic sensitization toward the target antigen [20, 35]. At present, such toxicity and other technical problems have kept many adjuvants, including CT, from becoming available for use in humans [13]. Alum is essentially the only adjuvant in clinical use today. It is relatively weak, does not work with a number of antigens, does not induce CTL activity, and because it must be delivered systemically, does not induce mucosal IgA [13]. A safe and effective mucosal adjuvant would be of great value in the development of better vaccines against mucosal pathogens. ISS-ODN is a potent adjuvant, which works with a wide range of protein antigens, and generally induces a Th_1-biased immune response with CTL activity [9, 31, 32, 41]. Administration of protein with ISS-ODN by i. n. and i. d. routes leads to vigorous and equivalent Th_1-biased systemic immune responses, while only i.n. delivery induces a mucosal immune response [15]. Therefore, i.n. delivery of relevant antigens with ISS-ODN may well prove superior to i.d. delivery for the induction of protective immunity against mucosal pathogens.

The concept of ISS-ODN pre-priming has some interesting implications with regards to clinical applications. Given the prolonged adjuvant effect provided by ISS-ODN, it is conceivable that ISS-ODN could be given without antigen to modulate the course of ongoing infections. This has already been suggested in a model of leishmaniasis [41]. By activation of the innate immune system with ISS-ODN it may also be possible to prevent infection. These considerations are under active investigation in our laboratory at the present time.

Conclusions

ISS-ODN are easy to manufacture, stable, and without identified toxicity at immunogenic doses in mice and primates (unpublished observations). Additionally, use of antisense oligodeoxynucleotides in monkeys and human clinical trials have demonstrated no significant toxicity with daily doses of up to fivefold more per kilogram than those used in the present study [39]. Moreover, we and others have shown that human and mouse immunocytes display similar immunological responses to ISS-ODN ([4, 31] and personal observations). Because ISS-ODN can be utilized as an adjuvant for both mucosal and systemic Th_1-biased immune responses toward simple monomeric protein antigens, it may well prove to be a valuable reagent for the development of mucosal vaccines and as an immunomodulatory therapeutic for the prevention or treatment of ongoing infections. However, future investigations in primates and humans are needed to establish whether ISS-ODN has utility in the development of strategies for the induction of protective immune responses against mucosal pathogens.

Acknowledgements This work was supported in part by NIH grants AI01490 and AI40682, and grants from Dynavax Technologies Corporation and The Sam and Rose Stein Institute for Aging.

References

1. Ada GL, McElrath MJ (1997) HIV type 1 vaccine induced cytotoxic T cell responses: potential role in vaccine efficacy. AIDS Res Hum Retroviruses 13:205
2. Anitescu M, Chace JH, Tuetken R, Yi AK, Berg DJ, Krieg AM, Cowdery JS (1997) Interleukin-10 functions in vitro and in vivo to inhibit bacterial DNA induced secretion of interleukin-12. J Interferon cytokine Res 17:781
3. Assenmacher M, Schmitz J, Radbruch A (1994) Flow cytometric determination of cytokines in activated murine T helper lymphocytes: expression of interleukin-10 in interferon-γ and in interleukin-4 producing cells. Eur J Immunol 24:1097
4. Ballas ZK, Rasmussen WL, Krieg AM (1996) Induction of natural killer cell activity in murine and human cells by CpG motifs in oligodeoxynucleotides and bacterial DNA. J Immunol 157:1840
5. Berlin C, Berg EL, Briskin MJ, Andrew DP, Kilshaw PJ, Holzmann B, Weissman IL, Hamann A, Butcher EC (1993) α4β7 Integrin mediates lymphocyte binding to the mucosal vascular adressin MAdCAM-1. Cell 74:185
6. Carpenter EA, Rudy J, Ramshaw IA (1994) IFN-gamma, TNF, and IL-6 production by vaccinia virus immune spleen cells: an in vitro study. J Immunol 152:2652
7. Coffman RL, Mosmann TR (1988) Isotype regulation by helper T cells and lymphokines. Monogr Allergy 24:96
8. Czerkinsky C, Holmgren J (1995) The mucosal immune system and prospects for anti-infectious and anti-inflammatory vaccines. Immunologist 3:97
9. Davis HL, Weeranta R, Waldschmidt TJ, Tygrett L, Schorr J, Krieg AM (1998) CpG DNA is a potent enhancer of specific immunity in mice immunized with recombinant hepatitis B surface antigen. J Immunol 160:870
10. Defrance T, Vanbervliet B, Briere F, Durand I, Rousett F, Banchereau J (1992) Interleukin-10 and transforming growth factor β cooperate to induce anti-CD40-activated na human B cells to secrete immunoglobulin A. J Exp Med 175:671
11. Fuleihan R, Ramesh N, Loh R, Jabara H, Rosen FS, Chatila T, Fu SM, Stamenkovic I, Geha RS (1993) Defective expression of the CD40 ligand in X chromosome-linked immunoglobulin deficiency with normal or elevated IgM. Proc Natl Acad Sci USA 90:2170
12. Gallichan WS, Johnson DC, Graham FL, Rosenthal KL (1993) Mucosal immunity and protection after intranasal immunization with recombinant adenovirus expressing herpes simplex virus glycoprotein. J Infect Dis 168:622

13. Gutpa RK, Siber GR (1995) Adjuvants for human vaccines-current status, problems and future prospects. Vaccine 13:1263
14. Haneberg B, Kendell D, Amerongen HM, Apter FM, Kraehenbuhl JP, Neutra MR (1994) Induction of specific immunoglobulin A in the small intestine, colon-rectum, and vagina measured by a new method for collection of secretions from local mucosal surfaces. Infect Immun 62:15
15. Horner AA, Ronaghy A, Cheng PM, Nguyen MD, Cho HJ, Broide D, Raz E (1998) Immunostimulatory DNA is a potent mucosal adjuvant. Cell Immunol 190:77
16. Jakob T, Walker PS, Krieg AM, Udey MC, Vogel JC (1998) Activation of cutaneous dendritic cells by CpG-containing oligodeoxynucleotides: a role for dendritic cells in the augmentation of Th1 responses by immunostimulatory DNA. J Immunol 161:3042
17. Karlsson L, Castano AR, Peterson PA (1996) Principles of antigen processing and presentation. In: Kagnoff MF, Kiyono H (eds) Essentials of mucosal immunology. Academic Press, San Diego, pp 3–28
18. Klinman DM, Yi AK, Beaucage SL, Conover J, Krieg AM (1996) CpG motifs present in bacterial DNA rapidly induce lymphocytes to secrete interleukin 6, interleukin 12, and interferon-γ. Proc Natl Acad Sci USA 93:2879
19. Letvin NL (1998) Progress in the development of an HIV-1 vaccine. Science 280:1875
20. Marinaro M, Staats HF, Hiroi T, Jackson RJ, Coste M, Boyaka PN, Okahashi N, Yamamoto M, Kiyono H, Bluethmann H, Fujihashi K, McGhee JR (1995) Mucosal adjuvant effect of cholera toxin in mice results in the production of T helper 2 (Th2) cells and IL-4. J Immunol 155:4621
21. Marinaro M, Boyaka PN, Finkelman FD, Kiyono H, Jackson RJ, Jirillo E, McGhee JR (1997) Oral but not parenteral interleukin (IL)-12 redirects T helper 2 (Th2)-type responses to an oral vaccine without altering mucosal IgA responses. J Exp Med 185:415
22. Martin-Orozco E, Kobayashi H, Van Uden J, Nguyen MD, Kornbluth RS, Raz E (1999) Enhancement of antigen presenting cell surface molecules involved in cognate interactions by immunostimulatory DNA sequences. Int Immunol 7:1111
23. McCluskie MJ, Davis HL (1998) CpG DNA is a potent enhancer of systemic and mucosal immune responses against hepatitis B surface antigen with intranasal administration in mice. J Immunol 161:4463
24. Moldoveanu Z, Love-Homan L, Huang WQ, Kreig AM (1998) CpG DNA, a novel immune enhancer for systemic and mucosal immunization with influenza virus. Vaccine 16:1216
25. Mosmann TR, Coffmann RL (1989) Th_1 and Th_2 cells: differential patterns of lymphokine secretion lead to different functional properties. Annu Rev Immunol 7:145
26. Muraguchi A, Hirano T, Tang B, Matsuda T, Horii Y, Nakajima K, Kishimoto T (1988) The essential role of B cell stimulatory factor 2 (BSF-2/IL-6) for the terminal differentiation of B cells. J Exp Med 167:332
27. Okahashi N, Yamamoto M, Vancott JL, Chatfield SN, Roberts M, Bluethmann H, Hiroi H, H, Kiyono H, McGhee JR (1996) Oral immunization of interleukin-4 (IL-4) knockout mice with a recombinant Salmonella strain or cholera toxin reveals that $CD4^+$ Th_2 cells producing IL-6 and IL-10 are associated with mucosal immunoglobulin A responses. Infect Immun 64:1516
28. Pisetsky DS (1996) Immune activation by bacterial DNA: a new genetic code. Immunity 5:303
29. Quiding-Jarbrink M, Nordstrom I, Granstrom G, Kilander A, Jertborn M, Butcher EC, Lazarovits AI, Holmgren J, Czerkinsky C (1997) Differential expression of tissue-specific adhesion molecules on human circulating antibody-forming cells after systemic, enteric, and nasal immunizations. J Clin Invest 99:1281
30. Ramsey AJ, Husband AJ, Ramshaw IA, Bao S, Matthaei K, Kohler G, Kopf M (1994) The role of IL-6 in mucosal immune responses in vivo. Science 264:561
31. Roman M, Martin-Orozco E, Goodman JS, Nguyen MD, Sato Y, Ronaghy A, Kornbluth R, Richman DD, Carson DA, Raz E (1997) Immunostimulatory DNA sequences function as T helper-1-promoting adjuvants. Nat Med 3:849
32. Sato Y, Roman M, Tighe H, Lee D, Corr M, Nguyen MD, Silverman GJ, Lotz M, Carson DA, Raz E (1996) Immunostimulatory DNA sequences necessary for effective intradermal gene immunization. Science 273:352
33. Shahinian A, Pfeffer K, Lee KP, Kundig TM, Kishihara K, Wakeham A, Kawai K, Ohashi PS, Thompson CB, Mak TW (1993) Differential T cell costimulatory requirements in CD28-deficient mice. Science 261:609
34. Smith CB (1998) Influenza viruses. In: Gornbach SL, Bartlett JG, Blacklow NR (eds) Infectious diseases. Saunders, Philadelphia, pp 2120–2125

35. Snider DP, Marshal JS, Perdue MH, Liang H (1994) Production of IgE antibody and allergic sensitization of intestinal and peripheral tissues after oral immunization with protein antigen and cholera toxin. J Immunol 153:647
36. Sparwasser T, Koch ES, Vabulas RM, Heeg K, Lipford GB, Ellwart JW, Wagner H (1998) Bacterial DNA and immunostimulatory CpG oligonucleotides trigger maturation and activation of murine dendritic cells. Eur J Immunol 28:2045
37. Staats HF, McGhee JR (1996) Application of basic principles of mucosal immunity to vaccine development. In: Kiyono H, Ogra PL, McGhee JR (eds) Mucosal vaccines. Academic Press, San Diego, pp 15–40
38. VanCott TC, Kaminski RW, Mascola JR, Kalyanaraman VS, Wassef NM, Alving CR, Ulrich JT, Lowell GH, Birx DR (1998) HIV-1 neutralizing antibodies in the genital and respiratory tracts of mice intranasally immunized with oligomeric gp120. J Immunol 160:2000
39. Webb A, Cunningham D, Cotter F, Clarke PA, Stefano F di, Ross P, Corbo M, Dziewanowska Z (1997) BCL-2 antisense therapy in patients with non-Hodgkin lymphoma. Lancet 349:1137
40. Yamamoto S, Yamimoto T, Kataoka T, Kuramoto E, Yano O, Tokunaga T (1992) Unique palindromic sequences in synthetic nucleotides required to induce IFN and augment IFN-mediated natural killer cell activity. J Immunol 148:4072
41. Zimmermann S, Egeter O, Hausmann S, Lipford GB, Rocken M, Wagner H, Heeg K (1998) CpG oligodeoxynucleotides trigger protective and curative Th1 responses in lethal murine leishmaniasis. J Immunol 160:3627

Immunostimulatory DNA sequences help to eradicate intracellular pathogens

Hermann Wagner, Hans Häcker, Grayson B. Lipford

Institute of Medical Microbiology, Immunology and Hygiene, Technical University of Munich, Trogerstr. 9, 81675 Munich, Germany

Introduction

Primary immune responses to pathogens are initiated within secondary lymphoid organs by dendritic cells (DCs). Pathogen proteins are engulfed by DCs and processed into surface presented foreign peptides that serve as a stimulus for antigen-specific T cell receptors, thus informing reactive naive T cells about the invading pathogen. $CD8^+$ cytotoxic T lymphocytes (CTL) recognize peptide antigens presented by major histocompatibility complex (MHC) class I molecules, while $CD4^+$ T helper (Th) cells respond to peptide antigens presented by MHC class II molecules. CD4 Th cells provide help to CD8 T cells, however, help is indirect since Th cells do not engage CTL precursors. CD40 ligand (CD154) positive CD4 Th cells provide help by activation of antigen-presenting cells (APCs) via CD40 signaling; therefore, Th cell to CTL help is via APC activation [8, 18]. CD40 cross-linking on antigen-presenting DCs not only causes DC activation but also replaces CD4 Th in the priming of CD8 CTL responses [3, 24, 25].

DCs also bear receptors for conserved molecular patterns associated with pathogens, such as endotoxin (LPS), mannans, double-stranded RNA and immunostimulatory DNA sequences (CpG-DNA) [17]. In the case of LPS, microbial pattern recognition via Toll-like receptors (TLRs) triggers DCs to synthesize and up-regulate costimulatory molecules, cytokines and chemokines [12]. It thus appears that DCs can integrate stimuli either from antigen-reactive Th cells via CD40 cross-linking, or directly via recognition of pathogen-derived conserved molecular patterns.

As members of the innate immune system, DCs and macrophages not only control emanating adaptive immune responses but also represent an important first line defense against invading pathogens. Once activated, both macrophages and DCs can limit intracellular growth of pathogens via the generation of oxygen radicals and nitric oxide [4, 5]. Cellular activation can be initiated and/or augmented by proinflammatory and effector cytokines such TNF-α and IFN-γ, respectively [7]. It is less clear whether similar to LPS, recognition of other conserved molecular patterns of pathogen-derived constituents like CpG-DNA acutely activates innate immune cells to display bactericidal activity.

Correspondence to: H. Wagner

A potential breakthrough regarding LPS activation came with the identification of an LPS binding and signaling complex. The complex is assembled when members of the TLR family interact with LPS bound to CD14. The subsequent TLR signal is similar in many characteristics to the IL-1R signal transduction pathway [14, 22, 23]. In contrast, the mechanisms underlying CpG-oligodeoxynucleotide (ODN)-driven activation of APCs are not as well understood. Cellular uptake of CpG-ODN appears to be necessary for activation but is sequence nonspecific [10]. Upon translocation into early endosomes, inhibitors of endosomal maturation, such as chloroquine or bafilomycin A, block CpG-ODN sequence-specific downstream signaling events like the activation of JNK and p38 stress kinases [10]. Interestingly, in macrophages, but not in DCs, CpG-ODN additionally activates the ERK pathway, which negatively regulates the IL-12 promoter. This might explain why DCs but not macrophages produce high amounts of IL-12 upon CpG-ODN-driven activation [9].

There are differences and parallels between the activation of DCs and macrophages by LPS or CpG-DNA. For example, in contrast to LPS, CpG-ODN do not appear to signal via TLR4 or TLR2 (C. Kirschning, unpublished data and [22]). It has become apparent, however, that mammals, like Drosophila, have numerous TLR with remaining unknown ligand specificities, leaving the possibility open of one being a CpG-DNA receptor. Even though LPS and CpG-DNA may use distinct receptors to initiate signaling, the downstream events are remarkably similar. These events involve acute activation of the stress kinase and MAP kinase pathways that result in the activation of transcription factors like NF-κB and AP-1 [10, 19]. Upon activation, NF-κB translocates to the nucleus to activate genes with κB binding sites in their promoters and enhancers. These genes include TNF-α, IL-1β, IL-6, IL-8, IL-12p40, and the co-stimulatory molecules CD80, CD86 and MHC class II molecules. It is, thus, not surprising that CpG-DNA, similarly to LPS, activates in vitro and in vivo antigen-presenting immature DCs and macrophages to transit to professional APCs [28, 29].

A key feature of mammalian innate immunity is the ability to rapidly limit an infectious challenge. Initial constraint of infection is based on the capacity to discriminate, via pattern recognition, self from infectious non-self. The innate immune system thus bridges the time required to generate antigen-specific effectors by the emanating adaptive immune system. Here we will review the information available on the effect of CpG-DNA in model systems of infectious diseases.

CpG-DNA renders CD8 T cell peptides immunogenic: induction of protective antiviral CTL responses

Vaccines consisting of minimal peptide epitopes in adjuvants can induce protective viral CTL immunity, yet peptides alone often result in peripheral CTL tolerance [1, 2]. When H2-K^b mice are subcutaneously (s.c.) injected with the heterologous soluble protein ovalbumin (OVA), immature DC in the draining lymph nodes (LNs) constitutively engulf and process OVA to the immunodominant CD8 T cell epitope SIINFEKL [29]. These DCs are presentation competent; however, they fail to induce a protective CTL response. In contrast, s.c. challenge with an OVA/CpG-ODN mixture induces protective CTL responses. The CpG-DNA triggers in draining LNs antigen-presenting immature DCs to transit to professional APCs by inducing synthesis of co-stimulatory molecules (CD80, CD86, CD40, MHC class II) and to produce cytokines such as IL-12 [29]. Once activated, antigen-presenting DCs induce protective antigen-specific CTL responses.

Murine lymphocytic choriomeningitis virus (LCMV) infections are controlled by LCMV-specific CD8 CTL via perforin-dependent cytolysis of virus-infected cells [13, 33]. An immunodominant MHC class I-restricted T cell epitope in H-2^b mice is gp33, the peptide spanning residues 33–41 of the LCMV glycoprotein [21]. We vaccinated H-2^b mice s.c. once with a mixture of gp33-peptide plus immunostimulatory CpG-ODN. The vaccination not only triggered gp33 specific CTL responses, but also induced a protective T cell response against subsequent infection with LCMV [31]. For induction of cell-mediated protective antiviral immune responses with T cell peptides, CpG-ODN, if not better than, may be at least as efficient as the commonly used complete Freund's adjuvants (CFA), as has also been reported by Oxenius et al. [20].

CpG-DNA induces protection against intracellular bacterial infection

During the early phase of intracellular bacterial infections, neutrophils and macrophages play a critical role in limiting bacterial replication [30]. The cytokines IFN-γ and TNF-α, as well as reactive oxygen intermediates and NO produced by IFN-γ-activated macrophages, are critical for protection [7]. Late-phase primary infections and secondary infections are essentially controlled by effector functions of the adaptive immune system, such as antibodies and CTL [11]. Since bacterial CpG-DNA and i.s. CpG-ODN directly activate macrophages in vitro and in vivo [28, 29], we were not surprised to observe that CpG-ODN confer resistance against infection with *Listeria monocytogenes* [27]. Krieg et al. [15] reported that in CpG-ODN-challenged SPF-BALB/c mice, serum IL-12 was increased for at least 8 days and correlated with a state of IFN-γ-dependent resistance to infection with *L. monocytogenes*.

Interestingly, CpG-DNA induced sustained activation of innate immunity (1–2 weeks). Mice infected with *L. monocytogenes* during that period had much lower bacterial burdens in the spleen and liver [15, 20]. Essentially similar results have been reported in CpG-ODN-driven protection against *Francisella tularensis* live vaccine strain (LVS), with the exception that non-specific innate immunity appeared to somehow be dependent on B lymphocytes [6].

CpG-DNA conveys protection against intracellular *Leishmania major*

Epidemiological studies indicate an inverse relationship between Th1-promoting infections (mycobacteria, measles virus) and the propensity of individuals to develop atopic disorders [26]. This raised the question whether bacterial CpG-DNA and CpG-ODN mimic the Th1-promoting effect of bacterial infections. To address this issue, we investigated the CpG-DNA effect on *L. major*-infected BALB/c mice, a widely accepted model for Th2-driven disease. CpG-ODN sequence dependently promoted Th1 development in LNs draining the site of *L. major* challenge and conveyed NO-dependent protective immunity. Conversion from *the L. major*-susceptible Th2 phenotype to a Th1-resistant phenotype was associated with IL-12 production and sustained expression of the IL-12 receptor-β2 chain [32]. Strikingly, challenge with i.s. CpG-ODN prior to infection induced a sustained state of resistance to *L. Major* infection for up to 2 weeks [16]. This resistance correlated with sustained

IL-12 production in the draining LNs. Overall these data parallel, at least in part, those obtained in protection assays to *L. monocytogenes* and *F. tularensis*. These data indicate the power of CpG-DNA to remodel innate immune system function that ensures a sustained state of resistance to intracellular pathogens associated with a propensity to trigger Th1-polarized adaptive immune responses. In this regard, CpG-ODN appear to mimic the principle of Th1-promoting infections.

Conclusion

There has been a change in our view concerning the relationship and interplay between the innate and adaptive immune system. Bactericidal innate immunity represents an ancient defense mechanism, the principles of which were already operative in flies, and is dependent on pathogen pattern recognition. The adaptive immune system on the other hand appeared later and is dependent on the recombination of gene segments to create an abundance of novel antigen receptors, which allows memory to pathogens already encountered. Innate immune system cells like DCs and macrophages have acquired additional functions that serve as a bridge between the two immune systems. They not only process and present antigens but post activation stimulate and orient primary adaptive immune responses via cytokine production and expression of co-stimulatory molecules. Activation can be brought about by pattern recognition of pathogen-derived constituents. Prototypic examples of pattern recognition ligands are LPS and genomic bacterial CpG-DNA. Viewed from this perspective, CpG-DNA ought to enhance bactericidal activity of DCs and macrophages towards intracellular pathogens, promote transition of immature antigen presenting to professional APCs and polarize emanating T cell responses. Although a detailed picture is still incomplete, evidence is available that CpG-ODN trigger aspects of all these innate immune system functions in the various models of intracellular infections, such as challenge with LCMV, *L. monocytogenes*, *F. tularensis* and *L. major*. The change in function of innate immune cells that ensures a sustained state of resistance to intracellular pathogens, however, is one effect of CpG-DNA that was unexpected. How this 'remodeling' operates mechanistically is poorly understood. Speculating, one may hypothesize that innate immunity has at its disposal functional characteristics of the adaptive immune response, that is to develop a sustained state of resistance to pathogens.

References

1. Aichele P, Brduscha-Riem K, Oehen S, Odermatt B, Zinkernagel RM, Hengartner H, Pircher H (1997) Peptide antigen treatment of naive and virus-immune mice: antigen-specific tolerance versus immunopathology. Immunity 6:519
2. Aichele P, Brduscha-Riem K, Zinkernagel RM, Hengartner H, Pircher H (1995) T cell priming versus T cell tolerance induced by synthetic peptides. J Exp Med 182:261
3. Bennett SR, Carbone FR, Karamalis F, Flavell RA, Miller JF, Heath WR (1998) Help for cytotoxic-T-cell responses is mediated by CD40 signalling. Nature 393:478
4. Chatham WW, Turkiewicz A, Blackburn WDJ (1994) Determinants of neutrophil HOCl generation: ligand-dependent responses and the role of surface adhesion. J Leukoc Biol 56:654
5. Ding AH, Nathan CF, Stuehr DJ (1988) Release of reactive nitrogen intermediates and reactive oxygen intermediates from mouse peritoneal macrophages. Comparison of activating cytokines and evidence for independent production. J Immunol 141:2407

6. Elkins KL, Rhinehart-Jones TR, Stibitz S, Conover JS, Klinman DM (1999) Bacterial DNA containing CpG motifs stimulates lymphocyte-dependent protection of mice against lethal infection with intracellular bacteria. J Immunol 162:2291
7. Endres R, Luz A, Schulze H, Neubauer H, Futterer A, Holland SM, Wagner H, Pfeffer K (1997) Listeriosis in p47(phox–/–) and TRp55–/– mice: protection despite absence of ROI and susceptibility despite presence of RNI. Immunity 7:419
8. Grewal IS, Flavell RA (1996) A central role of CD40 ligand in the regulation of CD4+ T-cell responses. Immunol Today 17:410
9. Hacker H, Mischak H, Hacker G, Eser S, Prenzel N, Ullrich A, Wagner H (1999) Cell type-specific activation of mitogen activation protein kinases by CpG-DNA controls interleukin-12 release from antigen presenting cells. EMBO J 18:6973
10. Hacker H, Mischak H, Miethke T, Liptay S, Schmid R, Sparwasser T, Heeg K, Lipford GB, Wagner H (1998) CpG-DNA-specific activation of antigen-presenting cells requires stress kinase activity and is preceded by non-specific endocytosis and endosomal maturation. EMBO J 17:6230
11. Harty JT, Bevan MJ (1995) Specific immunity to *Listeria monocytogenes* in the absence of IFN gamma. Immunity 3:109
12. Hoffmann JA, Kafatos FC, Janeway CA, Ezekowitz RA (1999) Phylogenetic perspectives in innate immunity. Science 284:1313
13. Kagi D, Seiler P, Pavlovic J, Ledermann B, Burki K, Zinkernagel RM, Hengartner H (1995) The roles of perforin- and Fas-dependent cytotoxicity in protection against cytopathic and noncytopathic viruses. Eur J Immunol 25:3256
14. Kirschning CJ, Wesche H, Merrill AT, Rothe M (1998) Human toll-like receptor 2 confers responsiveness to bacterial lipopolysaccharide. J Exp Med 188:2091
15. Krieg AM, Love-Homan L, Yi AK, Harty JT (1998) CpG DNA induces sustained IL-12 expression in vivo and resistance to *Listeria monocytogenes* challenge. J Immunol 161:2428
16. Lipford GB, Sparwasser T, Zimmermann S, Heeg K, Wagner H (2000) CpG-DNA mediated transient lymphadenopathy is associated with a state of Th1 predisposition to antigen-driven responses. J Immunol (in press)
17. Medzhitov R, Janeway CA Jr (1997) Innate immunity: the virtues of a nonclonal system of recognition. Cell 91:295
18. Noelle RJ (1996) CD40 and its ligand in host defense. Immunity 4:415
19. O'Neill LA, Greene C (1998) Signal transduction pathways activated by the IL-1 receptor family: ancient signaling machinery in mammals, insects, and plants. J Leukoc Biol 63:650
20. Oxenius A, Martinic MM, Hengartner H, Klenerman P (1999) CpG-containing oligonucleotides are efficient adjuvants for induction of protective antiviral immune responses with T-cell peptide vaccines. J Virol 73:4120
21. Pircher H, Rohrer UH, Moskophidis D, Zinkernagel RM, Hengartner H (1991) Lower receptor avidity required for thymic clonal deletion than for effector T-cell function. Nature 351:482
22. Poltorak A, He X, Smirnova I, Liu MY, Huffel CV, Du X, Birdwell D, Alejos E, Silva M, Galanos C, Freudenberg M, Ricciardi-Castagnoli P, Layton B, Beutler B (1998) Defective LPS signaling in C3H/HeJ and C57BL/10ScCr mice: mutations in Tlr4 gene. Science 282:2085
23. Qureshi ST, Lariviere L, Leveque G, Clermont S, Moore KJ, Gros P, Malo D (1999) Endotoxin-tolerant mice have mutations in Toll-like receptor 4 (Tlr4) [published erratum appears in J Exp Med (1999) 189:following 1518]. J Exp Med 189:615
24. Ridge JP, Di Rosa F, Matzinger P (1998) A conditioned dendritic cell can be a temporal bridge between a CD4+ T- helper and a T-killer cell. Nature 393:474
25. Schoenberger SP, Toes RE, Voort EI van der, Offringa R, Melief CJ (1998) T-cell help for cytotoxic T lymphocytes is mediated by CD40-CD40L interactions. Nature 393:480
26. Shirakawa T, Enomoto T, Shimazu S, Hopkin JM (1997) The inverse association between tuberculin responses and atopic disorder. Science 275:77
27. Sparwasser T, Hultner L, Koch ES, Luz A, Lipford GB, Wagner H (1999) Immunostimulatory CpG-oligodeoxynucleotides cause extramedullary murine hemopoiesis. J Immunol 162:2368
28. Sparwasser T, Koch ES, Vabulas RM, Heeg K, Lipford GB, Ellwart J, Wagner H (1998) Bacterial DNA and immunostimulatory CpG oligonucleotides trigger maturation and activation of murine dendritic cells. Eur J Immunol 28:2045
29. Sparwasser T, Vabulas RM, Villmow B, Lipford GB, Wagner H (2000) Bacterial CpG-DNA activates dendritic cells in vivo: helper cell-independent cytotoxic T cell responses to soluble proteins. E J Immunol (in press)

30. Unanue ER (1997) Inter-relationship among macrophages, natural killer cells and neutrophils in early stages of *Listeria* resistance. Curr Opin Immunol 9:35
31. Vabulas RM, Lipford GB, Pircher H, Wagner H (2000) CpG-DNA activates in vivo T cell peptide presenting immature dendritic cells to trigger protective antiviral cytotoxic T cell responses. J Immunol 164:2372 (in press)
32. Zimmermann S, Egeter O, Hausmann S, Lipford GB, Rocken M, Wagner H, Heeg K (1998) CpG oligodeoxynucleotides trigger protective and curative Th1 responses in lethal murine leishmaniasis. J Immunol 160:3627
33. Zinkernagel RM, Althage A (1977) Antiviral protection by virus-immune cytotoxic T cells: infected target cells are lysed before infectious virus progeny is assembled. J Exp Med 145:644

The antigenic properties of bacterial DNA in normal and aberrant immunity

David S. Pisetsky

Division of Rheumatology, Allergy and Clinical Imunology,
Durham VA Medical Center and Duke University Medical Center, Box 151G, Room E-1008,
508 Fulton Street, Durham, NC 27705, USA

Introduction

DNA is a complex macromolecule whose antigenic properties reflect an interplay of sequence and structure. This molecule has occupied a singular place in immunology since, until recently, it was considered exclusively an autoantigen and a unique target of immune reactivity in systemic lupus erythematosus (SLE). In this prototypic autoimmune disease, antibodies to DNA (anti-DNA) occur prominently and serve as markers for diagnosis and prognosis. These autoantibodies bind sites on both single-stranded (ss) and double-stranded DNA (ds) and are part of a diverse group of autoantibodies directed to nuclear antigens (antinuclear antibodies or ANA) [28, 44].

In contrast to the study of other ANA responses, the analysis of anti-DNA long focused on the antibodies rather than the antigen. Indeed, DNA was viewed as an immunologically bland and inert macromolecule, a large polyanion devoid of activity outside the pathological setting. As shown by exciting and provocative investigation over the last decade, however, this conceptualization is incorrect. Many studies have now demonstrated clearly, that bacterial DNA, because of its base sequence, can cause potent immune activation and can induce specific antibody responses as well as nonspecific immunostimulation. By virtue of these activities, DNA from bacterial sources has the potential to drive the production of both pathogenic and non-pathogenic antibodies [30].

This review will consider the antigenic properties of bacterial DNA as they relate to the production of anti-DNA antibodies in both normal and aberrant immunity. As this account will indicate, the recognition of the immunological properties of bacterial DNA provides a new perspective on the anti-DNA response and directs attention to the possibility that foreign DNA can drive pathogenic antibody production in an individual predisposed in autoimmunity. Since initial studies on the anti-DNA response focused on SLE, the serology of this disease will be considered first to provide a context for understanding the antigenic properties of bacterial DNA.

Serology of SLE

The most notable serological disturbance in SLE is the production of ANA antibodies. These antibodies bind to a diverse array of antigens that includes DNA,

RNA, proteins and protein-nucleic acid complexes. Of ANA commonly found in SLE sera, two ANA have achieved the status of diagnostic markers. These antibodies are anti-DNA and anti-Sm. Antibodies to DNA are directed to structural determinants on DNA, while antibodies to Sm are directed to protein components of a complex called a snRNP (small nuclear ribonucleoprotein) [12, 40].

While anti-DNA and anti-Sm are both useful diagnostic markers, they nevertheless differ importantly in their expression. These ANA responses occur independently of each other and do not display linkage (i.e., the expression of anti-DNA does not predict the response to anti-Sm and vice versa). Furthermore, in individual patients who express both antibodies, the quantitative expression of the two responses differs. In patients with both anti-DNA and anti-Sm, the time course of antibody expression also varies. Whereas anti-DNA levels frequently fluctuate with disease activity, anti-Sm levels tend to be more static [23].

As shown by longitudinal studies of patients, levels of anti-DNA can parallel disease activity, in particular, glomerulonephritis. At times when renal disease activity is increased, levels of anti-DNA are frequently elevated. When renal disease subsides (often because of therapy), anti-DNA levels can fall and sometimes become undetectable. The dramatic decrease in anti-DNA levels with therapies such as corticosteroids and cytotoxic drugs contrasts with the much more modest changes in overall levels of immunoglobulin or other autoantibodies [2, 21].

The correlation between levels of anti-DNA and renal disease activity, while demonstrating a critical feature of this ANA response, also points to a direct role of these anti-DNA in immunopathogenesis. Additional evidence for this role comes from the isolation of anti-DNA antibodies in enriched form from glomerular eluates as well as the demonstration of glomerular deposition of infused anti-DNA into normal animals. Together, these data indicate a propensity for anti-DNA to localize in the kidney, mostly likely in the form of immune complexes, where they may incite inflammatory damage [2, 21].

Although anti-DNA antibodies can promote glomerulonephritis, studies on patients indicate many discrepancies between clinical and serological profiles. Thus, patients with anti-DNA may lack evidence of active renal disease, suggesting that the ability to cause glomerular disease is a property of only certain anti-DNA. These anti-DNA have been termed nephritogenic, although the properties that distinguish them from non-pathogenic antibodies remain unknown [7, 8, 17, 18, 26].

Specificity of SLE anti-DNA

The specificity of anti-DNA has been analyzed to understand the role of antigen drive in the etiology of this response as well as to define critical interactions promoting nucleic acid binding. Several major conclusions, relevant to subsequent studies on antibodies to bacterial DNA, arise from this analysis: (1) among anti-DNA, while some bind exclusively to either ss or dsDNA, most bind to sites present on both; (2) antibodies to dsDNA in the B conformation provide the most highly specific markers for diagnosis; (3) anti-DNA bind determinants that are conserved and widely present on natural DNA irrespective of species origin; (4) anti-DNA interactions with DNA have an important contribution from charge-charge interactions, most likely reflecting binding to sites on the phosphodiester backbone that can be present on both ss and dsDNA; and (5) anti-DNA may have preference for DNA with certain base sequences. Together, these observations suggest that, while bases may contribute to the antibody interaction, the backbone is the major source of binding energy [7, 13, 40, 42, 43].

The affinity of anti-DNA has been more difficult to evaluate, although this issue is important in defining the role of DNA antigen drive in this response and distinguishing pathogenic and non-pathogenic antibodies. A key difficulty in these determinations concerns the polymeric nature of DNA and the uncertainty in the concentration of antigenic sites along the extended macromolecule. If the major determinant bound by SLE anti-DNA is the backbone itself, the concentration of antigen is extremely large, with a given DNA molecule accommodating antibodies as long as they do not interfere with each other physically. On the other hand, if antigenic determinants involve bases as well as the backbone, the concentration of epitopes will be lower and depend on the frequency of those bases or base sequences: *a priori*, there is no way to make this assessment quantitatively.

One approach to defining affinity and epitope density has been the use of DNA antigens varying in molecular size. These sized antigens can be created by use of limit digests with DNase or restriction enzymes with frequent cutting sites. As shown by Papalian et al.[27], the binding of SLE serum anti-DNA is critically dependent on the size of the DNA antigen. In fluid phase assays, stable binding by SLE sera requires DNA pieces of the order of 40–50 bases in length. Among sera as well as monoclonal anti-DNA preparations, the minimal size for antigenicity varies since some antibody preparations need pieces of DNA several hundreds of bases long for appreciable binding. These results are notable since an antibody combining site can accommodate only a few bases [1, 27].

The most likely explanation for the size profile for antigenic DNA relates to the mechanisms by which antibody contacts DNA. As an extended macromolecule, DNA can bridge both Fab combining sites of an individual IgG. This bridging allows binding by a mechanism called monogamous or bivalent interaction. In this mechanism, stable binding requires simultaneous interaction with both Fab sites. Depending on the isotype and structure of the hinge region of an IgG, the distance between both Fab sites is greater than 10 nm, a distance corresponding to a nucleotide chain of 40–50 bases. The reason some antibodies require even longer DNA pieces most likely relates to the binding of antigenic determinants that are more rarely distributed along the DNA molecule.

In the solid phase, the size requirement for antigenic DNA is even greater than the fluid phase. As shown using *Hinf* restriction digests of DNA, ssDNA pieces of less than 1000–2000 bases are poorly antigenic in an ELISA, although they are nevertheless antigenic in the fluid phase and can effectively block the binding of SLE sera to high molecular weight DNA in an ELISA. These findings suggest that the binding of anti-DNA to DNA is constrained when DNA is fixed in the solid phase and that the antigenicity of DNA depends on its physical disposition [33].

Thus, for binding of anti-DNA to occur, the DNA and antibody may need to rearrange in space to bring antigenic determinants in contiguity with both Fab sites by processes such as looping or bending. These considerations indicate that, while the measured affinity of pathogenic anti-DNA is high, significant binding energy results from the polymeric nature of DNA and the capacity for cross-linking [25, 41].

Induction of pathogenic anti-DNA antibodies

Considerable evidence indicates that the immune response to DNA in SLE is an antigen-driven process with DNA the inciting antigen. This evidence includes the affinity and specificity of anti-DNA, the pattern of expression of anti-DNA during the course of SLE, and the molecular properties of anti-DNA. As shown most clearly with monoclonal products from lupus mice, anti-DNA antibodies bear variable (V) region sequences that are indicative of selection of DNA by a receptor-driven mechanism. These features include V region somatic mutations and heavy chain CDR3 regions with a high content of arginine residues as well as arginine residues in certain positions. Since arginine can bind DNA by charge-charge interactions as well as hydrogen bonding, the presence of this amino acid points to the selecting role of DNA [34, 35].

While the anti-DNA response in both human and murine SLE has features of DNA drive, it has been difficult to replicate this response in normal animals by immunization with mammalian DNA. Thus, immunization with DNA alone fails to induce a significant response although, when DNA is administered in the presence of a carrier such as methylated bovine serum albumin (mBSA), a limited response to ssDNA ensues. At least with this carrier, significant induction of antibodies to dsDNA, the serological hallmark of SLE, does not occur. Even in mice genetically determined to develop anti-DNA, immunization with DNA with mBSA fails to induce or accelerate an autoantibody response [22].

Although other carriers (e.g., Fus 1) may lead to greater anti-DNA responses than those obtained with mBSA [5], the poor immunogenicity of mammalian DNA in the classic double-stranded B conformation is, nevertheless, notable and stands in contrast to the immunogenicity of self proteins. When administered to normal animals, a variety of autoantigenic proteins can induce clinical and serological features of disease. The failure of DNA immunization to induce an SLE-like illness has suggested that DNA may differ from other macromolecules in its immunological capabilities and can induce immune responses only in certain forms or in the setting of immunoregulatory disturbances.

Immune properties of bacterial DNA

As this account indicates, studies on the origin of pathogenic anti-DNA in SLE have been guided by two key assumptions on the immunology of DNA: (1) anti-DNA responses occur exclusively in SLE and are antigen-driven responses; and (2) DNA is immunologically uniform. While these assumptions have received experimental support from a variety of systems, recent data suggest that they are oversimplified and fail to reflect the structural and immunological diversity of DNA. As shown now by many investigators and reviewed in this volume, DNA is heterogeneous in its immune activities, with DNA from bacteria displaying properties distinct from mammalian DNA [29].

The identification of the immunological properties of bacterial DNA came from a number of laboratories working on disparate issues, including the serology of anti-DNA. As now recognized, bacterial DNA has potent immunostimulatory activities that result from short sequence motifs that have the general structure of two 5' purines, an unmethylated CpG motif, and two 3' pyrimidines. Depending on the sequences of the 5' and 3' ends, this motif can exist as a palindrome. This sequence motif has been called an immunostimulatory sequence (ISS) or CpG motif [20, 47].

As currently conceptualized, CpG motifs can serve as a danger signal that, in code-like fashion, indicates the presence of foreign DNA. These motifs occur much more commonly in bacterial than mammalian DNA for two main reasons: CpG suppression and cytosine methylation. The combination of CpG suppression and cytosine methylation leads to a marked difference in the array of base sequences present in eukaryotic and prokaryotic DNA, with dramatic differences in the content of CpG motifs. Some investigators have suggested the differences in nucleic acid structure among species may have arisen as a mechanism of host defense [6, 15].

Using either natural or synthetic compounds as stimulants, DNA containing CpG motifs can cause B cell activation, including both proliferation as well as polyclonal antibody production. Furthermore, bacterial DNA is a potent inducer of cytokines and can elicit directly or indirectly TNF-α, IL-12, IL-6, IFN-α/β and IFN-γ. Although bacterial DNA or CpG oligonucleotides do not directly activate T cells, they may provide costimulatory signals for other activators (e.g., anti-CD3). Importantly, in the context of induction of antibodies to DNA, the outcome of these activities is an adjuvant effect and the stimulation of a Th1 response [4, 20, 24, 47].

Antibody responses to bacterial DNA

Although bacterial DNA has the potential to modify host defense non-specifically, the most compelling evidence that bacterial DNA affects the mammalian immune system comes from the study of specific antibody responses. As noted above, anti-DNA has long been considered a diagnostic marker of SLE and an exclusive feature of the autoimmune state. This conclusion has been based on studies of a limited number of mammalian and non-mammalian DNA, with dsDNA in the B conformation identified as the antigenic form most relevant for delineating mechanisms of autoreactivity. As now recognized, studies on the serology of anti-DNA were misleading and missed a normal pathway of anti-DNA production. Indeed, the expression of antibodies to certain antigenic sites on bacterial DNA appears to be a prominent feature of normal immunity [30].

The discovery of antibody responses to bacterial DNA came from an effort to define the contribution of base sequence to anti-DNA binding. As model antigens that bear diverse sequences, a panel of bacterial and mammalian DNA differing in base composition was tested for their ability to bind to sera from patients with SLE and normal human subjects (normal human sera, NHS) by ELISA. In these assays, ssDNA was used as antigen since this structural form provides more sensitive assays and allows detection of cross-reactive binding to dsDNA. Although previous studies suggested that SLE sera show variable levels of binding to DNA from different species origin, in these studies, the levels of binding to the different antigens was similar. These findings are consistent with a predominant recognition in SLE of a conserved antigenic determinant that is commonly expressed by DNA irrespective of base composition or species origin [16].

The study of control NHS, however, provided an unexpected result. Although NHS failed to bind to mammalian DNA as well as certain bacterial DNA in the panel, they showed high levels of binding to DNA from two bacterial species, *Micrococcus lysodeikticus* (MC) and *Staphylococcus epidermidis* (SE). The binding of

NHS was fully sensitive to DNase, suggesting that the antigenic moiety was nucleic acid rather than a contaminating macromolecule. The level of antibody binding of NHS and SLE sera to these antigens was similar, although the binding of NHS to other DNA was low, as anticipated from studies documenting the marker function of anti-DNA [16].

Studies on the specificity of anti-DNA in SLE sera and NHS indicate marked differences in cross-reactivity. As shown by inhibition binding assays, SLE sera bind to cross-reactive determinants found widely on DNA from mammalian and bacterial sources since all DNA tested could block binding to MC DNA. In contrast, NHS anti-DNA are highly specific for DNA from a single bacterial species since MC DNA does not inhibit binding to NHS to SE DNA and vice versa. These findings are consistent with the recognition in NHS of sequence-specific antigenic determinants that are variably present on DNA depending on species origin.

The simplest interpretation of these studies is that normal humans can generate an antibody response to bacterial DNA in a manner analogous to the response to protein antigens. As such, these antibodies would specifically target sequences that are absent from host DNA and therefore not subject to tolerance. While these sequences have not yet been defined, they appear to be different from CpG motifs. Thus, DNA from only certain bacteria are antigenic, although CpG motifs are widely present on bacterial DNA, albeit in varying concentrations [46].

At present, the reason that DNA from only some bacteria are antigenic is not known. These differences in response could result from the level or site of exposure during bacterial colonization or infection; immunogenicity of DNA because of sequence; or the existence of tolerance. Interestingly, NHS do not react well to DNA from *E. coli,* although the gut exposure of this organism is presumed high [46].

Further studies on the immunochemical properties of antibodies in DNA in normal humans and patients with SLE indicated important differences in the nature of these responses. Thus, the binding of antibodies to bacterial DNA in NHS is affected less by ionic strength and pH than the binding of SLE antibodies to either bacterial or mammalian DNA. With increasing ionic strength, the binding of SLE anti-DNA diminishes much more markedly than the binding of NHS anti-DNA. These findings suggest that NHS anti-DNA binding depends less on charge-charge interaction than SLE anti-DNA, consistent with a preference for base recognition in contrast to the backbone [37].

The preference for NHS anti-DNA for base sequence is also apparent in their ability to bind to low molecular weight DNA. As noted above, SLE anti-DNA is limited in its ability to bind to restriction fragments of DNA that are adherent to solid-phase supports. Even though these DNA antigens are active in soluble form, they show dramatically reduced activity with SLE sera in ELISA assays. In contrast, NHS sera show similar levels of binding to intact, high molecular weight bacterial DNA as well as restriction fragments. This result is consistent with binding of NHS anti-DNA to sequential determinants that do not have to undergo conformational changes or rearrangements in space to bind antibody [32]. Although studies have not been performed to evaluate directly monogamous or bivalent interaction, it appears likely that NHS will be able to interact monovalently with DNA, with Fab fragments active as well as an intact IgG.

Since NHS anti-DNA can discriminate among DNA molecules by sequence-specific binding, it is likely that their avidity for DNA is higher than SLE anti-DNA which are sequence nonspecific and bind by charge-charge interactions. As noted above, the assessment of anti-DNA avidity is complicated by uncertainty in epitope content and size, making any measurement of this value an approximation. Within the limits of this approach, it nevertheless appears that NHS anti-DNA binds to bacterial DNA with higher avidity than SLE anti-DNA. Thus, the concentrations of DNA required to inhibit binding of NHS anti-DNA to MC DNA are much lower than those required to inhibit SLE anti-DNA. SLE anti-DNA shows similar avidity with bacterial and mammalian DNA, consistent with the binding to a shared determinant [37].

Although NHS anti-DNA bind selectively to bacterial DNA, they nevertheless interact with both ss- as well as dsDNA. By ELISA, NHS bind to dsDNA from bacterial DNA. Furthermore, as shown by the inhibition binding assays using MC DNA as an antigen, ssDNA and dsDNA show cross-inhibition, indicating the existence of a shared determinant on both conformational forms [3]. These observations imply that NHS anti-DNA can interact with base sequences that are accessible even in dsDNA. Alternatively, dsDNA may open structurally to expose ss regions that are bound by antibodies. The idea that antibodies to dsDNA are specific for SLE must, therefore, be qualified in view of data that NHS anti-DNA bind to bacterial dsDNA, albeit without cross-reactivity.

Induction of anti-DNA by bacterial DNA immunization

The serological studies on NHS suggest that bacterial DNA can serve in vivo as an immunogen and induce specific antibody response comparable to other foreign antigens. This potential has been fully documented in animals. Thus, under conditions in which immunization with mammalian DNA elicits a limited response, bacterial DNA induces a robust IgG antibody response. With ssDNA from *E. coli* (EC) as an immunogen, the resulting antibodies cross-react with ssDNA from both mammalian and non-mammalian sources; some of the induced antibodies also bind to EC dsDNA but not dsDNA from mammalian sources. In contrast, immunization with EC dsDNA leads to the expression of antibodies that bind EC dsDNA but do not cross-react with mammalian dsDNA; these induced antibodies can also bind certain synthetic DNA duplexes (e.g., poly-dGC:poly-dGC) but not others (poly-dAT:poly-dAT). These findings suggest that the determinant bound by these antibodies, while present on dsDNA, is distinct from the B DNA conformation which is conserved on all DNA [10]. These immunization experiments therefore replicate key features of the NHS anti-DNA response.

As these considerations indicate, bacterial DNA contains at least three immunologically relevant determinants that include conserved and non-conserved epitopes as well as CpG motifs (Table 1). In bacterial DNA, CpG motifs may serve as internal

Table 1. Immunological determinants of bacterial DNA

Determinant	*Structure*	*Activity*
CpG motif	Base sequence	Immune activation (B cells, macrophages)
Non-conserved epitope	Base sequence	Bind antibodies in normal sera
Conserved epitope	Backbone	Bind antibodies in SLE sera

Table 2. Molecular differences between normal and SLE anti-DNA

Isotype
Light chain utilization
Affinity
Binding of sequence vs. backbone
Role of charge-charge interactions
Size requirement for antigenicity
CDR sequences

adjuvants and, in normal individuals, promote the production of antibodies to non-conserved DNA sites. In normal individuals, the antibodies to bacterial DNA display predominantly the IgG2 isotype, suggesting resemblance to the response to bacterial carbohydrates in induction mechanisms. In contrast, antibodies to bacterial DNA in SLE are primarily IgG1 and IgG3, suggesting that the autoimmune state is associated with altered isotype expression as well as cross-reactivity [36].

Another difference between SLE and NHS anti-DNA concerns utilization of light chains. As shown using MC DNA, NHS anti-DNA show disproportionate light chain utilization and are overwhelming κ. In constrast, SLE anti-DNA show a κ/λ utilization similar to that of serum Ig [36]. The basis of restriction in NHS is not known, although it could reflect regulatory interactions or the necessity of particular V region sequences to allow DNA binding. Whatever the basis of this finding, it serves as a further feature distinguishing antibodies to bacterial DNA in NHS and SLE patients. Table 2 summarizes differences between normal and SLE anti-DNA [16, 36, 37].

Although antibodies to bacterial DNA occur commonly in NHS, their physiological effects in normal immunity are not known. These antibodies could serve a protective function by binding bacterial DNA and promoting the elimination of this immunostimulatory molecule. In the absence of these antibodies, bacterial DNA could persist and promote nonspecific immunostimulation. While antibodies to bacterial DNA could promote DNA elimination, resulting immune complexes could theoretically deposit in the kidney similar to DNA-anti-DNA complexes in SLE. This occurrence may not be pathogenic, however, since the predominant isotype of antibodies to bacterial DNA is IgG2 which fixes complement poorly. Future investigation will be needed to define the functional properties of the antibodies specific for bacterial DNA.

The role of bacterial DNA in driving pathogenic anti-DNA production

Since anti-DNA levels fluctuate during disease course, the pathogenesis of SLE must involve profound changes in either the amount or form of DNA or the immunological capability of the host. As an essential cellular macromolecule, DNA is present ubiquitously, suggesting that differences in stimulation by DNA during flare could relate to cellular events that alter the accessibility of DNA to the immune system (e.g., cell injury or damage as well as the acceleration of processes such as apoptosis). The consequences of these processes would be release of DNA into the extracellular mileu or a redistribution of DNA from nucleus to cytoplasm where it may be more immunogenic [12].

The recognition of the immunological properties of bacterial DNA has suggested an alternative mechanism to explain the serology of SLE as well as the occurrence of flare. According to this new view, pathogenic anti-DNA production can result from an aberrant response to a foreign molecule (bacterial DNA) rather than solely an aberrant response to a self molecule (mammalian DNA). In this scenario, infection provides a vehicle for introducing a potent immunostimulatory molecule that bears self-antigen determinants. This dualism of bacterial DNA is possible because of the unique structure of DNA that comprises conserved and non-conserved determinants as well as an internal adjuvant.

Two lines of experimental evidence indicate that an aberrant pattern of antigen specificity underlies SLE and leads to the expression of cross-reactive anti-DNA autoantibodies in response to foreign DNA. The first line came from studies on the consequences of immunization of preautoimmune NZB/NZW mice with EC dsDNA as mBSA complexes in adjuvant. As noted above, although normal mice can generate antibodies to this immunogen, the induced antibodies are highly specific for non-conserved sites on bacterial DNA and do not cross-react with mammalian DNA. In contrast, NZB/NZW mice, when similarly immunized, produce antibodies that bind mammalian as well as bacterial dsDNA and resemble SLE autoantibodies in their specificity. Interestingly, mammalian DNA fails to stimulate production of cross-reactive anti-dsDNA autoantibodies in NZB/NZW mice, although these animals are destined to produce such autoantibodies after the onset of spontaneous disease [11].

In this model system, both the normal and autoimmune strain receive the same immunogen in conjunction with a foreign carrier protein (mBSA) that should serve as an adequate source of T cell help. Furthermore, since the immunogen itself is an adjuvant, the stage is set for a powerful immune response. The unique expression of autoantibodies by NZB/NZW mice in response to bacterial DNA would, therefore, appear to reside at the level of the B as opposed to the T cell. This situation could occur if the B cell compartment in SLE mice differs from that of normal mice and contains precursors that directly bind dsDNA or at least allow mutations that create this specificity. These B cells could result from defects in either peripheral or central tolerance.

Analysis of the sequences of monoclonal anti-DNA from immunized mice suggests that normal and autoimmune mice differ quantitatively, if not qualitatively, in their capacity to express pathogenic anti-DNA. Although anti-DNA induced in normal mice by bacterial DNA immunization can bind ssDNA from mammalian and bacterial sources as well as bacterial dsDNA, their CDR3 regions differ from spontaneous anti-DNA from SLE mice in their arginine content as well as occurrence of arginines at certain positions. In the absence of these amino acid sequences, the expression of anti-dsDNA may be constrained, thereby preventing the emergence of a cross-reactive anti-dsDNA response. Precursors with these sequences may be subject to tolerance because they bind sufficiently well to DNA even in the absence of somatic mutations, and are therefore subject to deletion or anergy. In the autoimmune mouse, however, tolerance defects would allow the presence of such precursors in the repertoire where they can be triggered by foreign DNA antigen [9].

The failure of mammalian DNA to induce cross-reactive antibodies in NZB/NZW mice is of interest in view of the spontaneous expression of these antibodies later in life as well as their induction by bacterial DNA. One possible explanation for the failure of mammalian DNA immunization to induce autoantibodies concerns the immune activity of mammalian DNA. Rather than being inert, this DNA may have immunological effects. These effects, however, may be suppressive rather than activating. As shown in vitro, mammalian DNA can block the induction of cytokines by bacterial DNA. Although this suppression may result from physical blockade of a receptor that binds CpG DNA, it may also reflect a direct inhibitory effect on immune cell function [19, 45]. If mammalian DNA caused generalized immunosuppressive effects, it could profoundly influence the immune properties of complexes with a carrier such as mBSA as well as endogenous nucleosomal complexes.

According to this model, bacterial DNA has an enhanced capacity to drive either anti-foreign or anti-self responses depending on the B cell repertoire, with its role as a molecular mimic depending on the host. A second line of evidence for this possibility comes from the study of the specificity of anti-DNA antibodies in SLE sera. Theoretically, SLE sera can contain two types of anti-DNA: a normal component that binds to non-conserved sites on bacterial DNA and an autoimmune component that binds to conserved sites on both foreign and self DNA. If autoimmune individuals had a disturbance in the composition of the B cell repertoire, their ability to generate these two classes of anti-DNA could be affected.

To determine the relative expression of classes of anti-DNA during autoimmune disease, SLE sera were absorbed with mammalian DNA [calf thymus (CT) DNA] to remove cross-reactive anti-DNA. Following this absorption, the SLE sera lacked antibodies to mammalian DNA as expected and, in addition, lacked antibodies to bacterial DNA, using as a model MC ssDNA. Under these conditions, absorption with CT DNA caused no loss of activity from NHS, indicating specificity of the treatment (Fig. 1). Furthermore, the absorption did not affect levels of antibodies to anti-Sm. These results indicate that the majority of SLE anti-DNA binds to conserved sites on DNA and that the normal response to non-conserved sites is reduced or lacking in this state of autoimmunity [31].

At least two mechanisms could account for these serological findings. The first concerns immunodeficiency. Thus, patients with SLE may be unable to produce a selective IgG2 response to bacterial DNA, perhaps reflecting an inherited or acquired immunodeficiency state. Although overall levels of IgG2 are intact in SLE, the existence of limited defects in anti-carbohydrate responses suggests that an antigen-specific deficiency is possible [14,38]. Such a deficiency state could predispose to autoimmune disease by allowing persistence of immunostimulatory DNA in the system.

The other mechanism to account for the serological findings relates to the observations on immunization of NZB/NZW mice. Because of an abnormal array of B cell precursors in the repertoire, the autoimmune individual may be predisposed to the expression of cross-reactive autoantibody specificities. These specificities, which could arise from abnormalities in peripheral or central tolerance, would cause a shift in the pattern of epitopes recognized during an immune response. This shift could lead to preferential recognition of conserved rather than non-conserved determinants. This shift could also influence binding of conformational as compared to sequential determinants. As a result of this shift, molecular mimicry would become a pervasive problem for the SLE-prone individual.

Studies on immune response to protein autoantigens also indicate that ANA in autoimmunity differ in fine specificity from that of antibodies induced to these antigens by immunization. In general, spontaneous ANA bind antigens from a variety of species (e.g., human, cow and rabbit in the case of anti-snRNP) indicating interaction with a conserved determinant. Binding to a conserved determinant is also demonstrated by the ability of spontaneous autoantibodies to inhibit the activity of self-antigens which are enzymes. Consistent with the binding to a conserved or conformational determinant, spontaneous ANA may bind less well to short peptide fragments predicted to be active by various paradigms for antigenicity [39, 44, 48].

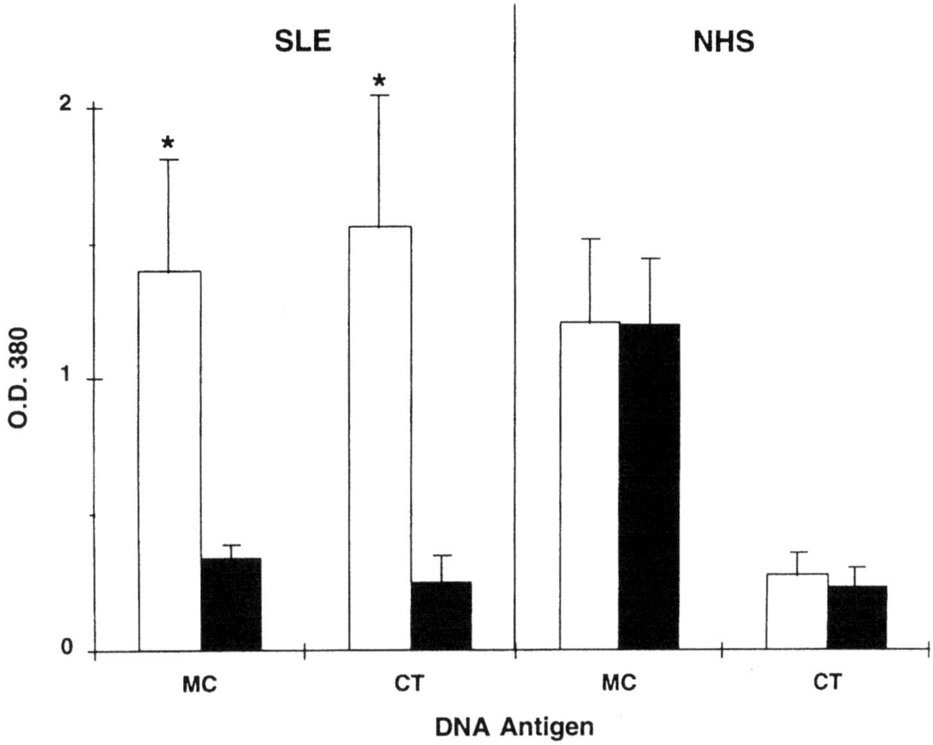

Fig. 1. Specificity analysis of anti-DNA antibodies in NHS and patients with SLE. A panel of sera of NHS and patients with SLE were absorbed with a control cellulose (*open bars*) or calf thymus DNA cellulose (*closed bars*) and then tested for binding to DNA from *Micrococcus lysodeikticus* (*MC*) or calf thymus (*CT*). As these data indicate, absorption of SLE sera with CT DNA leads to loss of activity for both mammalian and bacterial DNA (*NHS* sera from normal healthy subjects, SLE systemic erythematosus lupus). Reproduced with permission from [31]

In contrast to spontaneous autoantibodies, antibodies induced to these antigens by immunization of normal animals bind preferentially to non-conserved sites on these proteins. These antigenic sites are well represented by peptide fragments and appear to correspond to parts of molecules that should be antigenic by virtue of location, hydrophilicity or sequence. While many factors could account for these differences in epitope recognition, a skewing in the repertoire provides an encompassing explanation that unites the animal and human observations, on one hand, and the anti-DNA and anti-protein responses, on the other.

A role of foreign DNA in driving anti-DNA production does not preclude a contribution of self-DNA in the etiology of ANA responses. For example, foreign DNA could induce an initial wave of anti-DNA B cells which then bind the DNA component of nucleosomes. These B cells could serve as antigen-presenting cells and promote epitope spreading by presenting nucleosome proteins for the generation of B and T cell responses. Bacterial DNA could also function to stimulate anti-DNA production during flares since it represents a source of cross-reactive antigen that can quickly enter and exit the system, causing a spike in activity.

A final issue in pathogenicity concerns the ability of various classes of anti-DNA to modify the immunostimulatory properties of bacterial DNA. As noted above, bacterial DNA can cause polyclonal B cell activation as well as the induction of cytokines that could promote the inflammatory state. The effects of antibodies on these activities is unknown, although differences in normal and autoimmune anti-DNA could affect the in vivo disposition of foreign DNA as well as its ability to activate immune cells. If cross-reactive anti-DNA augmented immunostimulation by bacterial DNA, the pathogenicity of these antibodies could extend to overall immunoregulatory balance of the host.

Conclusions

DNA is a complex macromolecule whose immunological properties result from structural microheterogeneity. In normal immunity, antibodies to DNA can arise by stimulation by bacterial DNA because of the adjuvant properties of foreign DNA as well as the presence of non-conserved sequences that serve as B cell epitopes. In SLE, anti-DNA antibodies arise by a process of DNA antigen drive and could result from stimulation by either self or foreign DNA. Since foreign DNA is immunogenic, this antigen may have an enhanced ability to drive anti-DNA autoantibody production in the individual with functional abnormalities in the B or T cell compartment. Future research will define further the interaction of foreign DNA with the normal as well aberrant immune system and hopefully lead to strategies to eliminate the production of pathogenic anti-DNA autoantibodies.

References

1. Ali R, Dersimonian H, Stollar BD (1985) Binding of monoclonal anti-native DNA autoantibodies to DNA of varying size and conformation. Mol Immunol 22:1415
2. Berden JHM (1997) Lupus nephritis. Kidney Int 52:538
3. Bunyard MP, Pisetsky DS (1994) Characterization of antibodies to bacterial double-stranded DNA in the sera of normal human subjects. Int Arch Allergy Immunol 105:122
4. Cowdery JS, Chace JH, Yi A-K, Krieg AM (1996) Bacterial DNA induces NK cells to produce IFN-γ in vivo and increases the toxicity of lipopolysaccharides. J Immunol 156:4570
5. Desai DD, Krishnan MR, Swindle JT, Marion TN (1993) Antigen-specific induction of antibodies against native mammalian DNA in nonautoimmune mice. J Immunol 151:1614
6. Doerfler W (1991) Patterns of DNA methylation – evolutionary vestiges of foreign DNA inactivation as a host defense mechanism. A proposal. Biol Chem Hoppe Seyler 372:557
7. Eilat D, Anderson WF (1994) Structure-function correlates of autoantibodies to nucleic acids. Lessons from immunochemical, genetic and structural studies. Mol Immunol 31:1377
8. Gilkeson GS, Bernstein K, Pippen AMM, Clarke SH, Marion T, Pisetsky DS, Ruiz P, Lefkowith J (1995) The influence of variable-region somatic mutations on the specificity and pathogenicity of murine monoclonal anti-DNA antibodies. Clin Immunol Immunopath 76:59
9. Gilkeson GS, Bloom DD, Pisetsky DS, Clarke SH (1993) Molecular characterization of anti-DNA antibodies induced in normal mice by immunization with bacterial DNA. Differences from spontaneous anti-DNA in the content and location of V_H CDR3 arginines. J Immunol 151:1353
10. Gilkeson GS, Grudier JP, Karounos DG, Pisetsky DS (1989) Induction of anti-double stranded DNA antibodies in normal mice by immunization with bacterial DNA. J Immunol 142:1482
11. Gilkeson GS, Pippen AMM, Pisetsky DS (1995) Induction of cross-reactive anti-dsDNA antibodies in preautoimmune NZB/NZW mice by immunization with bacterial DNA. J Clin Invest 95:1398
12. Hardin JA (1986) The lupus autoantigens and the pathogenesis of systemic lupus erythematosus. Arthritis Rheum 29:457

13. Herrmann M, Winkler TH, Fehr H, Kalden JR (1995) Preferential recognition of specific DNA motifs by anti-double-stranded DNA autoantibodies. Eur J Immunol 25:1897
14. Jefferis R, Kumararatne DS (1990) Selective IgG subclass deficiency: quantification and clinical relevance. Clin Exp Immunol 81:357
15. Karlin S, Doerfler W, Cardon LR (1994) Why is CpG suppressed in the genomes of virtually all small eukaryotic viruses but not in those of large eukaryotic viruses? J Virol 68:2889
16. Karounos DG, Grudier JP, Pisetsky DS (1988) Spontaneous expression of antibodies to DNA of various species origin in sera of normal subjects and patients with systemic lupus erythematosus. J Immunol 140:451
17. Katz JB, Limpanasithikul W, Diamond B (1994) Mutational analysis of an autoantibody: differential binding and pathogenicity. J Exp Med 180:925
18. Kieber-Emmons T, Foster MH, Williams WV, Madaio MP (1994) Structural properties of a subset of nephritogenic anti-DNA antibodies. Immunol Res 13:172
19. Krieg AM, Wu T, Weeratna R, Efler SM, Love-Homan L, Yang L, Yi A-K (1998) Sequence motifs in adenoviral DNA block immune activation by stimulatory CpG motifs. Proc Natl Acad Sci USA 95:12631
20. Krieg AM, Yi A-K, Matson S, Waldschmidt TJ, Bishop GA, Teasdale R, Koretzky GA, Klinman DM (1995) CpG motifs in bacterial DNA trigger direct B-cell activation. Nature 374:546
21. Lefkowith JB, Gilkeson GS (1996) Nephritogenic autoantibodies in lupus. Current concepts and continuing controversies. Arthritis Rheum 39:894
22. Madaio M, Hodder S, Schwartz RS, Stollar BD (1984) Responsiveness of autoimmune and normal mice to nucleic acid antigens. J Immunol 132:872
23. McCarty GA, Bembe MB, Rice JR, Pisetsky DS (1982) Independent expression of autoantibodies in systemic lupus erythematosus. J Rheumatol 9:691
24. Messina JP, Gilkeson GS, Pisetsky DS (1991) Stimulation of in vitro murine lymphocyte proliferation by bacterial DNA. J Immunol 147:1759
25. Miyazaki S, Shimura J, Hirose S, Sanokawa R, Tsurui H, Wakiya M, Sugawara H, Shirai T (1997) Is structural flexibility of antigen-binding loops involved in the affinity maturation of anti-DNA antibodies? Int Immunol 9:771
26. Ohnishi K, Ebling FM, Mitchell B, Singh RR, Hahn BH, Tsao BP (1994) Comparison of pathogenic and non-pathogenic murine antibodies to DNA: antigen binding and structural characteristics. Int Immunol 6:817
27. Papalian M, Lafer E, Wong R, Stollar BD (1980) Reaction of systemic lupus erythematosus antinative DNA antibodies with native DNA fragments from 20 to 1,200 base pairs. J Clin Invest 65:469
28. Pisetsky DS (1992) Anti-DNA antibodies in systemic lupus erythematosus. Rheum Dis Clin NA 18:437
29. Pisetsky DS (1997) DNA and the immune system. Ann Intern Med 126:169
30. Pisetsky DS (1998) Antibody responses to DNA in normal immunity and aberrant immunity. Clin Diagn Lab Immunol 5:1
31. Pisetsky DS, Drayton DM (1997) Deficient expression of antibodies specific for bacterial DNA by patients with systemic lupus erythematosus. Proc Assoc Am Physicians 109:237
32. Pisetsky DS, Gonzalez TC (1999) The influence of DNA size on the binding of antibodies to DNA in the sera of normal human subjects and patients with systemic lupus erythematosus. Clin Exp Immunol 116:354
33. Pisetsky DS, Reich CF (1994) The influence of DNA size on the binding of anti-DNA antibodies in the solid and fluid phase. Clin Immunol Immunopath 72:350
34. Radic MZ, Mackle J, Erikson J, Mol C, Anderson WF, Weigert M (1993) Residues that mediate DNA binding of autoimmune antibodies. J Immunol 150:4966
35. Radic MZ, Weigert M (1994) Genetic and structural evidence for antigen selection of anti-DNA antibodies. Annu Rev Immunol 12:487
36. Robertson CR, Gilkeson GS, Ward MM, Pisetsky DS (1992) Patterns of heavy and light chain utilization in the antibody response to single-stranded bacterial DNA in normal human subjects and patients with systemic lupus erythematosus. Clin Immunol Immunopathol 62:25
37. Robertson CR, Pisetsky DS (1992) Specificity analysis of antibodies to single-stranded micrococcal DNA in the sera of normal human subjects and patients with systemic lupus erythematosus. Clin Exp Rheumatol 10:589
38. Siber GR, Santosham M, Reid GR, Thompson C, Almeido-Hill, J, Morell A, deLange G, Ketcham JK, Callahan EH (1990) Impaired antibody response to *haemophilus influenzae* type b polysaccharide and low IgG2 and IgG4 concentrations in Apache children. N Engl J Med 323:1387

39. St. Clair EW, Kenan D, Burch J, Keene JD, Pisetsky DS (1990) Fine specificity of anti-La antibodies induced in mice by immunization with recombinant human La antigen. J Immunol 144:3868
40. Stevens SY, Glick GD (1999) Evidence for sequence-specific recognition of DNA by anti-single-stranded DNA autoantibodies. Biochemistry 38:560
41. Stevens SY, Swanson PC, Voss EW Jr, Glick GD (1993) Evidence for induced fit in antibody-DNA complexes. J Am Chem Soc 115:1585
42. Stollar BD (1994) Molecular analysis of anti-DNA antibodies. FASEB J 8:337
43. Swanson PC, Ackroyd C, Glick GD (1996) Ligand recognition by anti-DNA autoantibodies. Affinity, specificity, and mode of binding. Biochemistry 35:1624
44. Tan EM (1989) Antinuclear antibodies: diagnostic markers for autoimmune diseases and probes for cell biology. Adv Immunol 44:93
45. Wloch MK, Pasquini S, Ertl HCJ, Pisetsky DS (1998) The influence of DNA sequence on the immunostimulatory properties of plasmid DNA vectors. Hum Gene Ther 9:1439
46. Wu ZQ, Drayton D, Pisetsky DS (1997) Specificity and immunochemical properties of antibodies to bacterial DNA in sera of normal human subjects and patients with systemic lupus erythematosus (SLE). Clin Exp Immunol 109:27
47. Yamamoto T, Yamamoto S, Kataoka T, Komuro K, Kohase M, Tokunaga T (1994) Synthetic oligonucleotides with certain palindromes stimulate interferon production of human peripheral blood lymphocytes in vitro. Jpn J Cancer Res 85:775
48. Yamanaka H, Willis EH, Carson DA (1989) Human autoantibodies to poly(adenosine diphosphate-ribose) polymerase recognize cross-reactive epitopes associated with the catalytic site of the enzyme. J Clin Invest 83:180

The role of immunostimulatory CpG-DNA in septic shock

Hermann Wagner, Grayson B. Lipford, Hans Häcker

Institute of Medical Microbiology, Immunology and Hygiene, Technical University of Munich, Trogerstr. 9, 81675 Munich, Germany

Introduction

Septic shock is the most severe manifestation of infection, and in the intensive care unit (ICU) appears increasingly commonly (reviewed in [20]). As in other forms of acute circulatory failure, septic shock is best described as an imbalance between oxygen demand and oxygen delivery [18]. Older studies suggested that gram-negative bacteria are more commonly associated with septic shock; however, more recent studies have shown that gram-positive bacteria are just as common. Septic shock develops when specific microbial components gain access to the circulation and are recognized by the immune system which generates exaggerated mediator and cytokine responses. Cell wall constituents, such as LPS in gram-negative bacteria, or peptidoglycan and teichoic acid in gram-positive bacteria, or proteins liberated during growth (exotoxins) are considered as the principal microbial components responsible. Exotoxins are a group of bacterial proteins that have been termed superantigens (Sag) because of their unique mechanism to interact with antigen-presenting cells (APCs) and T lymphocytes [14]. All Sag share the ability to bind to MHC class II molecules outside the peptide binding groove as intact proteins. Once bound to MHC class II molecules Sag bind to certain regions of the T cell receptor (TCR) β chain encoded by Vβ gene segments. Consequently a trimolecular TCR-Sag-MHC complex is formed which causes cross-linking and immobilization of the TCR and activation of the respective T cells [17]. Finally, pore-forming bacterial exotoxins may also contribute to the pathogenesis of sepsis syndrome and septic shock [1].

With the realization that the vertebrate immune system has evolved the ability to detect and to be activated by microbial CpG-DNA, the list of microbial constituents linked to septic shock may now be extended [10, 13, 19, 27]. In contrast to the codon-based nucleotide triplets used to translate amino acid sequences, innate immune cells sense as 'danger code' CpG dinucleotides in a particular base sequence context, termed "CpG motif" or immunostimulatory CpG sequences.

Correspondence to: H. Wagner

Sensing of pathogen DNA: evolutionary vestige of foreign DNA

Antimicrobial host defense relies both on innate and adaptive components of the immune system. Microbial constituents display molecular patterns that are recognized by pattern recognition receptors (PRRs) expressed constitutively on cells of the innate immune system, such as dendritic cells (DCs) and macrophages [4, 15]. Molecular patterns seem to be shared among groups of pathogens. Representative examples are the LPS of gram-negative bacteria, the lipoteichoic acids of gram-positive bacteria and the mannans of yeast. Genomic DNA rich in CpG motifs, however, is also found in gram-positive, gram-negative bacteria, some large DNA viruses and even in flies [2, 26]. CpG dinucleotides are suppressed in the vertebrate genome (CpG suppression) and constitute only about 25% of the level expected from random base usage [9]. An additional difference is the degree of C5 methylation, which is uncommon in bacteria but common in vertebrates [2]. This suggests that the structural characteristics of bacterial DNA not present in mammalian DNA have been adopted by vertebrate immune cells to recognize pathogens on the basis of CpG motifs. In support, methylation of bacterial DNA and CpG inversion to GpC abolishes the immunobiology of CpG-DNA [7, 11].

CpG methylation is involved in the silencing of genes during mammalian development [12]. In vertebrates, CpG suppression may have evolved due to the mutability associated with methylated cytosine residues [3]. Of note, silencing of integrated foreign and thus genotoxic DNA, via methylation, may also represent a key mechanism of cellular defense to foreign DNA [5]. We speculate, however, that prevention of infection (before they cause accumulation of genotoxic foreign DNA) may be a strategy adopted by mammalian innate immune cells. Accordingly, mammalian cells of the innate immune system may have adapted DNA-binding proteins as receptors to recognize sequence specific bacterial CpG motifs.

By iteratively changing the sequences of immunostimulating single-stranded CpG motifs, it was concluded that a consensus DNA-motif requires an unmethylated CpG dinucleotide flanked by two 5' purines and two 3' pyrimidines [11]. Such CpG-DNA motifs within thioate-stabilized oligonucleotides of 8- to 20 base length mimic bacterial CpG-DNA. CpG-ODN are sequence-nonspecifically translocated into early endosomes. Once translocated they sequence-dependently cause immediate early activation of the p38 and JNK stress kinases in DCs and of p38/JNK stress kinases plus ERK kinases in macrophages, similar to LPS [6, 7]. Whether activation of DCs and macrophages is associated with increased bactericidal activity has not been studied in detail and is subject of ongoing experimentation. However, CpG-DANN-mediated activation causes transition of antigen-presenting immature DCs to professional APCs via induction of cytokine synthesis and expression of co-stimulatory molecules, both in vitro and in vivo [21, 24].

Despite intensive efforts, CpG sequence-discriminating CpG receptors have not yet been identified. Interestingly, there exist parallels between LPS- and CpG-ODN-initiated signal transduction pathways. Recent experiments indicate that mammalian Toll like receptors (TLRs) are critical in LPS-mediated signaling in association with LPS-binding protein (LBP) and CD14 [8]. TLRs have a cytoplasmic TIR (Toll-IL-1 receptor) homology domain to activate the Il-1 receptor signal pathway via MyD88 and TRAF6, thus resulting in NF-κB and stress kinase activation [16]. In preliminary experiments we noted that the adapter molecule MyD88 not only controls LPS signaling in macrophages but also intracellular signaling initiated by CpG motifs [6]. If, however, LPS and CpG-ODN were to use the same signal pathway for cell activation one may ask whether CpG-ODN is recognized via a not-yet-defined TLR. We believe that several arguments refute such reasoning. First, the biochemical organization of the extracytoplasmic region from known TLRs do not favor sequence-specific DNA binding. Second, the conserved pathways of innate immunity in flies and mammals, as illustrated with the transmembrane receptor Toll and vertebrate TLRs, respectively, point out a common ancestry of these receptors. Yet the postulated CpG receptors appear to have evolved in vertebrates, that is late in phylogeny. We thus consider it unlikely that the postulated CpG receptor will turn out to be a member of the expanding TLR family. Alternatively, it is possible that CpG-DNA discriminating proteins have been adopted to use the IL-1/TLR signal pathway. If so, the functional outcome of LPS signaling would mirror that of CpG signaling.

Macrophages and DCs sense pathogens via DNA motifs: induction of TNF-α mediated toxic shock

Two groups independently demonstrated that macrophages ingest and are activated by bacterial DNA. Stacey et al. [25] described that TNF-α mRNA was induced in macrophages by plasmid DNA. Importantly they showed that plasmid DNA is taken up by macrophages and remains sufficiently intact to code for luciferase protein. Sparwasser et al. [22, 23] reported that genomic DNA of gram-positive and gram-negative bacteria activate macrophages in vitro to produce TNF-α, as does LPS. Macrophages from LPS-resistant C3H/HeJ mice, however, responded to bacterial DNA but lacked responsiveness to LPS. CpG-oligonucleotides with CpG motif sequence specifically mimicked the immunostimulating effects of bacterial DNA. Both LPS and CpG-ODN caused activation of NF-κB. When mice were challenged i.p. with CpG-ODN, high but transient serum concentrations of TNF-α, IL-12, IL-1β and IL-6 were recorded, as was the case with LPS.

Like others we have sensitized mice to LPS or bacterial superantigens using liver-specific inhibitors such as D-GalN [17]. An essential feature of this in vivo model is that systemically released TNF-α causes liver damage due to TNF-α-mediated apoptotic liver cell death. This has been scored by measuring serum levels of liver enzymes, or lethality. Challenge of D-GalN-sensitized wild-type or LPS-resistant C3HeJ mice with DNA from gram-positive or gram-negative bacteria or with immunostimulating CpG-ODN not only caused high TNF-α levels in blood within 1–2 h, but also lethal shock within 12–14 h. In vivo, LPS and bacterial CpG-DNA motifs synergized for the induction of TNF-α. Thus, even though the recognition structures for LPS and CpG-DNA may be distinct, these early experiments already provided evidence that downstream the signaling pathways triggered may converge. Subsequently, it became clear that DCs grown from bone marrow in GM-CSF-conditioned medium were 10- to 20-fold more sensitive to the immunostimulating effects of CpG-DNA, and that they produce, besides TNF-α, very high amounts of IL-12 [21]. In vivo, CpG-DNA triggers antigen presenting immature DCs to synthesize co-stimulatory molecules (CD80, CD86, CD40, MHC class II) and cytokines (IL-12) and thus to transit to professional APCs. At this stage activated DCs trigger CTL responses to soluble proteins in a T helper cell-independent manner [24]. Finally, the signal pathways triggered by CpG-DNA were remarkably similar to those triggered by LPS. In macrophages, CpG-DNA activates stress and ERK kinases within minutes, as does LPS [6].

Conclusion

During septic shock the host produces an excess of proinflammatory cytokines in response to pathogen-derived constituents, including LPS and bacterial CpG-DNA. A distinction has to be made between local effects and the consequences of their systemic levels. If formed in small amounts, proinflammatory cytokines remain local and are important for the proper functioning of the immune system and its struggle with invading pathogens. If invading pathogens or pathogen-derived constituents gain systemic access, exuberant inflammation and septic shock may be the price to be paid. Under such conditions systemic inflammation occurs and large amounts of, for example, IL-1 and TNF are released into circulation. This in turn induces hypotension and, as worst outcome, lethal shock.

The delineation of the immunostimulatory effects on macrophages and DCs of bacterial CpG-DNA and i.s. CpG-ODN raises the question whether CpG motifs from bacterial DNA need to be regarded as a virulence factor of bacterial pathogenesis. The physiological and pathophysiological relevance of bacterial CpG-DNA ultimately depends on the demonstration that it indeed becomes liberated at a site of infection and is able to exert its immunobiology on macrophages and DCs. Alternatively, it will depend on experimental evidence to prove that bacterial CpG-DNA of phagocytosed bacteria becomes biologically active within macrophages/DCs thereby causing their activation. Recently, we succeeded in growing *E. coli* transformed with inducible cytosine methyl- transferase-encoding plasmids. Since genomic DNA from transformed *E. coli* appears largely methylated, we will attempt to discover whether bacterial pathogenesis in LPS non-responder mice is at variance to that of mock transformed *E. coli*.

References

1. Bhakdi S, Muhly M, Korom S, Schmidt G (1990) Effects of *Escherichia coli* hemolysin on human monocytes. Cytocidal action and stimulation of interleukin 1 release. J Clin Invest 85:1746
2. Burge C, Campbell AM, Karlin S (1992) Over- and under-representation of short oligonucleotides in DNA sequences. Proc Natl Acad Sci USA 89:1358
3. Coulondre C, Miller JH, Farabaugh PJ, Gilbert W (1978) Molecular basis of base substitution hotspots in *Escherichia coli*. Nature 274:775
4. Dempsey PW, Allison ME, Akkaraju S, Goodnow CC, Fearon DT (1996) C3d of complement as a molecular adjuvant: bridging innate and acquired immunity. Science 271:348
5. Doerfler W (1991) Patterns of DNA methylation-evolutionary vestiges of foreign DNA inactivation as a host defense mechanism. A proposal. Biol Chem Hoppe Seyler 372:557
6. Hacker H, Mischak H, Hacker G, Eser S, Prenzel N, Ullrich A, Wagner H (1999) Cell type-specific activation of mitogen activation protein kinases by CpG-DNA controls interleukin-12 release from antigen presenting cells. EMBO J (in press)
7. Hacker H, Mischak H, Miethke T, Liptay S, Schmid R, Sparwasser T, Heeg K, Lipford GB, Wagner H (1998) CpG-DNA-specific activation of antigen-presenting cells requires stress kinase activity and is preceded by non-specific endocytosis and endosomal maturation. EMBO J 17:6230
8. Hoffmann JA, Kafatos FC, Janeway CA, Ezekowitz RA (1999) Phylogenetic perspectives in innate immunity. Science 284:1313
9. Karlin S, Doerfler W, Cardon LR (1994) Why is CpG suppressed in the genomes of virtually all small eukaryotic viruses but not in those of large eukaryotic viruses? J Virol 68:2889
10. Krieg AM (1996) Lymphocyte activation by CpG dinucleotide motifs in prokaryotic DNA. Trends Microbiol 4:73
11. Krieg AM, Yi AK, Matson S, Waldschmidt TJ, Bishop GA, Teasdale R, Koretzky GA, Klinman DM (1995) CpG motifs in bacterial DNA trigger direct B-cell activation. Nature 374:546

12. Li E, Beard C, Jaenisch R (1993) Role for DNA methylation in genomic imprinting. Nature 366:362
13. Lipford GB, Heeg K, Wagner H (1998) Bacterial DNA as immune cell activator. Trends Microbiol 6:496
14. Marrack P, Kappler J (1990) The staphylococcal enterotoxins and their relatives [published erratum appears in Science (1990) 248:1066]. Science 248:705
15. Medzhitov R, Janeway CA Jr (1997) Innate immunity: the virtues of a nonclonal system of recognition. Cell 91:295
16. Medzhitov R, Preston-Hurlburt P, Janeway CA Jr (1997) A human homologue of the Drosophila Toll protein signals activation of adaptive immunity. Nature 388:394
17. Miethke T, Wahl C, Heeg K, Echtenacher B, Krammer PH, Wagner H (1992) T cell-mediated lethal shock triggered in mice by the superantigen staphylococcal enterotoxin B: critical role of tumor necrosis factor. J Exp Med 175:91
18. Parrillo JE (1993) Pathogenetic mechanisms of septic shock. N Engl J Med 328:1471
19. Pisetsky DS (1996) Immune activation by bacterial DNA: a new genetic code. Immunity 5:303
20. Rietschel ET, Wagner H (1996) Pathology of septic shock. Springer, Berlin Heidelberg New York, p 261
21. Sparwasser T, Koch ES, Vabulas RM, Heeg K, Lipford GB, Ellwart J, Wagner H (1998) Bacterial DNA and immunostimulatory CpG oligonucleotides trigger maturation and activation of murine dendritic cells. Eur J Immunol 28:2045
22. Sparwasser T, Miethke T, Lipford G, Borschert K, Hacker H, Heeg K, Wagner H (1997) Bacterial DNA causes septic shock. Nature 386:336
23. Sparwasser T, Miethke T, Lipford G, Erdmann A, Hacker H, Heeg K, Wagner H (1997) Macrophages sense pathogens via DNA motifs: induction of tumor necrosis factor-alpha-mediated shock. Eur J Immunol 27:1671
24. Sparwasser T, Vabulas RM, Villmow B, Lipford GB, Wagner H (1999) Bacterial CpG-DNA activates dendritic cells in vivo: helper cell independent cytotoxic T cell responses to soluble proteins (in press)
25. Stacey KJ, Sweet MJ, Hume DA (1996) Macrophages ingest and are activated by bacterial DNA. J Immunol 157:2116
26. Sun S, Kishimoto H, Sprent J (1998) DNA as an adjuvant: capacity of insect DNA and synthetic oligodeoxynucleotides to augment T cell responses to specific antigen. J Exp Med 187:1145
27. Wagner H (1999) Bacterial CpG DNA activates immune cells to signal infectious danger. Adv Immunol 73:329

Activation of the innate immune system by CpG oligodeoxynucleotides: immunoprotective activity and safety

Dennis M. Klinman, Soren Kamstrup, Daniela Verthelyi, Ihsan Gursel, Ken J. Ishii, Fumihiko Takeshita, Mayda Gursel

Section of Retroviral Research, Center for Biologics Evaluation and Research, Food and Drug Administration, Bldg 29A Rm 3 D 10, Bethesda, MD 20892

Immunostimulatory properties of CpG motifs

Immunostimulatory activity of bacterial DNA

The mammalian immune system responds to bacterial infection by rapidly initiating an inflammatory reaction that limits the early spread of the pathogen and facilitates the emergence of antigen-specific immunity (reviewed in [29]). Microorganisms have evolved to avoid such recognition by altering expression of their protein and lipid products [29]. Yet DNA is an indispensable and highly conserved component of all bacteria. Indeed, the genomes of otherwise diverse prokaryotes share DNA motifs that are rare in the genomes of higher vertebrates [3, 11, 30]. Yamamoto et al. [50, 51] were the first to show that bacterial but not mammalian DNA boosted the lytic activity of NK cells, inducing them to secrete IFN-γ. They attributed this effect to palindromic sequences present in bacterial DNA [51]. Other investigators showed that bacterial DNA stimulated B cells to proliferate and secrete Ig (especially if the DNA was complexed to a DNA-binding protein) [10–12, 30, 34, 49]. We were interested in defining the precise sequence motifs in bacterial DNA responsible for this immune activation, and to establish the breadth and nature of such activation.

Bacterial DNA and synthetic oligodeoxynucleotides elicit IgM and cytokine production

We examined the ability of bacterial DNA, and of synthetic oligonucleotides (ODN) patterned after sequences present in bacterial DNA, to stimulate cells of the immune system in vitro. Splenocytes from BALB/c mice were exposed to bacterial DNA, mammalian DNA or synthetic ODN in culture. The number of cells activated to secrete Ig or cytokine by these different types of DNA was monitored by ELIspot assay. As seen in Table 1, bacterial DNA induced the production of IgM, IL-6, IFN-γ and IL-12 [24, 26]. By testing hundreds of different synthetic ODN (in collaboration

Correspondence to: D. Klinman

Table 1. Immunostimulatory effects of CpG ODN in vitro

DNA	*Fold increase in secreting cell number*			
	IL-6	*IL-12*	*IFNγ*	*IgM*
E.coli DNA	3.2±0.2	3.8±0.4	4.7±2.3	3.9±1.1
Calf thymus DNA	0.8±0.2	1.1±0.2	0.8±0.3	0.7±0.2
xxPuPu*CG*PyPy	5.5±1.1	8.3±1.7	4.7±1.1	4.2±1.6
PuPu*CG*PyPyxx	3.4±0.6	5.0±1.2	5.2±0.9	3.1±0.7
xPuPu*CG*PyPy	1.1±0.1	1.1±0.2	0.8±0.1	1.2±0.2
xxPuPuGCPyPy	1.2±0.3	1.3±0.3	1.2±0.3	1.3±0.3
xxPuPuC*GPyPy	0.9±0.2	1.2±0.3	0.8±0.2	1.1±0.2
xxPuPy*CG*PyPy	1.5±0.3	1.6±0.4	1.3±0.3	0.8±0.2
xxPuPu*CG*PuPy	1.3±0.4	1.4±0.4	1.2±0.2	1.0±0.1
Plasmid vector		2.9±0.4	3.1±0.4	
Methylated vector	1.2±0.2	0.9±0.1		
DNA vaccine	3.2±0.7	3.4±0.9		
CpG-enhanced vaccine	6.7±1.2	5.2±1.1		

BALB/c spleen cells were incubated with 1 μM pODN, 10 μg/ml of plasmid DNA or 50 μg/ml of heat-denatured genomic DNA for 8 h. The stimulation index is calculated as the fold increase in number of cytokine- or IgM-secreting cells over background, as determined by ELIspot assay [24, 31]. The data shown are representative of more than 200 ODN studied

ODN, Oligodeoxynucleotide; x, any bp; Pu, purine; Py, pyrimidine; C*, methylated cytosine

with Dr. Art Krieg), we found that sequences containing a CpG dinucleotide tended to trigger the release of IgM and cytokine, whereas ODN lacking this motif did not. Multiple CpG generally stimulated larger numbers of spleen cells, although CpG located at the terminus of an ODN were ineffective.

The latter finding suggested that sequences flanking the CpG dinucleotide might contribute to the stimulatory capacity of an ODN. To define the size and composition of the stimulatory motif, additional ODN were examined. Optimal activation was induced when the central CpG was flanked by two 5' purines (GpA or ApA) and two 3' pyrimidines (TpC or TpT). Immune stimulation persisted despite purine/purine or pyrimidine/pyrimidine replacements, even if these substitutions eliminated a palindromic sequence. In contrast, stimulation was significantly reduced when a purine was substituted for pyrimidine, or vice versa, even if a palindromic sequence was maintained or created (Table 1) [24, 26]. If either base of the CpG was eliminated, or the cytosine methylated, stimulatory activity was lost, whereas optimization of the flanking region or incorporation of multiple CpG into a single ODN increased stimulation. These findings provided evidence that a 6-bp motif, consisting of an unmethylated CpG dinucleotide flanked by two 5' purines and two 3' pyrimidines, contributed to the immune stimulation elicited by bacterial DNA. Of note, these immunostimulatory CpG motifs are expressed nearly 20 times more frequently in bacterial than mammalian DNA [5, 36], due to a combination of CpG suppression and CpG methylation [11, 26, 30, 36].

The cytokines induced by CpG motifs perform critical immunomodulatory functions. IL-12 and IFN-γ promote type 1 cytokine production [4, 47, 54] and play important roles in the elimination of human pathogens and opposing the pro-allergenic effects of Th2 cytokines [4, 16, 19, 35, 45, 54]. IL-6 is a type 2 cytokine that facilitates the growth/differentiation of T and B lymphocytes [17, 27, 33, 48] and stimulates Ig production [18]. TNF-α and IL-18, which other laboratories showed to be activated by CpG ODN, improve antigen presenting cell (APC) function [15, 21, 28, 41].

CpG ODN enter cells within seconds, up-regulate cytokine mRNA within minutes, and induce the release of cytokines within hours of administration [24]. In vivo, CpG ODN mediate considerably more complex effects, initiating an "immunomodulatory cascade" involving multiple cell types, including some that are not directly responsive to ODN. For example, B cells are directly stimulated to proliferate by CpG ODN yet their production of IgM is dependent upon the release of IL-6, and thus requires several days to peak [53]. Similarly, CpG ODN stimulate the release of cytokines from macrophages, dendritic cells and NK cells that in turn activate T lymphocytes that are unresponsive to ODN alone (although pre-activated T cells may be stimulated by ODN) [2, 15, 24, 43, 44].

Whereas CpG ODN-dependent immune stimulation is polyclonal in nature, a degree of specificity is maintained by the strong Th1 bias of the resultant response. Indeed, while IL-6, IL-12, IL-18, IFN-γ and TNF-α are induced by these motifs, a number of other cytokines including IL-2, IL-3, IL-4, IL-5 or IL-10 are not [24]. Moreover, the finding that macrophages, NK, dendritic and B cells but not T cells are directly triggered by CpG-containing ODN suggests that there is selectivity in the immune recognition of this motif. We therefore examined the strength and persistence of the resultant response through a series of studies designed to determine whether CpG motifs could be of therapeutic benefit.

Immune protection mediated by CpG ODN

Rationale for the use of CpG ODN to prevent infection

Infectious organisms are a major source of morbidity and mortality worldwide. The innate immune system plays a critical role in controlling the early spread of pathogens in vivo. Recognizing that CpG ODN activate a rapid innate immune response, we postulated that immune recognition of CpG motifs might improve host resistance to such organisms [26]. Consistent with that hypothesis, the array of cytokines elicited by CpG ODN are known to limit the early spread of intracellular pathogens (such as *Francisella tularensis, Listeria monocytogenes* and *Salmonella typhimurium)* [7, 8, 20].

Protection against infection is induced by CpG ODN

We injected normal BALB/c, C3H and C57BL/6 mice with CpG ODN. Animals treated with these ODN, or with bacterial DNA, survived when subsequently challenged with $\geq 10^3$ LD_{50} of *F. tularensis* or *L. monocytogenes* (Table 2 and data not shown [9]). In contrast, mice treated with mammalian DNA, or ODN in which the CpG motif was inverted or methylated, succumbed to pathogen challenge (Table 2). Protection was not dependent on the route of DNA administration, as mice injected intramuscularly, intraperitoneally, intradermally, or intravenously were all resistant to infection [9].

Mice were challenged at various intervals after ODN administration to examine the time course over which protection was elicited and maintained. Mice treated with

Table 2. Impact of repeated CpG ODN administration on survival

Treatment	Duration of *treatment (weeks)*	Day of challenge *post treatment*	*% survival*
Bacterial DNA	1	3	100
Mammalian DNA	1	3	0
PBS	1	3	0
CpG ODN	1	1	0
CpG ODN	1	2	60
CpG ODN	1	3	100
CpG ODN	1	14	90
CpG ODN	1	21	0
GpC ODN[a]	1	3	0
C^{meth}pG ODN[a]	1	3	0
CpG ODN	10	1	100
CpG ODN	10	14	100
CpG ODN	20	2	100
CpG ODN	20	13	100
CpG ODN	20	21	30
CpG ODN	20	28	0
GpC ODN[a]	20	1	0
GpC ODN[a]	20	14	0

BALB/c mice were injected i. p. every 2 weeks for up to 4 months with 50 μg ODN, and challenged with 10^3 LD_{50} of *L. monocytogenes* on the day shown after the last treatment. Data represent the percentage of mice surviving for >3 weeks. Each group shown consists of 5–15 animals. All cases of 90–100% survival are statistically significant ($P<0.05$)

[a] Control GpC ODN

ODN at the time of infection did not survive. When CpG ODN were administered 2 days prior to challenge, 60% of mice survived 10^3 LD_{50} of *L. monocytogenes*. Survival reached 100% when mice were treated during the period from 3 to 14 days prior to challenge (Table 2). Protection waned by 21 days post treatment. These findings suggest that the protective response elicited by CpG DNA takes several days to develop, and persists for approximately 2 weeks.

We have observed partial or complete protection against a number of infectious agents, including anthrax, Ebola virus, murine AIDS virus, malaria and *Leishmania* [22]. Slow growing pathogens, such as leishmania, respond to CpG ODN even if therapy is initiated after the infectious process is well underway [55]. In contrast, challenge by rapidly lethal organisms (or very high LD_{50}) require that the innate immune system be pre-activated. Thus, the timing of protection varies as a function of the pathogenicity (and dose) of the microorganism.

Efficacy of long-term CpG ODN treatment

To determine whether repeated administration of CpG ODN could extend the duration of protection, mice were treated every 2 weeks with 50 μg ODN and then challenged with 10^3 LD_{50} of *L. monocytogenes*. Complete protection was maintained throughout the 4-month treatment period and for 2 weeks after the cessation of therapy (Table 2). In contrast, mice injected with PBS or control ODN (in which the CpG dinucleotide was inverted to a GpC) were not protected. Susceptibility to infection returned 3–4 weeks after the cessation of therapy (Table 2).

Table 3. Long-term antigen-specific protection in CpG ODN protected mice

Treatment	*Challenge*	*Re-challenge*	*% survival*[a]
PBS	*L. monocytogenes*		0
	F. tularensis		10
CpG ODN	*L. monocytogenes*		100
	F. tularensis		100
CpG ODN	*L. monocytogenes*	*L. monocytogenes*	100
	L. monocytogenes	*F. tularensis*	0
CpG ODN		*L. monocytogenes*[b]	0
		F. tularensis[b]	0

BALB/c mice were treated by i. p. injection with PBS or 50 µg CpG ODN every 2 weeks for two months (5 injections). At 1–14 days after the last injection, animals were challenged with 10^3 LD_{50} of *L. monocytogenes* or *F. tularensis*. Mice that survived *L. monocytogenes* challenge were then re-challenged 45 days later (after the cessation of CpG ODN therapy)

[a] Percentage of mice surviving >3 weeks post challenge

[b] Animals were challenged only once, 45 days after initial treatment with CpG ODN

PBS, Phosphate-buffered saline

Effect of CpG DNA on the induction of long-term pathogen-specific immunity

We examined whether treatment with CpG ODN also fostered the development of pathogen-specific immunity. Consistent with earlier studies, BALB/c mice treated with CpG ODN survived challenge 3 days later with 10^3 LD_{50} of *L. monocytogenes.* These mice were re-challenged more than a month later (after the protective effects of the ODN had worn off) with 10^4 LD_{50} of *L. monocytogenes* or 10^2 LD_{50} of *F. tularensis*. All of these animals survived *L. monocytogenes* challenge, while none survived *F. tularensis* (Table 3). Thus, long-term pathogen-specific immunity was induced when a lethal challenge was rendered sublethal by CpG ODN treatment.

Summary: therapeutic potential of CpG ODN

Identifying agents that boost antigen-specific immune responses is an important goal of vaccine research. We and others found that CpG motifs act as immune adjuvants, boosting the response elicited by both protein-based and DNA-based vaccines [23, 37, 38]. The preferential induction of a Th1-biased immunity by CpG ODN also supports their use to inhibit the development of Th2-dependent allergic asthma [46]. In this work, we focused on the ability of CpG ODN to stimulate an innate immune response that can protect mice from a variety of lethal infections, including *Listeria*, *Francisella*, malaria, *Leishmania*, Ebola and anthrax, indicating the therapeutic potential of CpG ODN. As in the case of allergic asthma, CpG ODN-dependent production of immunoregulatory cytokines appears to play a role in this protective process. The time course of the protection induced by CpG DNA is of interest. Zimmermann et al. [55] showed that a CpG-containing ODN protected susceptible mice from leishmania infection when administered several weeks *after* infection. Since leishmania parasites proliferate slowly, considerable time is available to induce a protective Th1-driven immune response. High doses of *Francisella* and *Listeria*, in contrast, cause death within 1 week. To prevent this mortality, CpG DNA had to be administered 3–14 days prior to infection. Thus, the immune cascade initiated by CpG motifs appears to takes several days to peak, but persists for approximately 2 weeks. Consistent with this conclusion, the anti-allergic Th1 response elicited by CpG motifs also required several days for optimal effect.

In overview, our results demonstrate that CpG ODN, administered once or on multiple occasions, can significantly improve the host's immune response to vaccines, increase resistance to infectious agents, and reduce susceptibility to allergic inflammation. These effects could be maintained for weeks to months if multiple doses of ODN were delivered. We consider it likely that lifelong effects can be achieved by repeated ODN administration, and that the additional benefits for CpG ODN will be identified.

Safety of foreign DNA

Introduction

The risks of using CpG ODN to improve the host's innate or adaptive immune response must be considered. While the immunostimulatory effects of CpG DNA have been studied using cells from species ranging from mouse to man, their long-term safety and efficacy in vivo are less well characterized. Of concern is the possibility that CpG ODN may (1) induce autoimmune disease, (2) trigger a persistent alteration in immune homeostasis by skewing the Th1:Th2 cytokine balance or (3) have direct toxic effects on the host.

Effect of CpG ODN on the development of autoimmunity

It is well established that CpG motifs in bacterial DNA can (1) stimulate the production of anti-DNA autoantibodies, (2) induce the production of pro-inflammatory cytokines, and (3) block the apoptotic death of activated lymphocytes, all of which can accelerate the development of autoimmune disease [12, 13, 24, 25, 32, 42, 52]. To determine whether CpG ODN impact the development of autoimmunity, we repeatedly injected ODN or bacterial DNA into BALB/c and NZB/W mice. The latter animals were selected because they develop a syndrome similar to systemic lupus erythematosus in humans.

One day after the fourth injection of ODN, the number of IL-6- and IFN-γ-secreting cells was increased in the spleen of both normal and lupus prone mice (Table 4). This was accompanied by an approximately twofold rise in serum IgG anti-DNA autoantibody levels in both groups. However, antibody and cytokine production returned to normal within 1 month after the cessation of therapy. Thus, while ODN have short-term immunostimulatory effects they do not appear to permanently alter immune homeostasis. Moreover, repeated administration of CpG ODN did not accelerate the development of autoimmune glomerulonephritis in NZB/W mice, or alter the survival of BALB/c or NZB/W mice. Consistent with these observations, Gilkeson et al. [14] found that the changes in immune reactivity induced by bacterial DNA did not accelerate the development of autoimmune disease in lupus prone mice.

Table 4. Safety Studies Involving CpG ODN

Mice	Treatment	Cytokine secreting cells ($\times 10^{-6}$)	IgG anti-DNA		Histology
		IL-6	*IFN-γ*	*Titer*	
NZB/W	Untreated	140±38	21±7	32±4	
	CpG ODN (1 day)	736±32	48±10	41±5	
	CpG ODN (1 month)	153±25	28±12	33±6	
BALB/c	Untreated	314±65	11±3	1±1	Normal
	CpG ODN (1 day)	816±130	22±5	2±1	Normal
	CpG ODN (1 month)	288±48	10±4	1±1	Normal

BALB/c or NZB/W mice were injected 3 or more times with 50 µg of CpG ODN at 2 to 6-week intervals. Cytokine-secreting spleen cells from these animals were monitored by ELIspot assay, while serum IgG anti-DNA autoantibody titers were determined by ELISA. Results reflect the average of at least three independently studied animals/group

The situation is somewhat more complex for organ-specific autoimmune diseases, which are promoted by the type of strong Th1 response induced by CpG ODN. In an IL-12-dependent model of experimental allergic encephalomyelitis (EAE), animals treated with CpG motifs and challenged with myelin basic protein generated autoreactive Th1 effector cells, triggering the development of EAE [39]. In a molecular mimicry model, CpG motifs acted as potent immune activators, inducing autoimmune myocarditis when co-injected with *Chlamydia*-derived antigens [1]. These findings indicate that CpG motifs may trigger deleterious autoimmune reactions under certain circumstances. There is also evidence that by altering the cytokine milieu (ratio of Th1- toTh2-secreting cells) of the host, CpG ODN can synergistically enhance the toxicity of other immunostimulatory agents [6, 40].

General safety

Several reports indicate that CpG ODN can be toxic if used in conjunction with lipopolysaccharide [6] or D-galactosamine [40, 41]. To examine whether ODN by themselves were harmful to normal animals, we repeatedly injected BALB/c mice with 50 µg CpG ODN, a dose that consistently induced protection against infectious organisms and inhibited the development of allergic asthma.

All animals injected with ODN ($n > 200$), including those injected weekly for up to 4 months, remained physically vigorous. None became sick, lost weight, or died. Cohorts of mice were killed 1 or 30 days after 20 weeks of treatment and their organs (spleen, lymph nodes, muscle, intestine, heart, lung, adrenal gland, kidney and liver) were fixed, stained, and examined histologically. Coded samples from ODN and control mice were analyzed by a pathologist. None of the organs showed macroscopic or microscopic evidence of damage or inflammation. Similarly, peripheral blood smears from all animals at all time points were normal. In addition, none of the animals developed proteinuria or other manifestations of lupus-like disease.

Thus, despite concern that CpG ODN might have adverse effects on the host, we find no evidence that even multiple doses of CpG ODN are directly toxic under normal situations. The chronic immune stimulation induced by these agents can potentially promote inflammatory, autoimmune or other type of toxicity in the host. Moreover, when co-administered with other pro-inflammatory agents, toxicity does occur. Yet our findings suggest that therapeutic doses of CpG ODN alone can be safely administered to normal animals.

Concluding remarks

The capacity of synthetic CpG-containing ODN to stimulate the mammalian immune system was first described 5 years ago. Since then, considerable insight has been gained into their mechanism of action, safety, and potential therapeutic value. Indeed, phase I clinical trials designed to examine the safety and activity of these agents in humans are planned. This rapid transition from the lab to the clinic was facilitated by advances in immunology and molecular biology that accelerated the production and testing of ODN with immunomodulatory properties. In vitro and in vivo analysis of rodents, primates, and other animals demonstrated that unmethylated CpG motifs reproducibly stimulated an innate immune response characterized by the production of IL-18 and TNF-α (which improve APC function), IL-6 (which facilitates B cell responses), and IFN-γ and IL-12 (which support the development of Th1-dependent immune responses and the generation of cytotoxic T lymphocytes). Additional animal models demonstrated the potential of CpG ODN to act as vaccine adjuvants, anti-allergens, and immunoprotective agents.

Only aluminum hydroxide gel is currently approved for human use as an immune adjuvant. This adjuvant primarily induces a strong Th2 response, yet protection against many infectious agents requires that the host generate Th1-dominated immunity. In this context, the ability of CpG ODN to stimulate a Th1 response (even when administered with Th2-inducing agents such as aluminum hydroxide or incomplete Freund's adjuvant) is of considerable interest. CpG ODN trigger IL-12 and IFN-γ production following both primary and secondary vaccination. Even in pre-sensitized mice where pathological Th2-mediated allergic responses already exist, CpG ODN can re-direct the allergen-specific response towards a Th1 profile. This alteration in the immune milieu persists for many weeks and is associated with a concomitant reduction in allergic manifestations, raising the possibility that CpG ODN might provide a long-lasting treatment for allergic asthma.

Perhaps the most remarkable activity of CpG ODN is their ability to stimulate an innate immune response that improves the host's ability to eliminate infectious pathogens while promoting the development of long-lasting antigen specific immunity. Exemplified by studies involving *F. tularensis* and *L. monocytogenes*, similar protection has been observed against a variety of bacterial, viral and parasitic diseases. We believe that CpG ODN will prove useful for the prevention and/or treatment of such infections, especially in situations where no vaccine is available or there is insufficient time to induce an antigen-specific response. The potential uses of CpG ODN are not limited to humans. In husbandry animals, serious infectious diseases are sometimes "treated" by slaughtering entire herds. For such diseases, monitoring for infection involves testing for the presence of pathogen-specific antibodies. This excludes the use of vaccines for disease control, since vaccination would interfere with antibody surveillance. Yet CpG ODN could prevent the spread of infection to neighboring herds without interfering with such surveillance.

We also envisage CpG ODN being combined with vaccines for use in post-exposure treatment/vaccination. In such a situation, the innate immune response triggered by the ODN would suppress the proliferation of the pathogen and provide an opportunity for the host to mount an antigen-specific response. The presence of ODN would then serve as an immune adjuvant, boosting the response elicited by the co-administered vaccine.

As technology improves and the motifs with optimal immunostimulatory activity in humans are identified, additional therapeutic uses for CpG ODN will almost certainly be described. We predict that classes of ODN will be defined that selectively promote specific types of immune response (i.e., biased towards Th1, Th2, or pro-inflammatory responses), and that such ODN will permit immune responses to be tailored to provide optimal protection against specific pathogens. Different ODN backbones and formulations will improve the uptake, stability, and in vivo distribution of these agents, and increase the likelihood that CpG ODN will contribute to disease prevention and treatment.

Acknowledgments The assertions herein are the private ones of the authors and are not to be construed as official or as reflecting the views of the Food and Drug Administration at large. This review was supported in part by a grant from the National Vaccine Program and by Military Interdepartmental Purchase Request no. MM8926.

References

1. Bachmaier K, Meu N, Maza LM, Pal S, Nessel A, Penninger JM (1999) *Chlamydia* infections and heart disease linked through antigenic mimicry. Science 283:1335
2. Bendigs S, Salzer U, Lipford GB, Wagner H, Heeg K (1999) CpG-ODN co-stimulate primary T cells in the absence of antigen-presenting cells. Eur J Immunol 29:1209
3. Bird AP (1987) CpG–rich islands and the function of DNA methylation. Trends Genet 3:342
4. Bohn E, Heesemann J, Ehlers S, Autenrieth IB (1994) Early gamma interferon mRNA expression is associated with resistance of mice against *Yersinia enterocolitica*. Infect Immun 62:3027
5. Cardon LR, Burge C, Clayton DA, Karlin S (1994) Pervasive CpG suppression in animal mitochondrial genomes. Proc Natl Acad Sci USA 91:3799
6. Cowdery JS, Chace JH, Yi A, Krieg AM (1996) Bacterial DNA induces NK cells to produce IFN-gamma in vivo and increases the toxicity of lipopolysaccharides. J Immunol 156:4570
7. Culkin SJ, Rhinehart-Jones T, Elkins KL (1997) A novel role for B cells in early protective immunity to an intracellular pathogen, *Francisella tularensis* strain LVS. J Immunol 158:3277
8. Elkins KL, Rhinethart-Jones TR, Culkin SJ, Yee D, Winegar RK (1997) Minimal requirements for murine resistance to infection with *Francisella tularensis* LVS. Infect Immun 64:3288
9. Elkins KL, Rhinehart-Jones TR, Stibitz S, Conover JS, Klinman DM (1999) Bacterial DNA containing CpG motifs stimulates lymphocyte-dependent protection of mice against lethal infection with intracellular bacteria. J Immunol 162:2991
10. Field AK, Tytell AA, Lampson GP, Hilleman MR (1967) Inducers of IFN and host resistance. II. Multistranded synthetic polynucleotide complexes. Proc Natl Acad Sci 58:1004
11. Gilkeson GS, Grudier JP, Karounos DG, Pisetsky DS (1989) Induction of anti-double stranded DNA antibodies in normal mice by immunization with bacterial DNA. J Immunol 142:1482
12. Gilkeson GS, Pippen AM, Pisetsky DS (1995) Induction of cross-reactive anti-dsDNA antibodies in preautoimmune NZB/NZW mice by immunization with bacterial DNA. J Clin Invest 95:1398
13. Gilkeson GS, Riuz P, Howell D, Lefkowith JB, Pisetsky DS (1993) Induction of immune-mediated glomerulonephritis in normal mice immunized with bacterial DNA. Clin Immunol Immunopathol 68:283
14. Gilkeson GS, Ruiz P, Pippen AM, Alexander AL, Lefkowith JB, Pisetsky DS (1996) Modulation of renal disease in autoimmune NZB/NZW mice by immunization with bacterial DNA. J Exp Med 183:1389
15. Halpern MD, Kurlander RJ, Pisetsky DS (1996) Bacterial DNA induces murine interferon-gamma production by stimulation of IL-12 and tumor necrosis factor-alpha. Cell Immunol 167:72

16. Heinzel FP, Sadick MD, Mutha SS, Locksley RM (1991) Production of IFN gamma, IL-2, IL-4 and IL-10 by CD4+ lymphocytes in vivo during healing and progressive murine leishmaniasis. Proc Natl Acad Sci USA 88:7011
17. Hirano T, Akira S, Taga T, Kishimoto T (1990) Biological and clinical aspects of IL-6. Immunol Today 11:443
18. Hirano T, Yasukawa K, Harada H, Taga T, Watanabe Y, Matsuda T, Kashiwamura S, Nakajima K, Koyama K, Iwamatsu A, Tsunasawa S, Sakiyama F, Matsui H, Takahara Y, Taniguchi T, Kishimoto T (1986) Complementary DNA for a novel human interleukin (BSF-2) that induces B lymphocytes to produce Ig. Nature 324:73
19. Iwanoto I, Hakajima H, Endo H, Yoshida S (1993) IFN-γ regulates antigen-induced eosinophil recruitment into the mouse airways by inhibiting the infiltration of CD4+ T cells. J Exp Med 177:537
20. Izzo AA, North RJ (1997) Evidence for an alpha/beta T cell-independent mechanism of resistance to mycobacteria. J Exp Med 176:581
21. Jakob T, Walker PS, Krieg AM, Udey MC, Vogel JC (1998) Activation of cutaneous dendritic cells by CpG containing oligodeoxynucleotides: a role for dendritic cells in the augmentation of Th1 responses by immunostimulatory DNA. J Immunol 161:3042
22. Klinman DM (1998) Therapeutic applications of CpG-containing oligodeoxynucleotides. Antisense Nucleic Acid Drug Dev 8:181
23. Klinman DM, Yamshchikov G, Ishigatsubo Y (1997) Contribution of CpG motifs to the immunogenicity of DNA vaccines. J Immunol 158:3635
24. Klinman DM, Yi A, Beaucage SL, Conover J, Krieg AM (1996) CpG motifs expressed by bacterial DNA rapidly induce lymphocytes to secrete IL-6, IL-12 and IFN-γ. Proc Natl Acad Sci USA 93:2879
25. Krieg AM (1995) CpG DNA: a pathogenic factor in systemic lupus erythematosus? J Clin Immunol 15:284
26. Krieg AM, Yi A, Matson S, Waldschmidt TJ, Bishop GA, Teasdale R, Koretzky GA, Klinman DM (1995) CpG motifs in bacterial DNA trigger direct B-cell activation. Nature 374:546
27. Le JM, Vilcek J (1989) IL-6: a multifunctional cytokine regulating immune reactions and the acute phase protein response. Lab Invest 61:588
28. Lipford GB, Sparwasser T, Bauer M, Zimmermann S, Koch E, Heeg K, Wagner H (1997) Immunostimulatory DNA: sequence-dependent production of potentially harmful or useful cytokines. Eur J Immunol 27:3420
29. Marrack P, Kappler J (1994) Submersion of the immune system by pathogens. Cell 76:323
30. Messina JP, Gilkeson GS, Pisetsky DS (1991) Stimulation of in vitro murine lymphocyte proliferation by bacterial DNA. J Immunol 147:1759
31. Mor G, Klinman DM, Shapiro S, Hagiwara E, Sedegah M, Norman JA, Hoffman SL, Steinberg AD (1995) Complexity of the cytokine and antibody response elicited by immunizing mice with *Plasmodium yoelii* circumsporozoite protein plasmid DNA. J Immunol 155:2039
32. Mor G, Singla M, Steinberg AD, Hoffman SL, Okuda K, Klinman DM (1997) Do DNA vaccines induce autoimmune disease? Hum Gene Ther 8:293
33. Muraguchi A, Hirano T, Tang B, Matsuda T, Horii Y, Nakajima K, Kishimoto T (1988) The essential role of B cell stimulatory factor 2 (BSF-2/IL-6) for the terminal differentiation of B cells. J Exp Med 167:332
34. Oehler JR, Herverman RB (1978) Natural cell-mediated cytotoxicity in rats. III. Effects of immunopharmacologic treatments on natural reactivity and reactivity augmented by polyinosinic-polycytidylic acid. Int J Cancer 21:221
35. Paul WE, Seder RA, Plaut M (1993) Lymphokine and cytokine production by FcεRI+ Cells. Adv Immunol 53:1
36. Razin A, Friedman J (1981) DNA methylation and its possible biological roles. Prog Nucleic Acid Res Mol Biol 25:33
37. Roman M, Martin-Orozco E, Goodman JS, Nguyen M, Sato Y, Ronaghy A, Kornbluth RS, Richman DD, Carson DA, Raz E (1997) Immunostimulatory DNA sequences function as T helper-promoting adjuvants. Nat Med 3:849
38. Sato Y, Roman M, Tighe H, Lee D, Corr M, Nguyen M, Carson DA, Raz E (1996) Immunostimulatory DNA sequences necessary for effective intradermal gene immunization. Science 273:352
39. Segal BM, Klinman DM, Shevach EM (1997) Microbial products induce autoimmune disease by an IL-12-dependent process. J Immunol 158:5087
40. Sparwasser T, Meithke T, Lipford G, Borschert K, Hicker H, Heeg K, Wagner H (1997) Bacterial DNA causes septic shock. Nature 386:336

41. Sparwasser T, Miethke T, Lipford G, Erdmann A, Hacker H, Heeg K, Wagner H (1997) Macrophages sense pathogens via DNA motifs: induction of tumor necrosis factor-α-mediated shock. Eur J Immunol 27:1671
42. Steinberg AD, Krieg AM, Gourley MF, Klinman DM (1990) Theoretical and experimental approaches to generalized autoimmunity. Immunol Rev 118:129
43. Sun S, Beard C, Jaenisch R, Jones P, Sprent J (1997) Mitogenicity of DNA from different organisms for murine B cells. J Immunol 159:3119
44. Sun S, Zhang X, Tough DF, Sprent J (1998) Type I interferon-mediated stimulation of T cells by CpG DNA. J Exp Med 188:2335
45. Sur S, Lam F, Bouchard A, Sigounas A, Holbert D, Metzger WJ (1996) Immunomodulatory effects of IL-12 on allergic lung inflammation depend on timing of doses. J Immunol 157:4173
46. Sur S, Wild JS, Choudhury BK, Alam R, Sur N, Klinman DM (1999) Long-term prevention of allergic lung inflammation in a mouse model of asthma by CpG oligodeoxynucleotides. J Immunol 162:6284
47. Trinchieri G (1994) IL-12: a cytokine produced by antigen-presenting cells with inmmunoregulatory functions in the generation of T-helper cells type 1 and cytotoxic lymphocytes. Blood 84:4008
48. Uyttenhove C, Couli PG, Van Snick J (1988) T cell growth and differentiation induced by IL-6, the murine hybridoma plasmacytoma growth factor. J Exp Med 167:1417
49. Vilcek J, Ny MH, Friedmann-Kien AE, Krawciw T (1968) Induction of IFN synthesis by synthetic double-stranded polynucleotides. J Virol 2:648
50. Yamamoto S, Katoaka T, Yano O, Kuramoto E, Shimada S, Tokunaga T (1989) Antitumor effect of nucleic acid fraction from bacteria. Proc Jpn Soc Immunol 48:272
51. Yamamoto S, Yamamoto T, Shimada S, Kuramoto E, Yano O, Kataoka T, Tokunaga T (1992) DNA from bacteria, but not vertebrates, induces interferons, activates NK cells and inhibits tumor growth. Microbiol Immunol 36:983
52. Yi A, Hornbeck P, Lafrenz DE, Krieg AM (1996) CpG DNA rescue of murine B lymphoma cells from anti-IgM induced growth arrest and programmed cell death is associated with increased expression of c-myc and bcl-xl. J Immunol 157:4918
53. Yi A, Klinman DM, Martin TL, Matson S, Krieg AM (1996) Rapid immune activation by CpG motifs in bacterial DNA. J Immunol 157:5394
54. Zhan Y, Cheers C (1995) Endogenous IL-12 is involved in resistance to *Brucella abortus* infection. Infect Immun 63:1387
55. Zimmermann S, Egeter O, Hausmann S, Lipford GB, Rocken M, Wagner H, Heeg K (1998) CpG oligodeoxynucleotides trigger protective and curative Th1 responses in lethal murine leishmaniasis. J Immunol 160:3627

MIX
Papier aus verantwortungsvollen Quellen
Paper from responsible sources
FSC® C105338

If you have any concerns about our products,
you can contact us on
ProductSafety@springernature.com

In case Publisher is established outside the EU,
the EU authorized representative is:
Springer Nature Customer Service Center GmbH
Europaplatz 3, 69115 Heidelberg, Germany

Printed by Libri Plureos GmbH
in Hamburg, Germany